SPRINGER PROTOCOLS HANDBOOKS

For further volumes:
http://www.springer.com/series/8623

Advances and Clinical Practice in Pyrosequencing

Editors

Guohua Zhou

*Jinling Hospital, State Key Laboratory of Analytical Chemistry for Life Science,
Medical School of Nanjing University, Nanjing, Jiangsu, China*

Qinxin Song

*Key Laboratory of Drug Quality Control and Pharmacovigilance, Ministry of Education,
China Pharmaceutical University, Nanjing, Jiangsu, China*

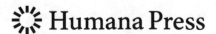

Humana Press

Editors
Guohua Zhou
Jinling Hospital
State Key Laboratory of Analytical
    Chemistry for Life Science
Medical School of Nanjing University
Nanjing, Jiangsu, China

Qinxin Song
Key Laboratory of Drug Quality Control
    and Pharmacovigilance
Ministry of Education
China Pharmaceutical University
Nanjing, Jiangsu, China

ISSN 1949-2448   ISSN 1949-2456   (electronic)
Springer Protocols Handbooks
ISBN 978-1-4939-8017-8   ISBN 978-1-4939-3308-2   (eBook)
DOI 10.1007/978-1-4939-3308-2

Dedication

The book is specially dedicated to Professor Hideki Kambara, an unsung hero of the human genome project.

Preface

The high-throughput DNA sequencing method based on Sanger's principle provided an efficient tool for the sequencing of the whole human genome. With the help of capillary array platform invented by Professor Kambara, the human genome project was finished two years earlier than expected. In the post-genomic era, many biomarkers related to early disease diagnosis and personalized medicine have been found by the use of next-generation DNA sequencers. Although there are several DNA sequencing tools available for clinical detection of these biomarkers, pyrosequencing has an especially important role in identifying microbial genotypes, as well as in sequencing a short fragment containing the biomarkers related to personalized medicine.

Pyrosequencing is a sequencing-by-synthesis method based on the bioluminometric detection of by-products of inorganic pyrophosphates (PPi) during primer extension reaction. Although only several tens of bases can be sequenced during a run, it is enough for clinical routine use in detecting known biomarkers. As pyrosequencing is very suitable to the sequencing of short DNA sequence, the CFDA approved pyrosequencing technology for clinical use. Pyrosequencing is becoming the most popular DNA sequencing tool for personalized medicine in hospitals.

I have engaged in pyrosequencing research since 1999 when I came to Professor Kambara's research group in Central Research Laboratory of Hitachi. Professor Kambara directed me to perform pyrosequencing research in developing new chemistry for increasing the sensitivity, simplifying protocols for SNP typing, and miniaturizing the instrumentation. Professor Kambara, who is honored as an unsung hero of the human genome project by Science, is a highly reputed scientist in the DNA sequencing research field. I am very fortunate to have had his supervision in the research of DNA detection. Even after my return to China from Japan, he supported me in following pyrosequencing research for many years.

The aim of this book is to improve pyrosequencing protocols as well as instrumentation for better clinical use. Due to our continuous contributions, pyrosequencing is greatly improved in terms of template preparation, sensitivity, instrumentation, and detectable target species. We simplified the protocols of pyrosequencing by skipping the ssDNA preparation step. We enabled pyrosequencing to quantify the expression levels of mRNA and microRNA by coupling base barcodes into pyrosequencing. We adapted pyrosequencing to prenatal diagnosis of trisomy 21 by quantitatively pyrosequencing heterozygotes of fetal genomic DNA. We miniaturized the pyrosequencer by using a photodiode array as the light sensor. This book describes all of these improvements and novel applications of pyrosequencing technology.

There are 34 chapters in the book, and they are grouped as five parts: Part I is Advances in Pyrosequencing Template Preparation; Part II explores Pyrosequencing Technology Innovations; Part III delves into Multiplex Pyrosequencing based on barcodes; Part IV looks at Miniaturizing Pyrosequencing Equipment; and Part V examines Applications.

Now we are progressing toward precision medicine. To allow the right drug with the right dose at the right time, genotyping of an individual patient is required before prescribing a drug. I believe that pyrosequencing would be a useful tool in this progress. This book should be useful for people who are engaged in personalized medicine, disease control, and DNA diagnosis in other fields.

Professor Kambara, my teacher, retired from Hitachi in March 2015. I would like to dedicate this book to him, a great contributor to DNA sequencing technology.

Nanjing, China   *Guohua Zhou*

Contents

Contributors

YING CHEN • *China Pharmaceutical University, Nanjing, China*

ZHIYAO CHEN • *Department of Pharmacology, Jinling Hospital, Medical School of Nanjing University, Nanjing, China*

SIJIA CHENG • *Department of Pharmaceutical Analysis, China Pharmaceutical University, Nanjing, Jiangsu, China*

YANAN CHU • *Department of Pharmacology, Jinling Hospital, Medical School of Nanjing University, Nanjing, China*

GAO CHUAN • *Central Research Laboratory, Hitachi, Ltd., Tokyo, Japan*

MARI GOTOU • *Central Research Laboratory, Hitachi, Ltd., Tokyo, Japan*

KUNIO HARADA • *Central Research Laboratory, Hitachi, Ltd., Tokyo, Japan*

HUAN HUANG • *Department of Pharmaceutical Analysis, China Pharmaceutical University, Nanjing, Jiangsu, China*

HUNING JIA • *Key Laboratory of Drug Quality Control and Pharmacovigilance, Ministry of Education, School of Pharmacy, China Pharmaceutical University, Nanjing, China*

YIRU JIN • *China Pharmaceutical University, Nanjing, China*

HUA JING • *Department of Pharmaceutical Analysis, China Pharmaceutical University, Nanjing, Jiangsu, China*

TOMOHARU KAJIYAMA • *Central Research Laboratory, Hitachi, Ltd., Tokyo, Japan*

MASAO KAMAHORI • *Central Research Laboratory, Hitachi, Ltd., Tokyo, Japan*

HIDEKI KAMBARA • *Central Research Laboratory, Hitachi, Ltd., Tokyo, Japan*

AKIHIKO KISHIMOTO • *Central Research Laboratory, Hitachi, Ltd., Tokyo, Japan*

JINHENG LI • *China Pharmaceutical University, Nanjing, China*

CHAO LIANG • *Department of Pharmaceutical Analysis, China Pharmaceutical University, Nanjing, China*

XIQUN LIU • *Department of Pharmaceutical Analysis, China Pharmaceutical University, Nanjing, Jiangsu, China*

YUNLONG LIU • *Department of Pharmacology, Jinling Hospital, Medical School of Nanjing University, Nanjing, China*

ZUHONG LU • *State Key Laboratory of Bioelectronics, Southeast University, Nanjing, China*

JUAN LUO • *Department of Pharmaceutical Analysis, China Pharmaceutical University, Nanjing, China*

YINJIAO MA • *China Pharmaceutical University, Nanjing, China*

KEIICHI NAGAI • *Central Research Laboratory, Hitachi, Ltd., Tokyo, Japan*

KAZUNORI OKANO • *Central Research Laboratory, Hitachi, Ltd., Tokyo, Japan*

XIEMIN QI • *Department of Pharmacology, Jinling Hospital, Medical School of Nanjing University, Nanjing, China*

ZONGTAI QI • *Department of Pharmaceutical Analysis, China Pharmaceutical University, Nanjing, China*

JIANZHONG RUI • *Department of Pharmacology, Jinling Hospital, Medical School of Nanjing University, Nanjing, China*

YIYUN SHEN • *China Pharmaceutical University, Nanjing, China*
HIROMI SHIRAKURA • *Central Research Laboratory, Hitachi, Ltd., Tokyo, Japan*
QINXIN SONG • *Key Laboratory of Drug Quality Control and Pharmacovigilance, Ministry of Education, China Pharmaceutical University, Nanjing, Jiangsu, China*
SHIGEYA SUZUKI • *Central Research Laboratory, Hitachi, Ltd., Tokyo, Japan*
JIANPING WANG • *China Pharmaceutical University, Nanjing, China*
WEIPENG WANG • *China Pharmaceutical University, Nanjing, China*
GUIJIANG WEI • *Department of Pharmaceutical Analysis, China Pharmaceutical University, Nanjing, China*
HAIPING WU • *Huadong Research Institute for Medicine and Biotechnics, Nanjing, China*
WENJUAN WU • *Department of Pharmaceutical Analysis, China Pharmaceutical University, Nanjing, China*
ZHENG XIANG • *China Pharmaceutical University, Nanjing, China*
PENGFENG XIAO • *China Pharmaceutical University, Nanjing, China*
XIAOQING XING • *China Pharmaceutical University, Nanjing, China*
SHU XU • *Department of Pharmacology, Jinling Hospital, Medical School of Nanjing University, Nanjing, China*
HUIYONG YANG • *China Pharmaceutical University, Nanjing, China*
HUI YE • *Key Laboratory of Drug Quality Control and Pharmacovigilance, Ministry of Education, School of Pharmacy, China Pharmaceutical University, Nanjing, China*
XIAODAN ZHANG • *Huadong Research Institute for Medicine and Biotechnics, Nanjing, China*
GUOHUA ZHOU • *Department of Pharmacology, Jinling Hospital, State Key Laboratory of Analytical Chemistry for Life Science, Medical School of Nanjing University, Nanjing, China*
SHUHUI ZHU • *China Pharmaceutical University, Nanjing, China*
BINGJIE ZOU • *Department of Pharmacology, Jinling Hospital, Medical School of Nanjing University, Nanjing, China*

Part I

Technology Preparation

Chapter 1

Preparation of Single-Stranded DNA for Pyrosequencing by LATE-PCR

Huiyong Yang, Chao Liang, Zhiyao Chen, Bingjie Zou, Qinxin Song, and Guohua Zhou

Abstract

To establish a simple method for preparing single-stranded DNA templates for pyrosequencing, the Linear-after-the-exponential (LATE)-PCR technology on the basis of Taq DNA polymerase without hot-start capacity was applied to amplify a 78-bp sequence (containing the SNP6 site), and the PCR-enhancing reagents (glycerol and BSA) were used to increase the efficiency and specialization, much more before the reagents A and B were designed to eliminate the impurity (limited primers, PPi, dNTPs, and so on), and 1–2 μL LATE-PCR products with simply treatment can be used in pyrosequencing directly. Then, five SNPs related with human breast-cancers in the BRCA1 gene were investigated, and the programs had no nonspecific signals that were made of theoretic sequences. Moreover, the genotyping of the SNPs could also be distinguished easily. The results indicated that this method can be used to prepare high quality single-stranded DNA templates for pyrosequencing and allows pyrosequencing be lower in cost, simpler in operation, and easier in automation, and the cross-contamination from sample preparation was also reduced.

Key words Pyrosequencing, Linear-after-the-exponential amplification, Preparation of single-stranded DNA template, Single nucleotide polymorphism

---

1 Introduction

Pyrosequencing is a novel sequencing technology that is based on single-stranded DNA (ssDNA) templates and different from Sanger technology, and this technique uses three enzymes (DNA polymerase, luciferase and ATP sulfurlyase) to catalyze the reactions from their corresponding substrates, such as adenosine 5′-phosphosulfate (APS), luciferin, and the added nucleotides, which was complementary to the template, to produce a flash of light signal with an intensity that is proportional to the number of incorporated bases. dNTPs that fail to incorporate with the template are degraded by apyrase and do not produce light signal. Pyrosequencing can provide the information of DNA sequences in

Guohua Zhou and Qinxin Song (eds.), *Advances and Clinical Practice in Pyrosequencing*, Springer Protocols Handbooks, DOI 10.1007/978-1-4939-3308-2_1, © Springer Science+Business Media New York 2016

a short time [1, 2], whereas it does not require labeled primers or electrophoresis. The pyrosequencing technique has become an ideal platform for sequencing short DNA sequences and has a wide range of applications in the fields of single-nucleotide polymorphism (SNP) detection [3], microbial genotyping [4, 5], CpG methylation analysis [6], and so on. The pyrosequencing technique has also been used in the large-scale DNA sequencing and brings a revolutionary advancement in the field of DNA sequencing [7].

Now, the preparation of single-stranded DNA material generally is dependent on solid-phase beads (streptavidin-coated) method, which has characters of multistep process, low efficiency, and high cost for the using biotinylated primers and streptavidin beads [8, 9], and moreover, the multistep process of samples preparation also increases the risk of contamination in PCR products, so that the application of pyrosequencing in clinical is limited. The asymmetric PCR method can produce ssDNA [10–12], but the method has not been widely used for the low efficiency in amplifying ssDNA. Linear-after-the-exponential-polymerase chain reaction (LATE-PCR) developed asymmetric amplifications by introducing the concentration to compute primers melting temperature (Tm) [13–15]. Under the condition of the Tm of limited primer (PL) being higher than that of excess primers (PX) (Tm (PL) – Tm(PX) ≥ 0 °C) and optimizing the concentration, and Tm of the primers, LATE-PCR can generate large amount of ssDNA, which is sufficient for reaction of probe hybridization, real-time fluorescence PCR detection, and so on [16–19].

Wangh et al. [16] used the LATE-PCR products to pyrosequencing directly with a satisfying result. However, the application of the AmpliTaq Gold Taq polymerase and commercial PyroGold kit increased the cost as well as ignored the cases of the residual PL, and not fully extended dsDNA products that could confuse the results of pyrosequencing. In this experiment, a system of LATE-PCR that is based on Taq DNA polymerase, which was introduced without hot-start capacity and one tube method was carried out for preparing the single-stranded template for pyrosequencing. The two reagents (A and B) were designed to eliminate the interfering components in PCR products. This method was applied to pyrosequence the 78-bp sequence (including SNP6 site) LATE-PCR product, and the five SNPs site in the brca1 gene (one of breast cancer susceptibility gene [20]) were detected.

2 Materials

1. PTC-225 PCR engine (MJ Research, Inc., USA).
2. PowerPac 1000 HV power supply (BIO-RAD, Inc, USA).
3. GenGenius gel imaging system (Syngene, Inc, UK).

4. The apparatus for pyrosequencing were set up according to reference [21]: R6335 photomultiplier (Hamamatsu Photonics K.K, Inc., Japan) and BPCL Ultra-Weak Chemiluminescence Analyzer System (Institute of Biophysics of Chinese Academy of Sciences).

5. Taq DNA polymerase, Deoxynucleotide (dNTPs, 10 mM), 1 × buffer (Mg_2+ free), and $MgCl_2$ (25 mM) were purchased from TaKaRa BioTech (Dalian, China).

6. AmpliTaq Gold DNA polymerase was purchased from Applied Biosystems (Foster City, USA).

7. Klenow Fragment (Exonuclease Minus), polyvinylpyrrolidone (PVP), and QuantiLum recombinant luciferase were purchased from Promega (Madison, WI).

8. Apyrase, D-luciferin, bovine serum albumin (BSA), and adenosine 5′-phosphosulfate (APS) were obtained from Sigma (St. Louis, MO).

9. Sodium 2′-deoxyadenosine-5′-O-(1-triphosphate) (dATPαS), 2′-deoxyguanosine-5′-triphosphate (dGTP), 2′-deoxythymidine-5′-triphosphate (dTTP), and 2′-deoxycytidine-5′- triphosphate (dCTP) were purchased from Amersham Pharmacia Biotech.

10. ATP sulfurylase was produced in our lab [22].

11. The other chemicals were of a commercially extra-pure grade.

12. All solutions were prepared with deionized and sterilized water.

13. The blood samples (named g-1, g-2, and g-3) for pyrosequencing were obtained from healthy volunteers in our lab, and the genomes were extracted according to phenol–chloroform method.

14. The sequences containing the five SNPs were obtained from the database of NCBI (NT_010755.15), and the primers for LATE-PCR and sequencing were designed by primer 5.0, whereas the Tm of primers were calculated by OligoAnalyzer 3.0 (a Web-based program) (*see* **Notes 1–5**).

3 Methods

3.1 Conditions of Amplification

1. A total of 25 μL of PCR mixture contains 1×PCR buffer (50 mM KCl, 15 mM Tris–HCl, pH 8.0), 3 mM $MgCl_2$, 0.1 mM dNTP, 1.5 U of Taq DNA polymerase, 1 μL of DNA template (36 μg/l), 0.1 μM limited primer, 13 % glycerol, and 4 % BSA.

2. The reaction procedure consisted of incubation at 95 °C for 5 min, 60 cycles of denaturation at 87 °C for 10 s, the primer annealing at 66 °C for 10 s, extension at 72 °C for 20 s, exten-

sion at 72 °C for 10 min, and was lastly preserved at 4 °C (*see* **Notes 6** and **7**).

3. The annealing temperature of SNP2 and 4 were 64 °C.

4. The results were detected by agarose gel electrophoresis (the dye was Goldview and Agarose Gel was 2 %).

3.2 Preparation of Reaction Reagents

1. Reagent A contains 0.1 M tris-acetate (pH 7.7), 2 mM EDTA, 10 mM magnesium acetate, 0.1 % BSA, 1.0 mM dithiothreitol (DTT), 2 μM adenosine 5′-phospho sulfate (APS), 0.4 g/L PVP, 0.8 mM D-luciferin, 200 U/L ATP sulfurylase, 6 mg/L luciferase, and 18 U/mL Klenow fragment.

2. Reagent B contains reagent A and 1.6 U/mL apyrase.

3.3 Preparation of Single-Stranded DNA Templates

1. For pyrosequencing, ssDNA templates were prepared as the follows: 1–2 μL products of LATE-PCR and 1.2 μL APS (1 mM) were added in 30 μL reagent A, vortexed, and left for 10–15 min.

2. 40 μL reagent B was added, vortexed, and left for 3–5 min.

3. At last the sequencing primer was added (the final concentration was 0.3 PM) to anneal for 10–15 min.

3.4 Pyrosequencing

1. The pyrosequencing reaction used a 4-enzyme cascade system to produce a visible light that was detected by a photo-sensitive device PMT.

2. All the four dNTPs were dispensed individually, and the dispensing order of the dNTPs could be designed beforehand. The light signal was recorded by data BPCL Ultra-Weak Chemiluminescence Analyzer System (Institute of Biophysics of Chinese Academy of Sciences) and pyrograms were produced by Origin 7.5.

4 Method Validation

4.1 Detection of a 78-bp Sequence (Including SNP6 Site) LATE-PCR Product

To investigate the effect of the inexpensive Taq DNA polymerase without hot-start capacity for LATE-PCR, the 78-bp sequence (containing SNP6 site) with TaKaRa-Taq polymerase (without hot-start capacity) and AmpliTaq Gold Taq DNA polymerase were amplified. The results were shown in Fig. 1 (lanes 1 and 3), and the effect was more excellent than that of TaKaRa-Taq polymerase. To improve the amplified efficiency and specialization of the TaKaRa-Taq polymerase, PCR-enhancing reagents (glycerol and BSA) were applied, and the extended time were shortened in the thermal cycle (according to the length of Amplicon and the extended speed 1000 bp min^{-1}), and the denaturalization temperatures were fallen (according to Tm of amplicon by computing

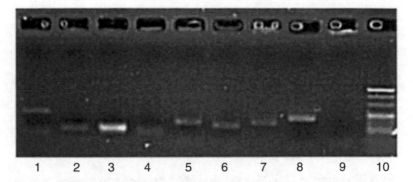

Fig. 1 Agarose electropherogram of amplicons from LATE-PCR at different conditions. Lane 1, the amplicon of the 78 bp sequence from TaKaRa-Taq DNA polymerase; lane 2, the amplicon of the 78-bp sequence from TaKaRa-Taq DNA polymerase (13 % of glycerol and 4 % of BSA); lane 3, the amplicon of the 78 bp sequence from AmpliTaq Gold DNA polymerase; lanes 4–9, the amplicons of 5 SNPs in BRCA1 gene from TaKaRa-Taq DNA polymerase (13 % of glycerol and 4 % of BSA); lane 4, SNP1 (64 bp); lane 5, SNP2 (121 bp); lane 6, SNP3 (102 bp); lane 7, SNP 4 (123 bp); lane 8, SNP 5 (171 bp); lane 9, blank control; lane 10, the DNA Maker (20–200 bp)

based on reference [25]). The lane 2 in Fig. 1 indicted that the amplified efficiency and specialization of the TaKaRa-Taq polymerase were improved obviously. The agarose electropherogram of the five SNP sites (brca1 gene, lane 4–8) also indicated that the Taq polymerase without hot-start capacity was available to be used in LATE-PCR by optimizing reaction condition.

Raw PCR products contain PPi, and dNTPs will consume the APS luciferin metabolized by the pyrosequencing enzymes, resulting in indiscriminant light emission, which not only interfered in the pyrosequencing reactions but also confused sequence determination. To obtain the ideal ssDNA templates, the LATE-PCR products were cleaned up by the followed steps: the PPi was converted to ATP using ATP sulfurylase and APS, and then the ATP and dNTPs were digested by apyrase to AMP and dAMP. However, the extended signals were detected from the PCR products without annealing with sequencing primers (after they were annealed by the two processes), see Fig. 2a. By analysis, the signals were brought on by the residual limited primers or not fully extended dsDNA products, and therefore, one process that used the Klenow DNA polymerase to extend the interfering matters was designed. The results of real-time monitoring the process of removing the interfering matters indicated that there were obvious extending reactions (as shown in Fig. 2b (I)). When the background signal descended and became stabilizing, the four dNTPs were dispensed individually and no obvious extended signals were observed, see Fig. 2b (II). By pyrosequencing the LATE-PCR product after annealing with sequencing primers, the pyrogram obtained was

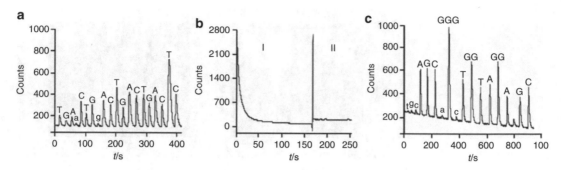

Fig. 2 Pyrograms of LATE-PCR products of 78 bp sequence treated by different ways. (**a**) directly pyrose-quenced without treatment by Klenow; (**b**) real-time background signals of the PCR products with treatment by Klenow (I) and the background signals after dispensed the four dNTPs individually (II); (**c**) pyrosequenced after treated according to the protocol in Sect. 3, item 3.3, the referenced sequence: AGCGGGTGGTAGGAGC; the dispensing order of dNTPs: TGCAGCAGTGTAG ATGC. The *capital letters* on the top of each peak indicated that the bases completed the extension reaction, the *small letters* indicated the background signals after adding the dNTPs that did not complete the extension reaction

shown in Fig. 2c. The results were consistent with the theoretical sequence, and it also indicated that the results of reference [16] could be obtained by LATE-PCR with TaKaRa Taq DNA polymerase (without hot-start capacity).

4.2 Detection of Five SNPs (brca1 Gene)

Under the optimized conditions, the five SNPs (brca1 gene), including base transition, insertion, and deletion, were detected. The pyrograms of the sample g-1 obtained were shown in Fig. 3. The heights of the signal peaks were effectively proportional to the number of bases in homopolymeric regions of the templates. However, no signals were observed after adding the dNTP that was not complementary to the template. It is reasonable that to say that introducing the methods that are based on the LATE-PCR products using into pyrosequencing is feasible.

The genotyping of SNPs by pyrosequencing were based on the signal peaks of the pyrograms. In Fig. 3, the genotyping carried out for SNP1, SNP2, SNP3, and SNP4 were wild-type, and the genotypes were AA, CT+/+, C–/–, and CC, respectively. However, when the SNPs locate homopolymeric regions, the results will have confusion to determine. For example, the genotyping of SNP5 from Fig. 3e was the confusion that the TT should be the output of the programs; however, the heterozygosis of CT was also logical according to the height of the signal peaks, and the sequence should be CT(C)1.5(T)0.5GTTTTC in all probability. The result of Sanger method also testified the CT genotyping. Because of this, we designed a new sequencing primer (Bs5b) that 3′-terminal was adjacent to SNP5 site, and the genotyping could be deter-mined easily (Fig. 4).

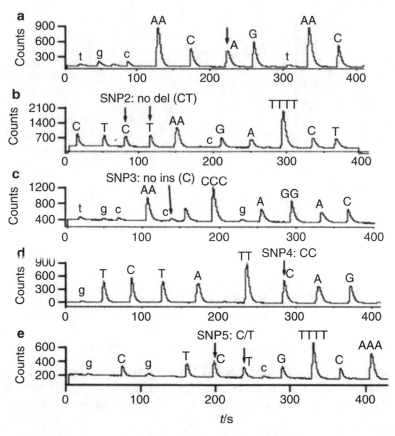

Fig. 3 Pyrograms of five SNPs in BRCA1 gene obtained. (**a**) SNP1: referenced sequence AAC[A > G]GAACT, the dispending order of dNTPs was TGGCACAGTAC and the measured genotyping was AA; (**b**), SNP2: referenced sequence CT[CT > del]AAGATTTTCT, the dispending order of dNTPs was CTCTACGATCT and the measured genotyping was CT+/+; (**c**) SNP3: referenced sequence was AA[C >ins]TCCCAGGAC, the dispending order of dNTPs was TGCACTCGAGAC and the measured genotyping was C–/–; (**d**) SNP4: referenced sequence was TCTATT[C > T]AG, the dispending order of dNTPs was GTCTAGTCAG and the measured genotyping was CC; (**e**) SNP5: referenced sequence was CTC[C > T]GTT TCAAA, the dispending order of dNTPs was GCGTCTCGTCA and the measured genotyping was CT; and others were the same as in Fig. 2)

5 Technical Notes

1. OligoAnalyzer 3.0 is available at http://scitools.idtdna.com/ analyzer/.The Tm of primers was estimated by the nearest neighbor formula, and the obtained Tm was closer to the real Tm than that obtained by Primer 5.0; and the Tm was different in a same primer for PCR amplification and for sequencing because the concentration of primers, and the reaction system were different [26].

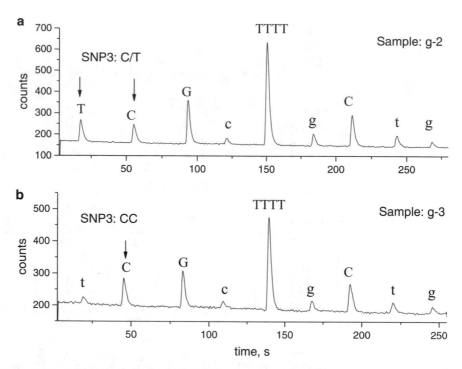

Fig. 4 Pyrograms of SNP5 with annealed by Bs5b sequencing primer. (**a**) the measured genotyping of sample g-2 was TC; (**b**) the measured genotyping of sample g-3 was CC; referenced sequence of SNP5 was [T > C] GTTTTC, the dispending order of dNTPs was TCGCTGCTG and the others were the same as in Fig. 2

2. The efficiency of the ssDNA produced by LATE-PCR is related to the Tm of the primers, so that the design of the primers is a key factor.

3. During the phase of exponential amplification, the limited primer has to be exhausted for pyrosequencing under the condition of $Tm(PL) - Tm(PX) \geq 5$ °C. During the phase of linear amplification, the one stranded DNA of PCR products and the excess primer will compete for hybridization to the limiting primer strand [23].

4. Sustained production of single stranded amplification is achieved under the condition of the $Tm(Amplicon) - Tm(PX) \leq 13–18$ °C [13, 23].

5. When the adequate Tm of primers cannot be designed to the actual DNA sequence of the target gene because the nucleotides A and T are abundant, the Tm can be increased by substituting one or two guanine bases for adenine near the 5′-end of the primer or adding of cytosine or guanidine to the 5′-end of the primer, irrespective of the target sequence [24]. According to this principle, one or three mismatched bases were introduced in the primers.

6. For LATE-PCR reactions, a higher anneal temperature of the thermal cycle is used during the phase of exponential amplification, and then, a lower anneal temperature is used during the phase of linear amplification. According to the results of the experiment, the ssDNA products will begin to amplify from 30 thermal cycle when the rate of PL:PX is 0.1:1 (the concentration of PX is 1 μM [16]), and the balance for pyrosequencing is required between maximizing the proportion of single-stranded material in the final product and minimizing the number of thermal cycles for minimizing the interfering PCR components.

7. According to the reference [16], the annealing temperatures were adjusted to below 1–2 °C to the Tm of the limited Primers in all thermal cycles.

References

1. Zhang XD, Wu HP, Zhou GH (2006) Pyrosequencing and its application in genetical analysis. Chinese J Anal Chem 34:582–586

2. Ronaghi M (2001) Pyrosequencing sheds light on DNA sequencing. Genome Res 11:3–11

3. Huang XQ, Roder MS, Roder J (2005) Development of SNP assays for genotyping the puroindoline b gene for grain hardness in wheat using pyrosequencing. J Agric Food Chem 53:2070–2075

4. Pai R, Limor J, Beall B (2005) Use of pyrosequencing to differentiate Streptococcus pneumoniae serotypes 6A and 6B. J Clin Microbiol 43:4820–4822

5. Pourmand N, Diamond L, Garten R, Erickson JP, Kumm J, Donis RO, Davis RW (2006) Rapid and highly informative diagnostic assay for H5N1 influenza viruses. PLoS ONE 1, e95

6. Tost J, Gut IG (2007) DNA methylation analysis by pyrosequencing. J Nat Protoc 2:2265–2275

7. Margulies M, Egholm M, Altman WE, Attiya S, Bader JS, Bemben LA (2005) Genome sequencing in microfabricated high-density picolitre reactors. Nature 437:376–380

8. Diggle MA, Clarke SC (2003) Pyrosequencing™. Mol Biotechnol 24:221–224

9. Royo JL, Hidalgo M, Ruiz A (2007) Pyrosequencing protocol using a universal biotinylated primer for mutation detection and SNP genotyping. Nat Protoc 2:1734–1739

10. Fujii T, Ohta M, Kono M, Hoshina S, Fukuhara K, Tsuruoka M (1999) Rapid detection of the gene of Legionella pneumophila using the fluorescence polarization with the asymmetric PCR. Nucleic Acids Symp Ser 42:59–60

11. Barratt K, Mackay JF (2002) Improving real-time PCR genotyping assays by asymmetric amplification. J Clin Microbiol 40:1571–1572

12. Wei Q, Liu S, Huang J, Mao X, Chu X, Wang Y, Qiu M, Mao Y, Xie Y, Li Y (2004) Comparison of hybridization behavior between double and single strand of targets and the application of asymmetric PCR targets in cDNA microarray. J Biochem Mol Biol 37:439–444

13. Pierce KE, Sanchez JA, Rice JE, Wangh LJ (2005) Linear-after-the-exponential (LATE)-PCR: primer design criteria for high yields of specific single-stranded DNA and improved real-time detection. J Proc Natl Acad Sci USA 102:8609–8614

14. Allawi HT, SantaLucia J Jr (1997) Thermodynamics and NMR of internal G.T mismatches in DNA. Biochemistry 36:10581–10594

15. Peyret N, Seneviratne PA, Allawi HT, SantaLucia J (1999) Nearest-neighbor thermodynamics and NMR of DNA sequences with internal A.A, C.C, G.G, and T.T mismatches. J Biochem 38:3468–3477

16. Salk JJ, Sanchez JA, Pierce KE, Rice JE, Soares KC, Wangh LJ (2006) Direct amplification of single-stranded DNA for pyrosequencing using linear-after-the-exponential (LATE)–PCR. J Anal Biochem 353:124–132

17. Abravaya K, Huff J, Marshall R, Merchant B, Mullen C, Schneider G, Robinson J (2003) Molecular beacons as diagnostic tools: technol-

ogy and applications. Clin Chem Lab Med 41:468–474

18. Sanchez JA, Abramowitz JD, Salk JJ, Reis AH Jr, Rice JE, Pierce KE, Wangh LJ (2006) Two-temperature LATE-PCR endpoint genotyping. J BMC Biotechnol 6:44

19. Hartshorn C, Eckert JJ, Hartung O, Wangh LJ (2007) Single-cell duplex RT-LATE-PCR reveals Oct4 and Xist RNA gradients in 8-cell embryos. J BMC Biotechnol 7:87

20. Starita LM, Parvin JD (2003) The multiple nuclear functions of BRCA1: transcription, ubiquitination and DNA repair. J Curr Opin Cell Biol 15:345–350

21. Zhou G, Kamahori M, Okano K, Harada K, Kambara H (2001) Miniaturized pyrose-quencer for DNA analysis with capillaries to deliver deoxynucleotides. Electrophoresis 22:3497–3504

22. Luo J, Wu WJ, Zou BJ, Zhou GH (2007) Expression and purification of ATP sulfurylase from saccharomyces cerevisias in escherichia coli and its application in pyrosequencing. Chinese J Biotech 23:623–627

23. Rice JE, Sanchez JA, Pierce KE, Reis AH Jr, Osborne A, Wangh LJ (2007) Monoplex/multiplex linear-after-the-exponential-PCR assays combined with PrimeSafe and dilute-'N'-Go sequencing. Nat Protoc 2:2429–2438

24. Thornhill A (2007) Single cell diagnostics, 7th edn. Humana Press Inc, Totowa, NJ, pp 65–85

25. Wetmur JG (1991) DNA probes: applications of the principles of nucleic acid hybridization. Crit Rev Biochem Mol Biol 26:227–259

26. Agah A, Aghajan M, Mashayekhi F, Amini S, Davis RW, Plummer JD, Ronaghi M, Griffin PB (2004) A multi-enzyme model for pyrose-quencing. Nucl Acids Res 32, e166

Chapter 2

A Simplified Protocol for Preparing Pyrosequencing Templates Based on LATE-PCR Using Whole Blood as Starting Material Directly

Yunlong Liu, Haiping Wu, Hui Ye, Zhiyao Chen, Qinxin Song, Bingjie Zou, Jianzhong Rui, and Guohua Zhou

Abstract

Pyrosequencing has been one of the most commonly used methods for genotyping; however, generally it needs single-stranded DNA (ssDNA) preparation from PCR amplicons as well as purified genomic DNA extraction from whole blood. To simplify the process of a pyrosequencing protocol, we proposed an improved linear-after-the-exponential (LATE)-PCR by employing whole blood as starting material. A successful LATE-PCR was achieved by using a common Taq DNA polymerase in high pH buffer (HpH-buffer). As amplicons from LATE-PCR contain a large amount of ssDNA, pyrosequencing can be performed on the amplicons directly. Since DNA extraction and ssDNA preparation are omitted, the labor, cost, and cross-contamination risk is decreased comparing to conventional pyrosequencing-based genotyping protocols. The results for typing three polymorphisms related to personalized medicine of fluorouracil indicate that the proposed whole-blood LATE-PCR can be well coupled with pyrosequencing, thus becoming a potential tool in personalized medicine.

Key words Pyrosequencing, Whole-blood PCR, Linear-after-the-exponential (LATE)-PCR, Genotyping, Fluorouracil

1 Introduction

Pyrosequencing is a sequencing-by-synthesis method which is based on the bioluminometric detection of inorganic pyrophosphate (PPi) coupled with cascade enzymatic reactions [1]. In addition to its good performance in quantification, no electrophoresis or fluorescence is required; thus various applications of pyrosequencing have been achieved, such as genotyping [2, 3], methylation detection [4], resequencing [5], gene expression analysis [6–8], micro RNA quantification [9], disease diagnosis [10], and microbial typing [11, 12]. For the moment, pyrosequencing has been widely used in clinical detection of genetic biomarkers related to personalized medicine.

Guohua Zhou and Qinxin Song (eds.), *Advances and Clinical Practice in Pyrosequencing*, Springer Protocols Handbooks, DOI 10.1007/978-1-4939-3308-2_2, © Springer Science+Business Media New York 2016

However, single-stranded DNA (ssDNA) preparation is needed to separate the immobilized strand before pyrosequencing. This step is tedious in operation, costly in the synthesis of biotinylated primers, and high in the risk of cross-contamination from amplicons. To overcome this shortcoming, we have proposed a method enabling pyrosequencing directly on double-stranded DNA (dsDNA) digested by nicking endonuclease [13], in which the recognition sequence of nicking endonuclease was introduced by a PCR primer. After a nicking reaction of the amplicons, pyrosequencing started at the nicked 3′ end, and extension reaction occurred when the added dNTP was complementary to the non-nicked strand. However, the strand-displacement activity of Klenow Fragment was limited. Although around ten bases can be accurately sequenced, the quality of pyrograms was no better than that from the template of ssDNA. In addition, nicking endonuclease is expensive.

In contrast to conventional asymmetric PCR with regular PCR primers at unequal concentrations, linear-after-the-exponential (LATE)-PCR could yield a large amount of ssDNA-amplicons directly [14]. The amount of ssDNA is enough for a successful pyrosequencing reaction after a simple pretreatment of amplicons from LATE-PCR [15]. However, a purified genomic DNA is needed for LATE-PCR. Although there are many commercial kits available for DNA extraction, several hundred microliters of blood sample have to be consumed for an extraction conventionally; so it is impossible to use a tiny amount of finger blood for detection. In addition, this labor-intensive step is a possible risk of cross-contamination. Consequently, it is preferable to directly employ a small amount of blood for PCR. Although our previous study showed that the change of PCR buffer could enable a successful PCR using finger blood or paper-dried blood as starting material [16], it is necessary to investigate whether or not this buffer condition is suitable to whole-blood LATE-PCR. Hence, three polymorphisms related to personalized medicine of fluorouracil (5-FU) were used as an example. The results indicate that our proposed whole-blood LATE-PCR significantly simplified the pyrosequencing-based genotyping protocol, decreasing the labor, cost, and cross-contamination risk.

2   Materials

1. rTaq DNA Polymerase (TaKaRa, China).

2. AmpliTaq Gold DNA Polymerase (Applied Biosystems, USA).

3. Bovine serum albumin (BSA), D-luciferin, adenosine 5′-phosphosulfate (APS), and apyrase VII (Sigma, USA).

4. ATP sulfurylase and Klenow fragment (obtained by gene engineering in our lab).

5. Polyvinylpyrrolidone (PVP) and QuantiLum Recombinant Luciferase (Promega, USA).

6. 2′-deoxyadenosine-5′-O-(1-thiotriphosphate) sodium salt (dATPαS), dGTP, dTTP, and dCTP (MyChem, USA).

7. Streptavidin Sepharose™ Beads (GE Healthcare, USA).

8. HpH buffer (1×): 100 mM Tris–HCl, 50 mM KCl, pH 9.3–9.5.

9. QIAamp DNA Blood Mini Kit (QIAGEN, Germany).

10. One Drop spectrophotometer (Shanghai, China).

11. Mastercycler PCR system (Eppendorf, Germany).

12. A portable bioluminescence analyzer (HITACHI, Ltd., Central Research Laboratory, Japan).

3 Methods

3.1 DNA Samples Extraction

1. Extract purified genomic DNA from whole blood samples by QIAamp DNA Blood Mini Kit.

2. Determine the DNA concentration by a One Drop spectrophotometer (*see* **Note 1**).

3.2 Primer Design

1. Primer sets were designed to amplify a 201-bp fragment containing the MTHFR C677T site, a 170-bp fragment containing the MTHFR A1298C site, and a 192-bp fragment containing the DPYD*2A site according to the principles of LATE-PCR [17] (*see* **Note 2**).

3.3 Whole-Blood LATE-PCR

1. Fifty microliters of PCR contained 1× HpH buffer, 2.0 mM MgCl₂, 100 μM dNTPs, 1 μM excessive primer, 0.1 μM limited primer, 2.5 U of rTaq DNA polymerase, 0.25 μL of Tween 20, 0.5 μL of whole blood (*see* **Notes 3** and **4**).

2. The PCR program was as follows: 94 °C for 3 min, followed by 60 cycles of (90 °C for 10 s; 60 °C for 10 s; 72 °C for 20 s); and finally 72 °C for 7 min.

3.4 Template Preparation for Pyrosequencing

1. Add 40 μL of self-prepared pyrosequencing mixture [18] (*see* **Note 5**) as well as 3 μL of APS (3 nmol) (*see* **Note 6**) into the tube having 3 μL of whole-blood LATE-PCR products.

2. Incubate the tube at room temperature for 5 min.

3. Add 10 pmol of sequencing primers anneal at room temperature for 5 min.

3.5 Pyrosequencing

1. We used a portable bioluminescence analyzer for pyrosequencing [14, 15] (*see* **Note** 7).

2. Pyrosequencing was carried out by the reported method [18]. The reaction volume was 40 μL, containing 0.1 M tris-acetate (pH 7.7), 2 mM EDTA, 10 mM magnesium acetate, 0.1 mg/mL BSA, 1 mM dithiothreitol, 2 μM APS, 0.4 mg/mL PVP, 0.4 mM D-Luciferin, 2 μM ATP sulfurylase, 5.7×10^8 RLU QuantiLum Recombinant Luciferase, 18 U/mL Klenow Fragment, and 1.6 U/mL apyrase.

4 Method Validation

4.1 Genotyping of SNPs Related to Personalized Medicine

As LATE-PCR needs more cycles than conventional PCR, AmpliTaq Gold polymerase, which belongs to a hot-start type with a good thermal stability, was routinely used for amplification [14]. To investigate whether or not this polymerase is suitable for PCR using blood as the starting material, AmpliTaq Gold polymerase-based LATE-PCR using kit-buffer and HpH-buffer (home-made) was carried out on purified genomic DNA and whole blood, respectively. As a proof-of-concept, three SNPs, C677T and A1298C in the MTHFR and DPYD IVS14+1G>A in the DPYD, were employed for the evaluation. These SNPs are related to personalized medicine of 5-FU [19]. As shown in Fig. 1, it is no problem to amplify genomic DNA by LATE-PCR with AmpliTaq Gold polymerase (Fig. 1a); however, it is problematic for AmpliTaq Gold polymerase-based LATE-PCR to directly amplify blood-DNA using either kit-buffer (Fig. 1b) or high pH buffer (HpH-buffer) (Fig. 1c). Therefore the AmpliTaq Gold polymerase which was used in conventional LATE-PCR is not suitable for LATE-PCR directly using blood as the starting material.

To enable LATE-PCR with blood directly, we tried to employ a regular Taq polymerase, named rTaq polymerase, for amplifying gDNA at first. As shown in Fig. 2, good pyrosequencing signals were observed from LATE-PCR using either kit-buffer (Fig. 2a) or HpH-buffer (Fig. 2b), suggesting that LATE-PCR based on rTaq polymerase could yield enough amounts of ssDNA amplicons although there are more heating-cooling cycles which may lower the activity of polymerase. Then, blood was employed as the starting material directly for LATE-PCR using both buffers. As shown in Fig. 2c, d, it is possible to use blood as the starting material for LATE-PCR, but ssDNA yield from kit-buffer-based PCR is much lower than that from HpH-buffer based PCR [20–21]. Most importantly, the intensities of peaks in the pyrogram from LATE-PCR using rTaq polymerase (Fig. 2d) are very close to those from LATE-PCR using AmpliTaq polymerase (Fig. 1a); thus, HpH-buffer previously developed for conventional blood-PCR is very

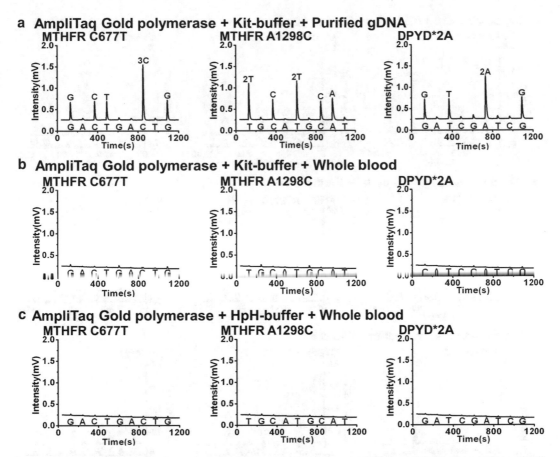

Fig. 1 Pyrograms of amplicons from AmpliTaq Gold polymerase-based PCR using kit-buffer (**a** and **b**) and HpH-buffer (**c**) for amplification as well as using purified gDNA (**a**) and whole blood (**b** and **c**) as starting materials. Three amplified fragments containing three SNPs (MT9HFR C677T, MTHFR A1298C, and DPYD IVS14+1G>A) were pyrosequenced

comparable to that used for LATE-PCR. This enables us to avoid the step of extracting gDNA from blood, greatly simplifying the pyrosequencing-based genotyping.

To demonstrate the feasibility of the proposed method, the three polymorphisms of MTHFR C677T, MTHFR A1298C, and DPYD IVS14+1G>A, which relate to the efficacy and toxicity of 5-FU, were used as the detection targets for the method evaluation. A total of 24 blood samples were obtained from people who voluntarily joined this study with an informed consent form, and the typing results are listed in Table 1. Pyrograms from typical genotypes of the 3 polymorphisms in 24 samples are shown in Fig. 3. As can be seen in the table, the inactive genotype DPYD*2A with the phenotype of DPYD enzyme deficiency was not found

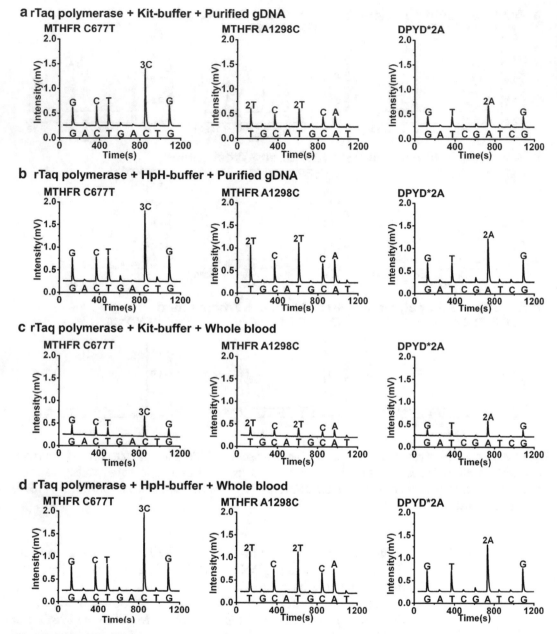

Fig. 2 Pyrograms of amplicons from rTaq polymerase-based LATE-PCR for amplifying purified gDNA (**a**, **b**) and whole blood (**c**, **d**) using kit-buffer (**a**, **c**) and HpH-buffer (**b**, **d**). Three amplified fragments containing three SNPs (MTHFR C677T, MTHFR A1298C, and DPYD*2A) were pyrosequenced

Table 1
Genotyping results of three SNPs in 24 clinical samples by the proposed method

Genes	Alleles/position	Genotype	Enzyme activity
MTHFR	C677T	CC: $n=8$	Normal
		CT: $n=8$	Decreased
		TT: $n=8$	Decreased
	A1298C	AA: $n=18$	Normal
		AC: $n=6$	Decreased
DPYD	*2A	GG: $n=24$	Normal

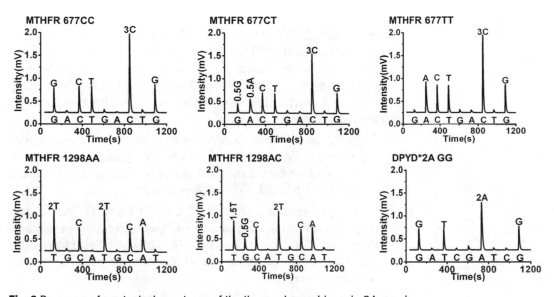

Fig. 3 Pyrograms from typical genotypes of the three polymorphisms in 24 samples

among 24 samples, indicating that the frequency of DPYD*2A is very low in the Chinese population. However, the frequency of MTHFR 677TT with the phenotype of decreased MTHFR activity is as high as 33.3 % in our study. Although the sample size is very small, the preliminary results did imply that it is necessary to detect the genotypes of the 3 polymorphisms in the Chinese population before the administration of 5-FU. MTHFR C677T in a set of 5 typical samples was typed in triplicate, showing a very good reproducibility of our proposed method.

5   Technical Notes

1. The DNA samples should be stored at –20 °C before use.

2. The Tm difference between the limiting primer and the excess primer is greater than 0 °C, the Tm difference between amplicon and the excess primer is less than 13 °C based on concentration-adjusted values. OligoAnalyzer 3.1 (http://www.idtdna.com/analyzer/Applications/OligoAnalyzer/) was used to calculate the primers' Tm values [22].

3. There is no obvious difference in signal intensity among three kinds of anticoagulated blood (EDTA, citrate, and heparin). Therefore, the protocol of the proposed LATE-PCR using HpH buffer is independent of anticoagulant types.

4. Good pyrograms can be obtained when the volume of a blood sample for an assay is larger than 0.1 μL.

5. As residue dNTPs, by-product PPi and incompletely-extended products in whole-blood LATE-PCR amplicons would affect pyrosequencing reactions, it is necessary to perform a cleanup step before pyrosequencing [23]. We can directly employ a conventional pyrosequencing mixture to clean up the amplicons.

6. To compensate for the consumed APS, further addition of APS is necessary. The amount of APS for the compensation is not critical, and we found that it is enough to compensate 1 nmol of APS for 1 μL of LATE-PCR products.

7. This apparatus has a portable size of 140 mm (W) × 158 mm (H) × 250 mm (D), with an array of 8 photodiodes (Hamamatsu Photonics K.K, Japan) to detect photo signals, and four separate capillaries to dispense small amounts of dNTPs into the reaction chamber.

References

1. Ronaghi M, Uhlen M, Nyren P (1998) A sequencing method based on real-time pyrophosphate. Science 281:363–365

2. Chen Z, Fu X, Zhang X, Liu X, Zou B, Wu H, Song Q, Li J, Kajiyama T, Kambara H, Zhou G (2012) Pyrosequencing-based barcodes for a dye-free multiplex bioassay. Chem Commun (Camb) 48:2445–2447

3. Huang H, Xiao P, Qi Z, Bu Y, Liu W, Zhou G (2009) A gel-based solid-phase amplification and its application for SNP typing and sequencing on-chip. Analyst 134:2434–2440

4. Brakensiek K, Wingen LU, Langer F, Kreipe H, Lehmann U (2007) Quantitative high-resolution CpG Island Mapping with Pyrosequencing™ reveals disease-specific methylation patterns of the CDKN2B gene in myelodysplastic syndrome and myeloid leukemia. Clin Chem 53:17–23

5. Schuster SC (2008) Next-generation sequencing transforms today's biology. Nat Methods 5:16–18

6. Song Q, Jing H, Wu H, Zhou G, Kajiyama T, Kambara H (2010) Gene expression analysis on a photodiode array-based bioluminescence analyzer by using sensitivity-improved SRPP. Analyst 135:1315–1319

7. Jia H, Chen Z, Wu H, Yan Z, Zhou G (2011) Pyrosequencing on templates generated by asymmetric nucleic acid sequence-based amplification (asymmetric-NASBA). Analyst 136:5229–5233

8. Zhang X, Wu H, Chen Z, Zhou G, Kajiyama T, Kambara H (2009) Dye-free gene expression detection by sequence-tagged reverse-transcription polymerase chain reaction coupled with pyrosequencing. Anal Chem 81: 273–281

9. Jing H, Song Q, Chen Z, Zou B, Chen C, Zhu M, Zhou G, Kajiyama T, Kambara H (2011) Dye-free microRNA quantification by using pyrosequencing with a sequence-tagged stem-loop RT primer. ChemBioChem 12:845–849

10. Ye H, Wu H, Huang H, Liu Y, Zou B, Sun L, Zhou G (2013) Prenatal diagnosis of trisomy 21 by quantitatively pyrosequencing heterozygotes using amniotic fluid as starting material of PCR. Analyst 138:2443–2448

11. Yang H, Huang H, Wu H, Zou B, Zhou G, Kajiyama T, Kambara H (2011) A pyrosequencing-based method for genotyping pathogenic serotypes of S. suis. Anal Methods 3:2517–2523

12. Wang WP, Wu WJ, Zhou GH (2008) Detection of avian influenza a virus using pyrosequencing. Chin J Anal Chem 36:775–780

13. Song Q, Wu H, Feng F, Zhou G, Kajiyama T, Kambara H (2010) Pyrosequencing on nicked dsDNA generated by nicking endonucleases. Anal Chem 82:2074–2081

14. Sanchez JA, Pierce KE, Rice JE, Wangh LJ (2004) Linear-after-the-exponential (LATE)-PCR: an advanced method of asymmetric PCR and its uses in quantitative real-time analysis. Proc Natl Acad Sci U S A 101:1933–1938

15. Salk JJ, Sanchez JA, Pierce KE, Rice JE, Soares KC, Wangh LJ (2006) Direct amplification of single-stranded DNA for pyrosequencing using linear-after-the-exponential (LATE)-PCR. Anal Biochem 353:124–132

16. Bu Y, Huang H, Zhou G (2008) Direct polymerase chain reaction(PCR) from human whole blood and filter-paper-dried blood by using a PCR buffer with a higher pH. Anal Biochem 375:370–372

17. Pierce KE, Sanchez JA, Rice JE, Wangh LJ (2005) Linear-After-The-Exponential (LATE)-PCR: primer design criteria for high yields of specific single-stranded DNA and improved real-time detection. Proc Natl Acad Sci U S A 102:8609–8614

18. Wu H, Wu W, Chen Z, Wang W, Zhou G, Kajiyama T, Kambara H (2011) Highly sensitive pyrosequencing based on the capture of free adenosine 5′ phosphosulfate with adenosine triphosphate sulfurylase. Anal Chem 83:3600–3605

19. Song Q, Yang H, Zou B, Kajiyama T, Kambara H, Zhou G (2013) Improvement of LATE-PCR to allow single-cell analysis by pyrosequencing. Analyst 138:4991–4997

20. Scartozzi M, Maccaroni E, Giampieri R, Pistelli M, Bittoni A, Del Prete M, Berardi R, Cascinu S (2011) 5-fluorouracil pharmacogenomics: still rocking after all these years? Pharmacogenomics 12:251–265

21. Jiang W, Lu Z, He Y, Diasio RB (1997) Dihydropyrimidine dehydrogenase activity in hepatocellular carcinoma: implication in 5-fluorouracil-based chemotherapy. Clin Cancer Res 3:395–399

22. Diasio RB, Harris BE (1989) Clinical pharmacology of 5-fluorouracil. Clin Pharmacokinet 16:215–237

23. Van Kuilenburg AB, Haasjes J, Richel DJ, Zoetekouw L, Van Lenthe H, De Abreu RA, Maring JG, Vreken P, Van Gennip AH (2000) Clinical implications of dihydropyrimidine dehydrogenase (DPD) deficiency in patients with severe 5-fluorouracil-associated toxicity: identification of new mutations in the DPD gene. Clin Cancer Res 6:4705–4712

Chapter 3

Improvement of LATE-PCR to Prepare Pyrosequencing Template

Qinxin Song, Huiyong Yang, Bingjie Zou, Hideki Kambara, and Guohua Zhou

Abstract

Nucleic acid analysis in a single cell is very important, but the extremely small amount of template in a single cell requires a detection method more sensitive than the conventional method. In this chapter, we describe a novel assay allowing a single cell genotyping by coupling improved linear-after-the-exponential-PCR (imLATE-PCR) on a modified glass slide with highly sensitive pyrosequencing. Due to the significantly increased yield of ssDNA in imLATE-PCR amplicons, it is possible to employ pyrosequencing to sequence the products from 1-µL chip PCR which directly used a single cell as starting material. As a proof-of-concept, the 1555A>G mutation (related to inherited deafness) on mitochondrial DNA and the SNP 2731 C>T of the BRCA1 gene on genome DNA from a single cell have been successfully detected, indicating that our single-cell-pyrosequencing method has high sensitivity, simple operation, and low cost. The approach has promise for efficient use in the fields of diagnosis of genetic disease from a single cell, for example, preimplantation genetic diagnosis (PGD).

Key words Single cell analysis (SCA), Pyrosequencing, imLATE (Improved linear-after-the-exponential-PCR), Low volume PCR, Nucleic acid analysis

1 Introduction

To achieve a sensitive PCR detection with a small amount of DNA template, a low volume (around 1 mL) PCR on a chemically structured chip was developed for the analysis of mitochondrial DNA at single cell levels. However, it is difficult to prepare a single-stranded DNA (ssDNA) from this low volume PCR product for pyrosequencing, which is a very suitable tool for genetic analysis. To allow pyrosequencing on this small amount of amplicons directly, it is necessary to escape the step of ssDNA preparation. If amplicons from PCR contains enough amount of ssDNA, no ssDNA-preparation is needed. Conventionally, ssDNA can be directly generated by asymmetric PCR with regular PCR primers at unequal concentrations. However, asymmetric PCR is inefficient, and it is

Guohua Zhou and Qinxin Song (eds.), *Advances and Clinical Practice in Pyrosequencing*, Springer Protocols Handbooks, DOI 10.1007/978-1-4939-3308-2_3, © Springer Science+Business Media New York 2016

difficult to get an optimized amplification condition for templates with different sequences.

A newly developed linear-after-the-exponential-PCR (LATE-PCR) is more efficient than asymmetric PCR in the generation of ssDNA products [1]. As the decrease of melting temperature of a limiting primer due to low concentration in asymmetric PCR was well compensated by the increased length of the primer, LATE-PCR could be optimized to give an amplification efficiency similar to that of symmetric PCR; linear amplification in LATE-PCR starts after the limiting primer decreased to a concentration which could not trigger a primer extension reaction. A high yield of ssDNA was generated without extensive PCR optimization, and signal strength in quantitative real-time analysis was increased by 80–250 % relative to symmetric PCR. It was proved that the yielded ssDNA could be a template of pyrosequencing just after a simple enzymatic treatment. However we found that the strict criteria for LATE-PCR primer design greatly limits the wide application of the method [2]. Most importantly, the length of amplicons should be short enough to ensure that Tm difference between the amplicon and the excess primer is less than 13 °C. Usually, an SNP loci of interest is fixed, so a difficulty may occur in designing qualified LATE-PCR primers at GC-rich or AT-rich regions. The main problem of low amplification efficiency of LATE-PCR is due to the competition of excess primer with the amplicon strand. As amplicon strand is increasing in the concentration along with the progress of PCR, while the excess primer is decreasing in the concentration, the yield of ssDNA should not be high if the amplicon is longer [3–6]. In this chapter, we describe a novel assay allowing a single cell genotyping by coupling improved linear-after-the-exponential-PCR (imLATE-PCR) (Fig. 1) on a modified glass slide with highly sensitive pyrosequencing.

2 Materials

1. AmpliTaq Gold DNA Polymerase (Applied Biosystems, CA).

2. TransStart Taq DNA Polymerase (TransGen Biotech, China).

3. Exo-Klenow Fragment, QuantiLum recombinant luciferase (Promega, WI).

4. ATP sulfurylase, apyrase, D-luciferin, and adenosine 5′-phosphosulfate (APS) (Sigma, MO).

5. 2′-Deoxyadenosine-5′-O-(1-thiotriphosphate) sodium salt (dATP-a-S) (Amersham Pharmacia Biotech, U.K.).

6. dGTP, dTTP, and dCTP (Amersham Pharmacia Biotech, NJ).

7. All the other reagents were analytical reagents or guaranteed reagents. All the solutions were prepared with deionized and sterilized H_2O.

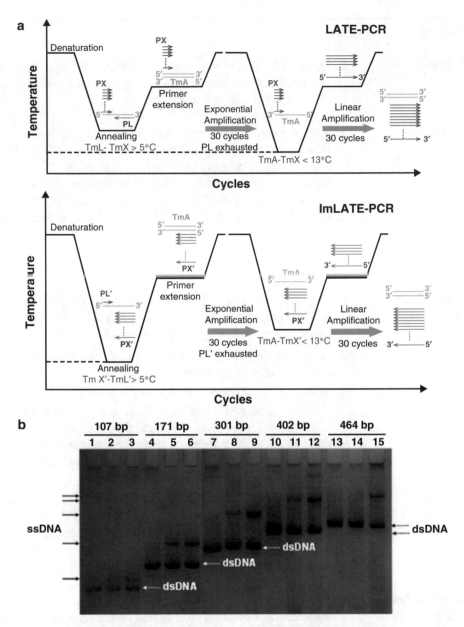

Fig. 1 (**a**) Comparison of principle between LATE-PCR and imLATE-PCR. (**b**) PAGE electropherogram of amplicons with different lengths from symmetry PCR (*lanes 1, 4, 7, 10,* and *13*), LATE-PCR (*lanes 2, 5, 8, 11,* and *14*), and imLATE-PCR (*lanes 3, 6, 9, 12,* and *15*) of the human BRCA1 gene

8. AmpliGrid AG480 (Fa. Advalytix, Brunnthal, Germany).

9. SMZ1000 dissection microscope (Nikon, Japan).

10. ECLIPSE TE2000-S inverted microscope (Nikon, Japan).

11. PTC-225 Peltier Thermal Cycler (MJ Research, Watertown, MA, USA).

12. Homemade PD array 8-channel pyrosequencer [7].

3 Methods

3.1 Cell Lines

1. Hep G2 Human liver cancer cell line, leucocyte in peripheral blood of nonsyndromic hearing impairment (NSHI) patients, ICR mice oocytes are used.

3.2 Primers

1. The sequences near the SNP (2731C>T) of human BRCA1 (breast cancer susceptibility gene 1) gene (NT_010755.15) are selected as examples to compare imLATE-PCR and LATE-PCR. The primers for 1555A>G mutation of inherited deafness on mitochondrial DNA are: excess primer 5′-TCGCCTGA GTGTAAGTTGGGTGCTTTGTGTT-3′ and limiting primer (anneal primer) 5′-AACCCCTACGCATTTATATAGAGG AG-3′, the amplicon length is 117 bp. All of the oligomers are synthesized and purified by Invitrogen (Shanghai, China).

3.3 Collect Single Cell by Using Glass Capillaries

1. The sterilized watch glass (or glass slides) is placed on microscope stage, and 30 μL of cell suspension is then added on the surface of the watch glass (*see* **Note 1**).

2. Let sit watch glass for 2 min to let cells precipitate completely to the surface of the watch glass.

3. With the SMZ1000 microscope under 4×10 magnifications (Nikon, Japan), the capillary tip is adjusted into the cell suspension and located at the central of the microscopic vision, and the pressure button of the manipulator is then manually and slightly adjusted to make a well-dispersed, full-membrane, and contour-cleared single cell [8].

4. Then, the capillary is lifted off the surface of cell suspension, and the captured single cell is transferred to the reaction locus of the AmpliGrid slides (AG480F). The image is obtained using ECLIPSE TE2000-S inverted microscope under 10 × 10 magnifications (*see* **Note 2**).

3.4 Single Cell Lysis and On-Chip imLATE-PCR

1. A volume of 0.5 μL of proteinase K (0.4 mg/ml) is pipetted to the reaction site of an AmpliGrid slide containing a single cell and covered immediately with 5 μL of sealing oil (*see* **Note 3**).

2. After complete loading, the AmpliGrid slide is incubated for 40 min at 56 °C and 10 min at 99 °C.

3. 0.5 μL of PCR master mix is added, piercing through the sealing oil. So a total volume of 1 μL PCR reaction mix, containing 0.1 μL AmpliTaq Gold (5 U/μL), 0.1 μL GeneAmp 10× PCR Gold Buffer (both: Applied Biosystems), 0.04 μL dNTPs

(2.5 mM each), 0.06 μL MgCl$_2$ (25 mM), 0.1 μL PX (10 μM), 0.1 μL PL (1 μM) is obtained.

4. On-chip imLATE-PCR program: initial heating step at 95 °C for 10 min, followed by 30 cycles (denaturation at 95 °C for 10 s, annealing at 54 °C for 10 s, elongation at 72 °C for 40 s), then followed by another 30 cycles (denaturation at 95 °C for 10 s, annealing at 65 °C for 10 s, elongation at 72 °C for 40 s), followed by a final 10 min elongation step at 72 °C. Negative controls are performed on different positions on the chip using the same reagent solutions without cell or DNA.

5. After the amplification, combine 1 μL aqueous phase and 4 μL loading dye (1.25×); a total 5 μL of each mixture is transferred to a 6 % PAGE gel and separated for 40 min at 100 V.

6. Silver staining is performed with 0.1 % AgNO$_3$ solution for 30 min, followed by a 10 s washing step in DI water and development in 2 % Na$_2$CO$_3$/0.1 % formaldehyde for 2 min.

3.5 Removal of PPi in dNTPs by Biotinylated Ppase

1. The biotinylated PPase is immobilized onto streptavidin-coated M280 Dynabeads (37 °C, 30 min) and washed with 1× annealing buffer (4 mM Tris–HCl, pH 7.5, 2 mM MgCl$_2$, 5 mM NaCl), then dissolved in 1× annealing buffer.

2. 10 mmol/L dNTPs (dATPαS, dCTP, dTTP, dGTP) are diluted by dNTPs diluent (5 mmol/L Tris-Ac, 25 mmol/L Mg(Ac)$_2$, pH 7.7) to 200 μmol/L.

3. Then 0.5 μL Beads-PPase is added to each kind of 200 μL dNTPs and incubated at room temperature for 5 min.

4. The beads is focused with a magnet, supernatant is aspirated carefully and added to the micro-dispenser of pyrosequencer separately. Using the pyrosequencer to detect the signal of biotinylated PPase treated dNTPs and the signal of untreated dNTPs.

3.6 Pyrosequencing

1. We constructed a prototype of 8-channel pyrosequencer by using a PD array sensor [7]. The reaction volume in every well for pyrosequencing is 40 μL, containing 0.1 M tris-acetate (pH 7.7), 2 mM EDTA, 10 mM magnesium acetate, 0.1 % BSA, 1 mM dithiothreitol (DTT), 2 μM adenosine 50-phosphosulfate (APS), 0.4 mg/mL PVP, 0.4 mM D-luciferin, 200 mU/mL ATP sulfurylase, 3 μg/mL luciferase, 18 U/mL Klenow fragment, and 1.6 U/mL apyrase.

2. Each of biotinylated PPase-treated dNTPs is added in the reservoir of the micro-dispenser, and pyrosequencing reaction starts when the dispensed dNTP is complementary to the template sequence.

4   Method Validation

4.1   Principle of the Improved Linear-After-the-Exponential (imLATE)-PCR

The difference in principle between LATE-PCR and improved LATE-PCR (imLATE-PCR) is displayed in Fig. 1a. In contrast to LATE-PCR, the annealing temperature in the phase of exponential amplification is lower than that of linear amplification. As the excess primer is longer in length, its Tm could be very close to Tm of amplicon, resulting in a very higher rate of linear amplification, which is a limiting process for yielding ssDNA. Therefore the length of amplicon could be longer, and the choice for primer sequences could be more. One potential issue of imLATE-PCR is the poor specificity due to a lower annealing temperature in the phase of exponential amplification.

To check this issue, and to verify whether or not imLATE-PCR is effective in the amplification of various lengths of amplicons, different primer sets are used to amplify the BRCA1 gene related to human breast cancer by symmetric PCR, LATE-PCR, and imLATE-PCR, respectively. The expected sizes of double-strand amplicons are 107 bp, 171 bp, 301 bp, 402 bp, and 464 bp. The electrophoresis results of amplicons from all PCRs are shown in Fig. 1b, indicating that all PCRs generated double-stranded amplicons with expected sizes and the yields of ssDNA from imLATE-PCR are much more than that from LATE-PCR in all the tested amplicons. In particular, when the size of amplicon is 464 bp, almost no ssDNA products are observed from conventional LATE-PCR, but ssDNA with a visible band in the figure is obtained for imLATE-PCR. Most importantly, the issue of poor specificity due to a low annealing temperature in the phase of exponential amplification in imLATE-PCR does not occur.

4.2   Evaluation of the imLATE-PCR Method

Before starting single cell pyrosequencing, 1 μL imLATE-PCR with various amounts of DNA templates (10, 10^3, 10^5 copies) diluted from amplicons is performed on the AmpliGrid chip. The amplicon is amplified from human mitochondrial DNA, and contains the mutation point of 1555A>G, which contributes to both amino glycoside-induced and non-syndromic hearing loss in families worldwide. After PCR, the amplicons are treated with pyrosequencing reaction mixture to extend all strands which are not fully extended during LATE-PCR, to degrade dNTPs, and to convert PPi to ATP [9, 10]. Then sequencing primer is added for hybridization before starting pyrosequencing reaction. A good quality pyrogram is observed even if the DNA template is as low as 10 copies (Fig. 2). This sensitivity is enough to detect the mutation point of 1555A>G in a single cell, because a single cell contains hundreds of copies of mitochondrial DNA.

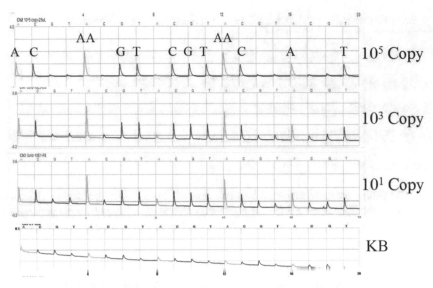

Fig. 2 Pyrograms of different amounts templates (10^5, 10^3, 10^1 copies, and blank) by 1 μL of imLATE-PCR products on slide. The expected sequence is indicated above peak

4.3 Evaluation of the Success Rate of Amplification and the Cross-Contamination on Chip

To check whether oil can closely seal the PCR mixture of each position, a series of single-cell PCR for detecting 1555A>G on mtDNA is performed at four lanes in a slide (Fig. 3). The positioning pattern of samples is single cancer cells (Hep G) at lanes A and C for positive control, water at lane B for blank control, and single mouse oocytes at lane D for negative control. As expected, no positive result is observed from all positions at the lanes C and D, suggesting that cross talk did not occur between positions in the slide. The negative results in the lane D also demonstrate a high specificity of the proposed method.

5   Technical Notes

1. For picking up and transferring individual cells, we usually use a mouth tube to control an attached micropipette (glass capillaries) under a dissection microscope, which permits swift and efficient control of individual cell collection and release. The glass pipette is connected by a flexible plastic pipe to the mouth of the researcher. If the pipette size is right it is readily feasible to control the pressure inside the pipette and collect individual cells with minimum volume of extracellular solution ($\ll 0.1$ μL).

2. As a control for contamination and inhibition of downstream reactions, 1 μL of the buffer or medium surrounding the cells should be collected and analyzed together with the single-cell samples.

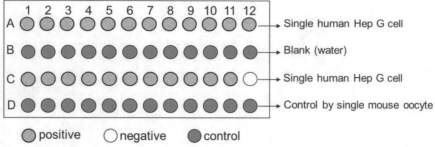

Fig. 3 Tests for evaluating cross-contamination between wells on the slide. The positioning pattern of samples is single cancer cells (Hep G) at *lanes a* and *c* for positive control, water at *lane b* for blank control, and single mouse oocytes at *lane d* for negative control. Pyrosequencing of the products from imLATE-PCR of the 1555A>G on mtDNA. About 95.8 % (23/24) wells are positively detected

3. Low volume-PCR is performed with chips (AG480F AmpliGrid slide) on PTC-225 Peltier Thermal Cycler Flat Block. These are chemically structured glass slides, originally developed for single cell analysis and quantification of single genome equivalents [11]. Biochemical reactions proceed on 48 lithographically defined hydrophilic anchor spots, each framed by a hydrophobic ring. Each of the reaction compartments can hold up to 2 μL of aqueous solution.

References

1. Kalisky T, Quake SR (2011) Single-cell genomics. Nat Methods 8:311–314
2. Schroeder T (2011) Long-term single-cell imaging of mammalian stem cells. Nat Methods 8:S30–S35
3. Zeevi DA, Renbaum P, Ron-El R, Eldar-Geva T, Raziel A, Brooks B, Strassburger DE, Margalioth J, Levy-Lahad E, Altarescu G (2013) Preimplantation genetic diagnosis in genomic regions with duplications and pseudogenes: long-range PCR in the single-cell assay. Hum Mutat 34:792–799
4. Kroneis T, Geigl JB, El-Heliebi A, Auer M, Ulz P, Schwarzbraun T, Dohr G, Sedlmayr P (2011) Combined molecular genetic and cytogenetic analysis from single cells after isothermal whole-genome amplification. Clin Chem 57:1032–1041
5. Sanchez JA, Pierce KE, Rice JE, Wangh LJ (2004) Linear-after-the-exponential (LATE)-PCR: an advanced method of asymmetric PCR and its uses in quantitative real-time analysis. Proc Natl Acad Sci U S A 101:1933–1938
6. Pierce KE, Sanchez JA, Rice JE, Wangh LJ (2005) Linear-After-The-Exponential (LATE)-PCR: primer design criteria for high yields of specific single-stranded DNA and improved real-time detection. Proc Natl Acad Sci U S A 102:8609–8614
7. Song Q, Jing H, Wu H, Zhou G, Kajiyama T, Kambara H (2010) Gene expression analysis on a photodiode array-based bioluminescence analyzer by using sensitivity-improved SRPP. Analyst 135:1315–1319
8. Ahmadian A, Ehn M, Hober S (2006) Pyrosequencing: history, biochemistry and future. Clin Chim Acta 363:83–94
9. Schmidt U, Lutz-Bonengel S, Weisser HJ, Sanger T, Pollak S, Schon U, Zacher T, Mann W (2006) Low-volume amplification on chemically structured chips using the PowerPlex16 DNA amplification kit. Int J Legal Med 120:42–48
10. Wu H, Wu W, Chen Z, Wang W, Zhou G, Kajiyama T, Kambara H (2011) Highly sensitive pyrosequencing based on the capture of free adenosine 5′ phosphosulfate with adenosine triphosphate sulfurylase. Anal Chem 83:3600–3605
11. Song Q, Wu H, Feng F, Zhou G, Kajiyama T, Kambara H (2010) Pyrosequencing on nicked dsDNA generated by nicking endonucleases. Anal Chem 82:2074–2081

Chapter 4

Pyrosequencing Templates Generated by Nicking PCR Products with Nicking Endonuclease

Qinxin Song, Haiping Wu, Guohua Zhou, and Hideki Kambara

Abstract

Although the pyrosequencing method is simple and fast, the step of ssDNA preparation increases the cost, labors, and cross-contamination risk. In this chapter, we proposed a method enabling pyrosequencing directly on dsDNA digested by nicking endonuclease (NEases). Recognition sequence of NEases was introduced by using artificially mismatched bases in a PCR primer (in the case of genotyping) or a reverse-transcription (RT) primer (in the case of gene expression analysis). PCR products were treated to remove excess amounts of primers, nucleotides, and pyrophosphate (PPi) prior to sequencing. After nicking reaction, pyrosequencing starts at the nicked 3′ end, and extension reaction occurs when the added dNTP is complementary to the non-nicked strand. Although the activity of strand displacement by Klenow is limited, ~10 bases are accurately sequenced; this length is long enough for genotyping and SRPP-based differential gene expression analysis. As the highly quantitative signals of two allele-specific bases in the pyrogram, DOWN'S syndrome diagnosis based on quantitative SNP typing and differential gene expression analysis of a breast cancer-related gene were successfully demonstrated. The results indicate that pyrosequencing using nicked dsDNA as templates is a simple, inexpensive, and reliable way in either quantitative genotyping or gene expression analysis.

Key words Pyrosequencing, Nicking endonuclease, Genotyping, Gene expression analysis

1 Introduction

Pyrosequencing is a well-developed technology for DNA sequencing that employs coupled enzymatic reactions to detect the inorganic pyrophosphate (PPi) released during dNTP incorporation [1]. For the advantages of accuracy, flexibility, and parallel processing [2–5], pyrosequencing has been widely used for DNA resequencing [6–8], genotyping [9, 10], DNA methylation [11], and gene expression analysis [12].

In conventional pyrosequencing protocol, a biotin-modified PCR primer and streptavidin-coated beads are required to prepare ssDNA template prior to pyrosequencing. Although very-high-quality sequence data are obtained with ssDNA, reagents used to

Guohua Zhou and Qinxin Song (eds.), *Advances and Clinical Practice in Pyrosequencing*, Springer Protocols Handbooks, DOI 10.1007/978-1-4939-3308-2_4, © Springer Science+Business Media New York 2016

prepare ssDNA are expensive [13] and multiple steps that are needed to prepare the template increase the risk of DNA contamination in the air. To eliminate the ssDNA preparation step, a method that enables pyrosequencing on double-stranded DNA template has been developed, using a combination of several enzymes to degrade PPi (a by-product produced in PCR) and residual PCR components, dNTPs, and primers [14]. This method was further simplified by employing blocking oligonucleotides to capture the free PCR primers [15]. A trial for realizing a robust pyrosequencing method using dsDNA templates has been achieved; however, the data quality for some templates was poor. The main reasons for the poor data quality were considered to be due to (a) the formation of primer dimers, (b) inefficient primer degradation, (c) ghost signals originated in undegraded PCR primers, and (d) low efficiency for a sequencing primer to hybridize to dsDNA.

An alternative method for simplifying the protocol is performed using an asymmetric PCR method, linear-after-the-exponential (LATE)-PCR [16, 17], where ssDNA is directly produced for pyrosequencing and, thus, a tedious ssDNA preparation step after PCR is avoided. Although it was demonstrated that the method could sequence DNA up to 50 bases or longer [18], our experiences using various DNA templates suggested that strict criteria for LATE-PCR primer design greatly limits the application of this method. In addition, a large number of thermal cycles (~60 cycles) in LATE-PCR significantly increase the risk of producing nonspecific amplicons, which cause false signals in a pyrogram, and decrease the amplification efficiency, because of the lower activity of DNA polymerase in the later cycles. Most importantly, the use of ssDNA as pyrosequencing templates may cause the self-priming of a template's 3′ end, resulting in undesired signals [19]. This becomes a serious concern when the template size is >300 bp as the possibility of self-priming of ssDNA's 3′ end increases with the template length. Although the formation of the secondary structure and self-priming of an ssDNA template were effectively prevented by blocking the template's 3′ end, this protocol is labor intensive and complex. Thus, the use of dsDNA instead of ssDNA as the templates for direct pyrosequencing is promising. Here, we describe a simple method for preparing a template DNA for pyrosequencing by nicking dsDNA. We used newly developed nicking endonucleases (NEases) [20–24], such as Nt.BstNBI and Nt.AlwI, which only cleave one specific strand of a duplex, instead of cleaving both strands. The cleaved DNA is still in a double-stranded state at room temperature, while the 3′ end at the nick is extendable, and can be extended by a polymerase that has strand displacement activity. For the moment, several polymerases with strand displacement activity are available in the market, including Sequence, Klenow, Phi-29 polymerase, and Bst DNA polymerases. Because

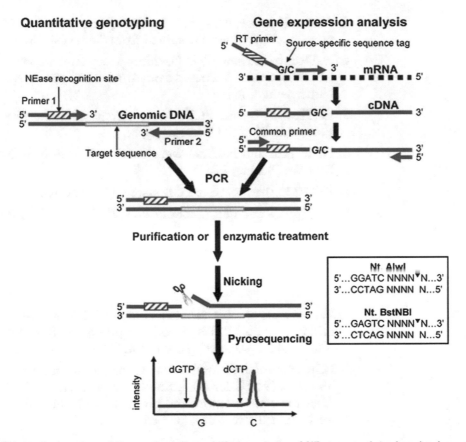

Fig. 1 Schematic overview of the method. Recognition sequence of NEases was introduced using artificially mismatched bases in a PCR primer (in the case of genotyping) or a reverse-transcription (RT) primer (in the case of gene expression analysis). PCR products were treated to remove excess amounts of primers, nucleotides, and pyrophosphate (PPi) prior to sequencing. After the nicking reaction, pyrosequencing starts at the nicked 3′ end, and extension reaction occurs when the added dNTP is complementary to the non-nicked strand. Inset shows the recognition sequences and nicking sites of two typical NEases. (The *superscripted inverted triangle symbol* in the sequence strands given in the *legend box* denotes the cleavage position of the NEase)

Klenow is the polymerase conventionally used in pyrosequencing, we employed nicked dsDNA template for pyrosequencing using the strand displacement activity of Klenow. We have successfully used this method for quantitative SNP typing and gene expression analysis. For a schematic overview, see Fig. 1.

2 Materials

1. HotStarTaq DNA polymerase was purchased from Qiagen (Qiagen GmbH, Hilden, Germany).

2. Exo-Klenow Fragment, QuantiLum recombinant luciferase was purchased from Promega (Madison, WI).

3. ATP sulfurylase, apyrase, D-luciferin, and adenosine 5′-phosphosulfate (APS) were obtained from Sigma (St. Louis, MO).

4. 2′-Deoxyadenosine-5′-O-(1-thiotriphosphate) sodium salt (dATP-R-S) was purchased from Amersham Pharmacia Biotech (Amersham, UK).

5. dGTP, dTTP, and dCTP were purchased from Amersham Pharmacia Biotech (Piscat-away, NJ).

6. Nt.BstNBI and Nt.AlwI were purchased from New England BioLabs (Beijing, PRC).

7. PTC-225 thermocycler PCR system (MJ research).

8. PCR purification kit (BioSpin PCR Purification Kit, BioFlux, PRC).

3 Methods

3.1 PCR

1. Each 50 μL of PCR mixture contained 1.5 mM MgCl$_2$, 0.2 mM of each dNTP, 0.3 μM of each primer, 1 μL of DNA template, and 1.25 unit of Hotstar Taq DNA polymerase.

2. PCR mixture denatured at 94 °C for 15 min and followed by 35 cycles (94 °C for 40 s; 55 °C for 40 s; 72 °C for 1 min). After the cycle reaction, the product was incubated at 72 °C for 10 min and held at 4 °C before use.

3.2 Treatment of dsDNA with Nicking Endonucleases

1. PCR products were purified by the commercially available PCR purification kit or enzymatically treated by apyrase coupled with ATP sulfurylase (see **Note 1**).

2. Incubate at 37 °C with Nt.AlwI or 55 °C with Nt.BstNBI in a 1× reaction buffer (see **Note 2**). Typically, the incubation was performed for 0.5–1 h with 5–10 U of nicking endonuclease (see **Note 3**).

3. The reactions were heat-killed at 80 °C for 20 min and stored at 4 °C until pyrosequencing.

4. Five microliters (5 μL) of the treated sample (see **Note 4**) were used for pyrosequencing.

3.3 Pyrosequencing

1. The reaction buffer of pyrosequencing was 100 μL, containing 0.1 M tris-acetate (pH 7.7), 2 mM EDTA, 10 mM magnesium acetate, 0.1 % BSA, 1 mM dithiothreitol (DTT), 2 μM adenosine 5′-phosphosulfate (APS), 0.4 mg/mL PVP, 0.4 mM D-LUCIFERIN, 200 mU/mL ATP sulfurylase, 3 μg/mL luciferase, 18 U/mL Klenow fragment (see **Note 5**), and 1.6 U/mL apyrase.

2. Pyrosequencing was performed at 28 °C on a commercialized Pyromark ID/PSQ 96 MA Pyrosequencer system or Prototype of Portable Bioluminescence Analyzer.

3. An initial dispensation of enzyme and substrate mixes.

4. Sequencing: A stepwise elongation of the primer strand through sequential additions of four types of deoxynucleotide triphosphates, degradation of nucleotides by apyrase, and simultaneous detection of the resulting light emission.

4 Method Validation

4.1 Pyrosequencing on Nicked dsDNA

Three individual regions (namely, M1, M2, and M3) from different parts of the Avian Influenza Virus M gene were investigated. The sequences from the pyrograms in Fig. 2 are read as 5'-AGTTAAG-3' (M1), 5'-ATTCACA-3' (M2), and 5'-GAGCAG GC-3' (M3), which are the same as those in NCBI.

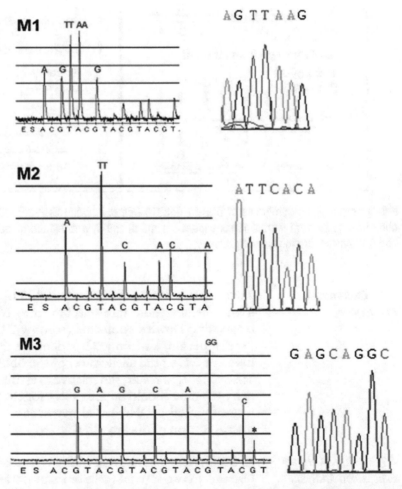

Fig. 2 Pyrograms of nicked dsDNA templates amplified from three different regions in the Avian Influenza Virus M Gene. Amplicons M1, M2, and M3 were amplified by the PCR primer having 1, 2, and 0 artificially mismatched bases, respectively

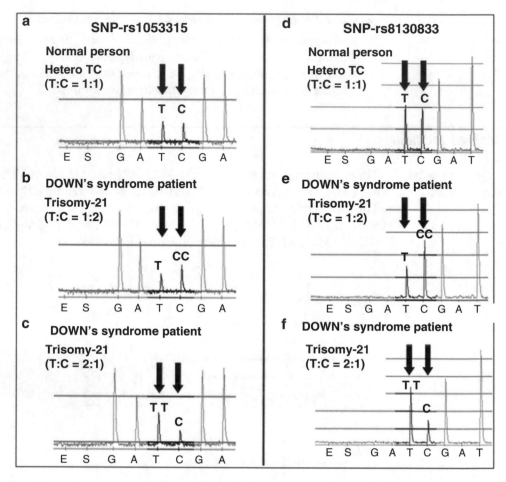

Fig. 3 Heterozygote pyrograms of SNP-rs1053315 (*left panel*) and SNP-rs8130833 (*right panel*) located in chromosome 21 from normal persons (panels **a** and **d**) and Down's syndrome patients (panels **b**, **c**, **e**, and **f**). The SNP types were indicated by *arrows*

4.2 Quantitative Genotyping

Two SNPs (rs1053315 and rs8130833 on chromosome 21) with a high heterozygote rate selected from NCBI were analyzed for diagnosing Down's syndrome (trisomy-21) *(25)*. In contrast to a normal person, a trisomy-21 patient has an additional third chromosome 21, so the allelic ratio of the SNPs in chromosome 21 is 1:2 or 2:1. As a result, the relative peak intensity of a heterozygote in a pyrogram should be 1:2 or 2:1 for the patient. The high accuracy of nicked dsDNA-based pyrosequencing gives unambiguous discrimination of trisomy-21 (Fig. 3).

4.3 Differential Gene Expression Analysis

In SRPP, the quantification of the expression levels of a given gene differing in two sources (cells or tissues) was achieved by comparing signal intensities of two peaks originated in the source-specific bases artificially introduced during reverse transcription. The logic of this assay is similar to an allele frequency analysis in genomic DNA

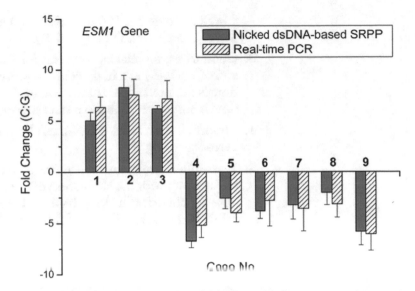

Fig. 4 Comparison between nicked dsDNA-based SRPP (*gray*) and real-time PCR (*white*) for the quantification of the expression levels of the ESM1 gene in nine cases suffering from breast cancer (*n*= 3). Differential expression levels between tumor tissue and normal tissue adjacent to tumor tissue were denoted by fold changes (tumor tissue/normal tissue)

pools; therefore, the quantification performance of nicked dsDNA-based pyrosequencing becomes a key issue of SRPP accuracy.

We have further applied the proposed SRPP to compare the expression levels of the ESM1 gene between breast cancer tissue and normal tissue in clinical samples. Fold changes of the expression levels of the ESM1 gene in nine cases were successfully detected by both SRPP and real-time PCR (see Fig. 4 for details), and we did not find any significant difference between the two methods, indicating reliable results of differential gene expression analysis by SRPP based on nicked dsDNA.

5   Technical Notes

1. The residual primers and nucleotides in PCR products should be removed prior to sequencing. It was found that there was no obvious sequencing signal for raw PCR products, while unambiguous sequencing data were observed when the PCR products were purified by a PCR purification kit or treated by enzymes.

2. The qualified NEases currently available are Nt.AlwI and Nt.BstNBI, both of which have a four-base distance between the recognition site and the nicking site. Nt.AlwI works in a buffer containing 50 mM NaCl, 10 mM Tris–HCl, 10 mM $MgCl_2$, and 1 mM DTT (pH 7.9), while Nt.BstNBI works in

a buffer containing 100 mM NaCl, 50 mM Tris–HCl, 10 mM MgCl$_2$, and 1 mM DTT (pH 7.9).

3. Conducting the nicking reaction for more than 1 h produces nicked dsDNAs at a high yield. However, a longer incubation time is not preferable, and we found that 30 min of incubation time is sufficient to obtain a satisfying pyrogram.

4. Almost all the nicked dsDNA can be the effective template of pyrosequencing.

5. The strand displacement activity of Klenow reduced significantly along with the elongation of the primer; thus, Klenow is not suitable for a long-base pyrosequencing on nicked dsDNA. However, this readable length is long enough for genotyping, as well as gene expression analysis.

References

1. Ronaghi M, Uhlen M, Nyren P (1998) A sequencing method based on real-time pyrophosphate. Science 281(363):365

2. Ahmadian A, Ehn M, Hober S (2006) Pyrosequencing: history, biochemistry and future. Clin Chim Acta 363:83–94

3. Zhou G, Kajiyama T, Gotou M, Kishimoto A, Suzuki S, Kambara H (2006) Enzyme system for improving the detection limit in pyrosequencing. Anal Chem 78:4482–4489

4. Pourmand N, Elahi E, Davis RW, Ronaghi M (2002) Multiplex Pyrosequencing. Nucleic Acids Res 30, e31

5. Zhou G, Kamahori M, Okano K, Harada K, Kambara H (2001) Miniaturized pyrosequencer for DNA analysis with capillaries to deliver deoxynucleotides. Electrophoresis 22:3497–3504

6. Duffy KJ, Littrell J, Locke A, Sherman SL, Olivier M (2008) A novel procedure for genotyping of single nucleotide polymorphisms in trisomy with genomic DNA and the invader assay. Nucleic Acids Res 36, e145

7. Gowda M, Li H, Alessi J, Chen F, Pratt R, Wang GL (2006) Robust analysis of 5′-transcript ends (5′-RATE): a novel technique for transcriptome analysis and genome annotation. Nucleic Acids Res 34, e126

8. Liu Z, Lozupone C, Hamady M, Bushman FD, Knight R (2007) Short pyrosequencing reads suffice for accurate microbial community analysis. Nucleic Acids Res 35, e120

9. Wang GP, Garrigue A, Ciuffi A, Ronen K, Leipzig J, Berry C, Lagresle-Peyrou C, Benjelloun F, Hacein-Bey-Abina S, Fischer A et al (2008) DNA bar coding and pyrosequencing to analyze adverse events in therapeutic gene transfer. Nucleic Acids Res 36, e49

10. Tost J, Gut IG (2007) DNA methylation analysis by pyrosequencing. Nat Protoc 2:2265–2275

11. Elahi E, Ronaghi M (2004) Pyrosequencing: a tool for DNA sequencing analysis. Methods Mol Biol 255:211–219

12. Elahi E, Pourmand N, Chaung R, Rofoogaran A, Boisver J, Samimi-Rad K, Davis RW, Ronaghi M (2003) Determination of hepatitis C virus genotype by Pyrosequencing. J Virol Methods 109:171–176

13. Gharizadeh B, Eriksson J, Nourizad N, Nordstrom T, Nyren P (2004) Improvements in Pyrosequencing technology by employing Sequenase polymerase. Anal Biochem 330:272–280

14. Nordstrom T, Alderborn A, Nyren P (2002) Method for one-step preparation of double-stranded DNA template applicable for use with Pyrosequencing technology. J Biochem Biophys Methods 52:71–82

15. Nordstrom T, Nourizad K, Ronaghi M, Nyren P (2000) Method enabling pyrosequencing on double-stranded DNA. Anal Biochem 282:186–193

16. Salk JJ, Sanchez JA, Pierce KE, Rice JE, Soares KC, Wangh LJ (2006) Direct amplification of single-stranded DNA for pyrosequencing using linear-after-the-exponential (LATE)-PCR. Anal Biochem 353:124–132

17. Pierce KE, Sanchez JA, Rice JE, Wangh LJ (2005) Linear-After-The-Exponential (LATE)-PCR: primer design criteria for high yields of specific single-stranded DNA and improved real-time detection. Proc Natl Acad Sci U S A 102:8609–8614

18. Rice JE, Sanchez JA, Pierce KE, Reis AH Jr, Osborne A, Wangh LJ (2007) Monoplex/multiplex linear-after-the-exponential-PCR assays combined with PrimeSafe and Dilute-'N'-Go sequencing. Nat Protoc 2:2429–2438

19. Kiesling T, Cox K, Davidson EA, Dretchen K, Grater G, Hibbard S, Lasken RS, Leshin J, Skowronski E, Danielsen M (2007) Sequence specific detection of DNA using nicking endonuclease signal amplification (NESA). Nucleic Acids Res 35, e117

20. Hosoda K, Matsuura T, Kita H, Ichihashi N, Tsukada K, Urabe I, Yomo T (2008) A novel sequence-specific RNA quantification method using nicking endonuclease, dual-labeled fluorescent DNA probe, and conformation-interchangeable oligo-DNA. RNA 14:584–592

21. Murakami T, Sumaoka J, Komiyama M (2009) Sensitive isothermal detection of nucleic acid sequence by primer generation-rolling circle amplification. Nucleic Acids Res 37, e19

22. Kuhn H, Frank-Kamenetskii MD (2008) Labeling of unique sequences in double-stranded DNA at sites of vicinal nicks generated by nicking endonucleases. Nucleic Acids Res 36, e40

23. Lo YM, Tsui NB, Chiu RW, Lau TK, Leung TN, Heung MM, Gerovassili A, Jin Y, Nicolaides KH, Cantor CR et al (2007) Plasma placental RNA allelic ratio permits noninvasive prenatal chromosomal aneuploidy detection. Nat Med 13:218–223

24. Zhang X, Wu H, Chen Z, Zhou G, Kajiyama T, Kambara H (2009) Dye-free gene expression detection by sequence-tagged reverse-transcription polymerase chain reaction coupled with pyrosequencing. Anal Chem 81:273–281

Chapter 5

Pyrosequencing Templates Generated by Asymmetric Nucleic Acid Sequence-Based Amplification (Asymmetric-NASBA)

Huning Jia, Zhiyao Chen, Haiping Wu, Hui Ye, Bingjie Zou, Qinxin Song, and Guohua Zhou

Abstract

Pyrosequencing is an ideal tool for verifying the sequence of amplicons. To enable pyrosequencing on amplicons from nucleic acid sequence-based amplification (NASBA), asymmetric NASBA with unequal concentrations of T7 promoter primer and reverse transcription primer was proposed. By optimizing the ratio of two primers and the concentration of dNTPs and NTPs, the amount of single-stranded cDNA in the amplicons from asymmetric NASBA was found increased 12 times more than the conventional NASBA through the real-time detection of molecular beacon specific to cDNA of interest. More than 20 bases have been successfully detected by pyrosequencing on amplicons from asymmetric NASBA using human para-influenza virus (HPIV) as amplification template. The primary results indicate that the combination of NASBA with pyrosequencing system is practical, and should open a new field in clinical diagnosis.

Key words Pyrosequencing, Asymmetric NASBA, Human parainfluenza virus

1 Introduction

Nucleic acid sequence-based amplification (NASBA) is a homogeneous, isothermal, in vitro amplification process involving three enzymes, reverse transcriptase, ribonuclease H (RNase H), and T7 RNA polymerase, as well as two target sequence-specific primers, resulting in the amplification of target sequences more than 109-fold within 120 min [1]. The main advantages of NASBA include the direct amplification of RNA targets, no need of thermal cycling equipments, and high sensitivity [2]; hence various applications were reported [3–5]. Currently, the detection methods include electrochemiluminescence (ECL), enzyme-linked immunosorbent assay (ELISA), and molecular beacons [6–8]. Unlike PCR, the main amplicons of NASBA are RNAs, so the detection method based on base sequencing has not yet been reported because the

Guohua Zhou and Qinxin Song (eds.), *Advances and Clinical Practice in Pyrosequencing*, Springer Protocols Handbooks, DOI 10.1007/978-1-4939-3308-2_5, © Springer Science+Business Media New York 2016

templates for the sequencing are always DNA. Obviously sequencing is the "gold standard" of the molecular diagnosis due to high accuracy. Therefore, combining NASBA with sequencing-based detection will extend the application scope of NASBA in various fields.

There are numerous technologies for DNA sequencing [9, 10]. Pyrosequencing is a well-developed dye-free technology for DNA sequencing using cascade enzymatic reactions to monitor the inorganic pyrophosphate released from dNTP incorporation [11]. With the good quantitative performance, pyrosequencing has been widely used for genotyping [12, 13], DNA methylation [14], and gene expression analysis [15]. Here we employed pyrosequencing technology to detect NASBA amplicons.

To enable pyrosequencing to sequence NASBA products, we modified the conventional NASBA protocol to increase the yield of single-stranded cDNA. As shown in Fig. 1, the main difference between the modified NASBA and the conventional NASBA is the cyclic phase in the amplification process. In conventional NASBA (Fig. 1a), primer-RT binds to the RNA first, and the action of reverse transcriptase extends it, thus generating RNA:DNA hybrid. RNase H now hydrolyzes the RNA stand to yield a single-stranded DNA intermediate. After annealing of primer-T7 to this strand and extension by reverse transcriptase, a transcriptionally active double-stranded DNA template is created. The template is then acted on by T7 RNA polymerase that results in the synthesis of yet more transcripts (RNA). A primer pair (primer-RT and primer-T7) with an equal concentration is employed, yielding the amplicons of single-stranded RNA, double-stranded DNA, and single-stranded cDNA. The majority of amplicon is ssRNA, which cannot be used as the templates for pyrosequencing reaction. While in asymmetric

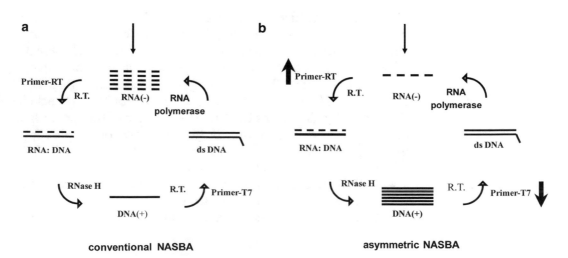

Fig. 1 Schematic illustration of the principle of asymmetric NASBA

NASBA (Fig. 1b), primer-RT with a concentration higher than that in the conventional NASBA would increase the amount of RNA:DNA hybrid; a larger amount of cDNA could thus be produced. On the other hand, a reduced amount of primer-T7 was used to decrease the yield of RNA (the main product of conventional NASBA). Due to the increase of primer-RT concentration in RT step, the accumulation of the RNA was further reduced. Therefore, cDNA from asymmetric NASBA was significantly increased, and reached to the amount required in pyrosequencing.

2 Materials

1. A 131 bp armored RNA fragment of HPIV (GenBank accession number NC_001796.2) was artificially prepared by biotechnology engineering method and was extracted according to the reported method [16].

2. The concentration of the extracted RNA was detected by the UV-Vis spectrophotometer (Gene SpeIII, Hitachi, Japan).

3. Bovine serum albumin (Sangon Biotech Co., Ltd, Nanjing, China).

4. RNase II (TaKaRa Biotechnology Co. Ltd., Dalian, China).

5. T7 RNA polymerase (Fermentas, USA).

6. AMV RT (Promega, USA).

7. RNasin (TaKaRa Biotechnology Co., Ltd., Dalian, China).

3 Methods

3.1 Primers and Probes

1. All the oligomers were synthesized and purified by Invitrogen Co. (Shanghai, China).

2. The fluorescence-labeled probe (molecular beacon) was synthesized by TaKaRa Biotechnology CO., Ltd. (Dalian, China).

3. Sequences of the oligomers used in this study are listed in Table 1.

3.2 Conventional NASBA Reaction

1. Add 2.5 µL of the extracted RNA (10^4 copies) into 5 µL of pre-mixture containing 80 mM Tris–HCl (pH 8.5), 32 mM $MgCl_2$, 80 mM KCl, 10 mM DTT (dithiothreitol), 2 mM each dNTP, 4 mM each NTP, 10 mM sorbitol, 16 % dimethyl sulfoxide, and 0.4 µM primer.

2. Reaction mixture was heated to 65 °C for 5 min and then cooled to 41 °C for 5 min.

3. After cooling, 2.5 µL enzyme mixture containing 1 µg of bovine serum albumin (Sangon Biotech Co., Ltd, Nanjing,

Table 1
Sequences of the oligomers

Name	Sequences (5′–3′)
Primer P1-1	[a]<u>AAT TCT AAT ACG ACTC ACT ATA GGG</u> **AGA GAG AGA** GCC TCC ATA CCC GAG AAA TA
Primer P1-2	ATG GCT CAA TCT CAA CAA CA
Primer P2-1	CCT CCA TAC CCG AGA AAT A
Primer P2-2	<u>AAT TCT AAT ACG ACT CAC TAT AGG G</u> **AG AGA GAG AG**G GCT CAA TCT CAA CAA CAA GAT T
MB probe[b]	CCG ATC CCT ATG CTG CAC TAT ACC CAG ATC GG

[a]Bases underlined represent T7 promoter sequence. Bold bases were added for improving amplification efficiency
[b]To detect both RNA and cDNA by the same molecular beacon probe, two similar pairs of primers (P1 and P2) were designed. The molecular beacon probe hybridizes to RNA in the amplicons when using P1-1 and P1-2 as NASBA primers, while the molecular beacon hybridizes to cDNA in the amplicons when using P2-1 and P2-2 as NASBA primers

China), 0.1 U of RNase H (TaKaRa Biotechnology Co. Ltd., Dalian, China), 20 U of T7 RNA polymerase (Fermentas, USA), 4 U of AMV RT (Promega, USA), and 20 U of RNasin (TaKaRa Biotechnology Co., Ltd., Dalian, China) was added to make up a final reaction volume to 10 μL before incubation at 41 °C for 120 min.

3.3 Asymmetric NASBA Coupled with Molecular Beacon-Based Real-Time Detection

1. cDNA in the asymmetric NASBA amplicons was detected by real-time molecular beacon assay (*see* **Note 1**).

2. The molecular beacon probe (0.4 μM) was added with the enzyme mix.

3. Then the reaction mixture was incubated at 41 °C for 120 min in a real-time PCR analyzer (MJ RESEARCH, Inc., USA); meanwhile fluorescence signals were measured at 522 nm with the excitation at 494 nm. The time interval between two measures was 120 s.

3.4 Template Preparation for Pyrosequencing

1. Firstly, 5 μL of beads were washed with water, and then 10 μL of binding buffer (10 mM Tris–HCl (pH 7.5), 1 mM EDTA, 2 M NaCl) and 10 μL of NASBA products were added before mixing (*see* **Note 2**).

2. The binding process was performed in a rotation way at 37 °C for 15 min. The products immobilized on the beads were washed four to five times with water, and then denatured with 0.1 M NaOH.

3. The supernatant was discarded, and the beads were washed with 100 μL of washing buffer (5 mM Tris–HCl (pH 7.5), 0.5 mM EDTA, 1 M NaCl) twice, and with 100 μL of annealing

buffer (40 mM Tris–HCl (pH 7.5), 20 mM $MgCl_2$, 50 mM NaCl) once.

4. The pyrosequencing primer (10 pmol) was added to the beaded strands and annealed at 94 °C for 30 s, and 55 °C for 3 min.

3.5 Pyrosequencing Reaction

1. Pyrosequencing was carried out by a portable Bioluminescence Analyzer (Hitachi Ltd., Japan).

2. The pyrosequencing reaction mixture contained 0.1 M Tris-acetate (pH 7.7), 2.0 mM EDTA, 10 mM $Mg(Ac)_2$, 0.1 % BSA, 1.0 mM dithiothreitol, 2.0 μM APS, 0.4 g/L PVP (MW 360,000), 0.4 mM D-luciferin, 1.6 mU/L ATP sulfurylase, 1.6 U/mL apyrase, 27 U/mL exonuclease-deficient Klenow DNA polymerase, and appropriate purified luciferase [17, 18].

3. After adding the template to the reaction mixture, the sequencing procedure was accomplished by a stepwise elongation of the primer strand through iteratively dispensing dNTPs.

4 Method Validation

4.1 Detecting of Human Parainfluenza Virus (HPIV) on Amplicons from Asymmetric NASBA

In conventional NASBA, the concentration of each primer is 0.2 μM [19, 20]. So firstly we kept the T7-primer with the same concentration of 0.2 μM, but increased the RT-primer concentration to 20 μM (100-fold) and 40 μM (200-fold), respectively (*see* **Note 3**). The amounts of cDNA and ssRNA were measured by real-time monitoring of the fluorescent signals from target-specific molecular beacons. The results were shown in Fig. 2. In comparison with conventional NASBA, the amount of cDNA (Fig. 2a) significantly increased with the increasing of RT-primer concentration, but the cDNA yield with the 40 μM RT-primer is less than that with 20 μM increase. On the other hand, the amount of ssRNA (Fig. 2b) relatively reduced with increasing RT-primer concentration. Therefore, as expected, a higher concentration of RT-primer produced a larger amount of cDNA.

From the results in Fig. 2, we also found that the yields of both cDNA (Fig. 2a) and ssRNA (Fig. 2b) were unexpectedly decreased when increasing RT-primer concentration from 20 to 40 μM. This indicates that excessively high concentration of RT-primer probably inhibits the generation of ssRNA. Therefore, we decreased the RT-primer concentration from 20 μM to 1.3 μM (around sevenfold increase) and 0.8 μM (around fourfold increase), respectively. To keep the difference in concentration between two primers, the concentration of T7-primer was reduced to 0.013 μM (around 15-fold decrease) and 0.008 μM (around 25-fold decrease), respectively. As shown in Fig. 2, we found that 1.3 μM of RT-primer and 0.013 μM of T7-primer yielded the largest amount of cDNA (Fig. 2a) in all the tested NASBA conditions.

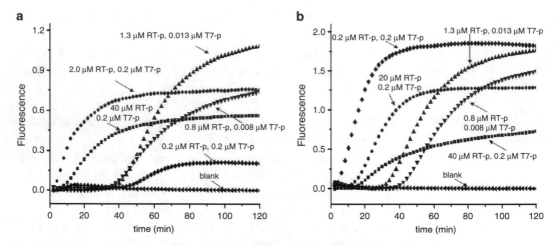

Fig. 2 Real-time quantification of cDNA (**a**) and ssRNA (**b**) yielded from NASBA with different concentrations of RT-primer and T7-primer. The concentrations of both primers labeled beside each curve. RT-p and T7-p mean reverse transcription primer and T7 promoter primer. The sequence of MB is listed in Table 1

Based on the process of NASBA, hence we infer that a lower NTP concentration and a higher dNTP concentration would produce more cDNA. Real-time quantification of cDNA in NASBA at the two- and fourfold decrease of NTP concentration as well as the two- and threefold increase of dNTP concentration was performed. As shown in Fig. 3a (▼, ■), the cDNA yield increased about 30 % when NTP concentration (1 mM) was two times lower than that (2 mM) in conventional NASBA; but no more increase of cDNA yield was observed at fourfold decrease of NTP concentration (♦, ▼ in Fig. 3a). So 1 mM NTPs was employed for the following experiments.

On the other hand, almost no cDNA was obtained from NASBA with dNTP concentrations two and three times higher than that in conventional NASBA (●, ▲ in Fig. 3a). The unexpected results suggest that NASBA at a lower dNTP concentration may be beneficial to the yield of cDNA. Further investigation by using two- and fourfold decreases of dNTP concentration for NASBA with 1 mM NTPs indicated that cDNA yield increased significantly; and NASBA at the fourfold decreases of dNTP concentration (0.25 mM) gave a cDNA yield two times higher than that at 1 mM (▲, ■ in Fig. 3b). The reason we believe is that the consumption of free Mg^{2+} by the increased dNTPs for dNTPs can form a complex with Mg^{2+}; thus the reduced concentration of Mg^{2+} slowed down the enzymatic reactions. Usually, an increase of 200 μM dNTPs needs an additional 1 mM Mg^2. As shown in Fig. 3c, cDNA yields of NASBA at high concentrations of dNTPs (2 mM and 3 mM) together with high concentrations of Mg^{2+} (21 mM and 26 mM) are higher than those in Fig. 3a (●, ▲), but still lower than that at the conventional dNTP concentration (1 mM, ■ in Fig. 3c).

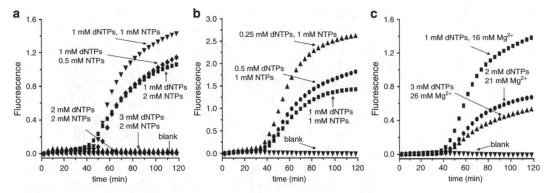

Fig. 3 Real-time quantification of cDNA on different conditions. (**a**) NASBA with a gradually increased dNTP concentration (from 1 to 3 mM) and a gradually decreased NTP concentration (from 2 to 0.5 mM). (**b**) NASBA with a constant NTP concentration (1 mM), and a gradually decreased dNTP concentration (from 1 to 0.25 mM). (**c**) NASBA with a constant NTP concentration (1 mM), and a gradually increased dNTP concentration (from 1 to 3 mM) together with a gradually increased Mg^{2+} concentration (from 16 to 25 mM). The concentration data were directly marked near each curve

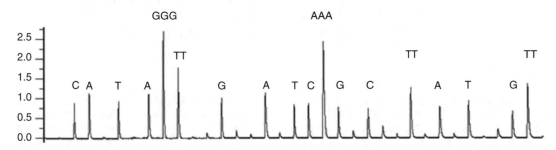

Fig. 4 Pyrogram of HPIV virus by pyrosequencing on cDNA from asymmetric NASBA

Consequently, the appropriate concentrations of dNTPs and NTPs in NASBA were 0.25 mM and 1 mM at the optimal primer concentrations, which yielded a 12-fold increase of cDNA amount over conventional NASBA.

Under the best conditions for yielding cDNA, NASBA was performed with RNA of 10^4 copies as the template. After NASBA, pyrosequencing on the single-stranded cDNA prepared from NASBA products was carried out with the pyrosequencing primer of Primer-P (5′-CAA CAG ATG GGT ATA GTG CAG-3′). As shown in Fig. 4, 25 bases can be detected. The results indicated that sample was HPIV virus (*see* **Note 4**).

5 Technical Notes

1. The protocol designed for asymmetric NASBA was the same as the conventional real-time NASBA [8, 18] except for the primer concentration.

2. To prepare high-quality templates for pyrosequencing, primer-RT was biotinylated, and streptavidin-coated sepharose beads were used to bind the biotinylated NASBA products [21].

3. In NASBA, the amplification step is T7 RNA polymerase-catalyzed transcription, which could yield 100–1000 copies of ssRNA from each T7-primer-DNA template duplex. In the reverse transcription step, the ssRNAs are captured by RT-primer, and generate cDNAs with an equal amount to the RT-primer by reverse transcription; then the cDNAs hybridize with the same amount of T7-primer to produce dsDNAs. As the concentration of two primers is equal in conventional NASBA, almost no cDNA exists in the amplicons theoretically. To allow the accumulation of cDNA, we should reduce the concentration of the T7-primer, or increase the concentration of the RT-primer [22–24].

4. Although there is some noise peaks appearing in the late cycles of the pyrogram, the comparison of the theoretical histograms and the obtained pyrograms indicated that these noise peaks had less impact on the base-calling accuracy. Therefore asymmetric NASBA coupled with pyrosequencing system is feasible.

References

1. Compton J (1991) Nucleic acid sequence-based amplification. Nature 350:91–92

2. Min J, Baeumner AJ (2002) Highly sensitive and specific detection of viable Escherichia coli in drinking water. Anal Biochem 303:186–193

3. Rutjes SA, Italiaander R, van den Berg HH, Lodder WJ, de Roda Husman AM (2005) Isolation and detection of enterovirus RNA from large-volume water samples by using the NucliSens miniMAG system and real-time nucleic acid sequence-based amplification. Appl Environ Microbiol 71:3734–3740

4. Mugasa CM, Laurent T, Schoone GJ, Kager PA, Lubega GW, Schallig HD (2009) Nucleic acid sequence-based amplification with oligo-chromatography for detection of Trypanosoma brucei in clinical samples. J Clin Microbiol 47:630–635

5. Lau LT, Reid SM, King DP, Lau AM, Shaw AE, Ferris NP, Yu AC (2008) Detection of foot-and-mouth disease virus by nucleic acid sequence-based amplification (NASBA). Vet Microbiol 126:101–110

6. D'Souza DH, Jaykus LA (2003) Nucleic acid sequence based amplification for the rapid and sensitive detection of Salmonella enterica from foods. J Appl Microbiol 95:1343–1350

7. Gill P, Ramezani R, Amiri MV, Ghaemi A, Hashempour T, Eshraghi N, Ghalami M, Tehrani HA (2006) Enzyme-linked immuno-sorbent assay of nucleic acid sequence-based amplification for molecular detection of M. tuberculosis. Biochem Biophys Res Commun 347:1151–1157

8. Landry ML, Garner R, Ferguson D (2005) Real-time nucleic acid sequence-based amplification using molecular beacons for detection of enterovirus RNA in clinical specimens. J Clin Microbiol 43:3136–3139

9. Swerdlow H, Zhang JZ, Chen DY, Harke HR, Grey R, Wu SL, Dovichi NJ, Fuller C (1991) Three DNA sequencing methods using capillary gel electrophoresis and laser-induced fluorescence. Anal Chem 63:2835–2841

10. Oetting WS (2008) Large scale DNA sequencing: new challenges emerge--the 2007 Human Genome Variation Society scientific meeting. Hum Mutat 29:765–768

11. Ronaghi M, Uhlen M, Nyren P (1998) A sequencing method based on real-time pyro-phosphate. Science 281:363–365

12. Duffy KJ, Littrell J, Locke A, Sherman SL, Olivier M (2008) A novel procedure for geno-typing of single nucleotide polymorphisms in trisomy with genomic DNA andthe invader assay. Nucleic Acids Res 36, e145

13. Elahi EN, Pourmand N, Chaung R, Rofoogaran A, Boisver J, Samimi-Rad K, Davis RW,

Ronaghi M (2003) Determination of hepatitis C virus genotype by Pyrosequencing. J Virol Methods 109:171–176

14. Irahara N, Nosho K, Baba Y, Shima K, Lindeman NI, Hazra A, Schernhammer ES, Hunter DJ, Fuchs CS, Ogino S (2010) Precision of pyrosequencing assay to measure LINE-1 methylation in colon cancer, normal colonic mucosa, and peripheral blood cells. J Mol Diagn 12:177–183

15. Soderback E, Zackrisson AL, Lindblom B, Alderborn A (2005) Determination of CYP2D6 gene copy number by pyrosequencing. Clin Chem 51:522–531

16. Hietala SK, Crossley BM (2006) Armored RNA as virus surrogate in a real-time reverse transcriptase PCR assay proficiency panel. J Clin Microbiol 44:67–70

17. Deiman B, van Aarle P, Sillekens P (2002) Characteristics and applications of nucleic acid sequence-based amplification (NASBA). Mol Biotechnol 20:163–179

18. Deiman B, Schrover C, Moore C, Westmoreland D, van de Wiel P (2007) Rapid and highly sensitive qualitative real-time assay for detection of respiratory syncytial virus A and B using NASBA and molecular beacon technology. J Virol Methods 146:29–35

19. Ovyn C, van Strijp D, Ieven M, Ursi D, van Gemen B, Goossens H (1996) Typing of Mycoplasma pneumoniae by nucleic acid sequence-based amplification, NASBA. Mol Cell Probes 10:319–324

20. Oehlenschlager F, Schwille P, Eigen M (1996) Detection of HIV-1 RNA by nucleic acid sequence-based amplification combined with fluorescence correlation spectroscopy. Proc Natl Acad Sci U S A 93:12811–12816

21. Henegariu O, Heerema NA, Dlouhy SR, Vance GH, Vogt PH (1997) Multiplex PCR: critical parameters and step-by-step protocol. Biotechniques 23:504–511

22. Wu H, Wu W, Chen Z, Wang W, Zhou G, Kajiyama T, Kambara H (2011) Highly sensitive pyrosequencing based on the capture of free adenosine 5′ phosphosulfate with adenosine alphosphate sulfurylase. Anal Chem 83:3600–3605

23. Song Q, Jing H, Wu H, Zhou G, Kajiyama T, Kambara H (2010) Gene expression analysis on a photodiode array-based bioluminescence analyzer by using sensitivity-improved SRPP. Analyst 135:1315–1319

24. Kambara H, Zhou G (2009) DNA analysis with a photo-diode array sensor. Methods Mol Biol 503:337–360

Chapter 6

Gel Immobilization of Acrylamide-Modified Single-Stranded DNA Template for Pyrosequencing

Pengfeng Xiao, Huan Huang, Bingjie Zou, Qinxin Song, Guohua Zhou, and Zuhong Lu

Abstract

A novel two-step process was developed to prepare ssDNA templates for pyrosequencing. First, PCR-amplified DNA templates modified with an acrylamide group and acrylamide monomers were copolymerized in 0.1 M NaOH solution to form polyacrylamide gel spots. Second, ssDNA templates for pyrosequencing were prepared by removing electrophoretically unbound complementary strands, unmodified PCR primers, inorganic pyrophosphate (PPi), and excess deoxyribonucleotides under alkali conditions. The results show that the 3-D polyacrylamide gel network has a high immobilization capacity and the modified PCR fragments are efficiently captured. After electrophoresis, gel spots copolymerized from 10 μL of the crude PCR products and the acrylamide monomers contain template molecules on the order of pmol, which generate enough light to be detected by a regular photomultiplier tube. The porous structure of gel spots facilitated the fast transportation of the enzyme, dNTPs, and other reagents, and the solution-mimicking microenvironment guaranteed polymerase efficiency for pyrosequencing. Successful genotyping from the crude PCR products was demonstrated. This method can be applied in any laboratory; it is cheap, fast, and simple, and has the potential to be incorporated into a DNA-chip format for high-throughput pyrosequencing analysis.

Key words Acrylamide-modified nucleic acids, Gel immobilization, Pyrosequencing, ssDNA

1 Introduction

Pyrosequencing is a sequencing-by-synthesis method that employs a set of enzymatic reactions to monitor the inorganic pyrophosphate (PPi) released during deoxyribonucleotide triphosphate (dNTP) incorporation [1–4]. The reaction starts when DNA polymerase incorporates a dNTP, releasing an equal molar amount of PPi. ATP sulfurylase subsequently converts the PPi to ATP, which in turn drives luciferase to oxidize luciferin to oxyluciferin, generating visible light in amounts proportional to the number of

Guohua Zhou and Qinxin Song (eds.), *Advances and Clinical Practice in Pyrosequencing*, Springer Protocols Handbooks, DOI 10.1007/978-1-4939-3308-2_6, © Springer Science+Business Media New York 2016

incorporated nucleotides. Pyrosequencing has advantages of accuracy, flexibility, and simple automation over traditional sequencing methods. It has been widely used in applications of SNP analysis [5], clone checking [6], identification of short DNA sequences used in bacterial typing [7], and recently in high-throughput genome sequencing [8]. Although the pyrosequencing chemistry itself is quite simple and straightforward, template preparation step involves tedious procedures. There are two widely used strategies for preparing ssDNA templates. One is directly preparing the templates from double-stranded PCR products with a set of enzymatic reactions that remove excess primers and nucleotides [9]. However, the template/primer complexes formed by the fast cooling of the denatured PCR products may be replaced by the reassociated complementary strands, further reducing the template/primer complex concentration and light generated during pyrosequencing. The alternate approach is solid-phase ssDNA preparation, which uses streptavidin-coated magnetic or Sepharose beads [2–5, 10–16] to capture biotinylated PCR products. Although this method is most widely used due to its high collection efficiency and capacity, and extensive automation [16], this method is comparatively expensive, although the streptavidin-coated magnetic beads can be reused [17, 18]. For parallel pyrosequencing, Biotage AB (Uppsala, Sweden) developed the PyroMark MD that features an integrated vacuum prep workstation for the fully automated preparation of ssDNA templates immobilized on streptavidin-coated beads. A recently reported third method to prepare ssDNA template involves immobilizing DNA targets, PCR-amplified by primers modified with different functional groups, onto an activated solid surface [19]. This method is effective in fluorescence assays as the sensitivity can be increased through the use of powerful lasers [20]. However, it is difficult to generate high-quality data in chemiluminescence-based pyrosequencing because the template immobilization capacity and efficiency on a planar surface limit signal intensity.

Recently, our group and other groups tried different 3-D hydrogel films for DNA and protein immobilization. Agarose and polyacrylamide films showed improved performance over standard preparation in protein arrays and molecular beacon arrays [21–24]. Rehman et al. [25] developed a new chemistry for copolymerizing acrylamide monomers and acrylamide-modified oligonucleotides to form stable DNA-containing polyacrylamide copolymers. We have successfully modified this method to fabricate high-quality DNA microarrays [26]. In this report, we tried to investigate the possibility of preparing ssDNA templates for pyrosequencing directly from the crude PCR products with these 3-D hydrogels pots. The results showed that ssDNA templates prepared by this cheap, fast, and simple method give a high-quality pyrosequencing

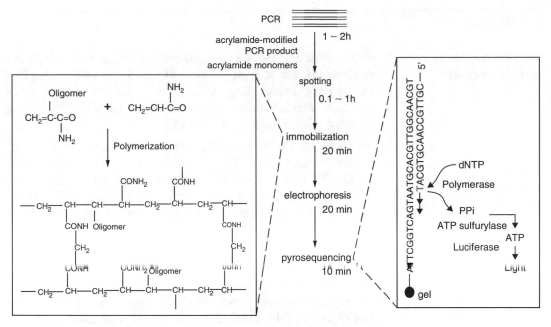

Fig. 1 Schematic illustration of gel immobilization of an ssDNA template for pyrosequencing. The immobilization step is illustrated in the *left panel*: PCR products amplified with a reverse primer, the 5'-end of which had been modified with an acrylamide group, and an unmodified forward primer are copolymerized with acrylamide monomers to form gel spots. The immobilized PCR products are denatured and interfering components are removed by electrophoresis. The pyrosequencing reaction is illustrated in the *right panel*: a sequencing primer is annealed to the gel-immobilized ssDNA template. When extension occurs, ATP sulfurylase catalyzes ATP production with the released PPi and photoemission is detected after luciferase reacts with ATP. The duration of each step is listed at the *middle panel*

data, indicating that a DNA-chip format for high-throughput pyrosequencing is possible by our method. For a schematic illustration of this technique, *see* Fig. 1.

2 Materials

1. Polyvinylpyrrolidone (PVP), dNTPs, DNA polymerase I Klenow fragment (exo–), and Quanti-LumTM recombinant luciferase (95 %) were purchased from Promega (Madison, WI, USA).

2. ATP disodium trihydrate salt was from WakoPure Chemical Industries (Osaka, Japan).

3. ATP sulfurylase, apyrase (Sigma, type V, VI, and VII), BSA (Takara), DTT (Invitrogen), D-luciferin, inorganic pyrophosphatase (PPase), and adenosine 5'-phosphosulfate (APS) were purchased from Sigma (St. Louis, MO, USA).

4. Sodium 2'-deoxy-adenosine 5'-O-(1-triphosphate) (dATPαS) was from Amersham Pharmacia Biotech (Amersham, UK).

3 Methods

3.1 Oligonucleotides and DNA Template

1. 5'-Terminal acrylamide group-modified oligonucleotides were synthesized on a Model 391 DNA Synthesizer (Applied Biosystems, Foster City, CA, USA), using a commercially available acrylamide phosphoramidite (Acrydite™; Matrix Technologies, Hudson, NH, USA).

2. Synthesized DNA template, oligonucleotide 50 (50 nt) (5'-acrylamide-TTT TTTTTG GGG TTT TCC CCA AAA GGG TTT CCC AAA GGTTCC AAG TCA CCC CGC CCG C-3'), and sequencing primer (5'-GCG GGC GGG G-3') were used for optimizing the reaction conditions. Biotinylated oligonucleotide 50 (50 nt) (5'-biotin-TTT TTT TTG GGG TTT TCC CCA AAAGGG TTT CCC AAA GGT TCC AAG TCA CCC CGC CCGC-3') was purchased from Invitrogen Biotechnology (Shanghai, China).

3. For sample analysis, DNA135 (135 bp), which includes the 14417 locus of the oxidized low-density lipoprotein receptor 1 gene (OLR-1; MIM 602601) polymorphisms, was amplified from the forward primer (5'-TAC TAT CCTTCC CAG CTC CT), and the acrylamide group-modified reverse prime (5'-acrylamide-TTTTCAGCAACTTGGCAT- 3'). The forward primer was also used as the sequencing primer. The genotyping primer of the 14417 locus was 5'-TTC ATT TAA CTG GGAAAA-3'.

3.2 Preparation of the Acryl-Modified Slides

Acryl-modified slides were prepared as described in [16]. The microscope slides (Shanghai Jinglun Industrial glass, China) were cleaned by soaking in 10 % aqueous nitric acid for 2 h. Slides were rinsed with water and acetone, and then dried by air. Cleaned slides were then soaked in 10 % 3-methacryloxy-propyltrimethoxysilane (Sigma) in acetone for 1 h, washed with acetone, and dried by air.

3.3 Immobilization of the Modified Oligonucleotides

1. Acrylamide-modified oligonucleotide (see **Note 1**) solutions containing 3 % w/w acrylamide monomer (see **Note 2**) (29:1 w/w acrylamide/bis-acrylamide), 30 % w/w glycerol, and 1 % w/v ammonium per-sulfate were prepared at the desired concentration.

2. One, two, four, and eight microliters of these mixtures were spotted on the acryl-modified slides, which were subsequently placed into a humid airtight chamber. The airtight chamber was vacuumed to about 1000 Pa and kept at this vacuum pressure for 15–20 min at room temperature to vaporize a droplet of TEMED preplaced into it.

3. Under this pressure, TEMED was vaporized and diffused onto the slide surfaces to induce the copolymerization between acrylamide groups and acryl groups, and then oligonucleotides

immobilized onto the gel were attached on the slide. Before being peeled off the slides for pyrosequencing, the gel spots were subjected to electrophoresis in 1× Tris-borate-EDTA (TBE) (40 V/cm, 10 min) buffer to remove the nonimmobilized oligonucleotide and other impurities.

3.4 Immobilization of the Acrylamide-Modified PCR Products

1. Three samples with known genotypes were amplified with the forward primer and the acrylamide-modified reverse primer. After purification of the crude PCR products with a QIAquick PCR Purification Kit, the concentrations of the dsDNA were determined to be around 11.8 mg/mL (0.133 μM) by detecting OD260 in Gene Spe III (Naka Instruments, Japan).

2. Three different immobilization conditions were investigated: (a) Immobilization under neutral condition: Crude PCR products were purified and preconcentrated four times by ethanol precipitation. The immobilization mixtures containing the acrylamide-modified PCR products, 1 % w/v ammonium persulfate, 30 % w/w glycerol, and 3 % w/w acrylamide monomers were prepared and immobilized onto the acryl-modified slide as described above. (b) Immobilization under alkali condition: Crude PCR products were purified and preconcentrated four times by ethanol precipitation process. The immobilization mixtures containing 3 % w/w acrylamide monomer, 30 % w/w glycerol, and 1 % w/v ammonium persulfate in 0.1 M NaOH were spotted on the acryl-modified slide and polymerized immobilized onto the slide as described above. (c) Direct immobilization of the crude acrylamide-modified PCR products: Immobilization mixtures containing crude PCR products (1–16 mL), 3 % w/w acrylamide monomer, 30 % w/w glycerol, and 1 % w/v ammonium persulfate in 0.1 M NaOH were spotted on the acryl-modified slide and polymerized onto the slide as described above.

3.5 Denaturing and Purifying the Immobilized PCR Products

Two methods (*see* **Note 3**) for preparing ssDNA template for pyrosequencing were performed: (a) for immobilization under neutral condition, the gel spots were put into a 95 °C water bath for 5 min to denature the dsDNA. They were then subjected to electrophoresis in 1× TBE (40 V/cm) for 10 min at room temperature; (b) for immobilization under alkali condition, the gel spots were directly subjected to electrophoresis in 0.1 M NaOH solution (100 mA) for 5 min, followed by an electrophoresis in 1× TBE (40 V/cm) for another 5 min.

3.6 Preparation of Sepharose Beads Immobilized with Biotinylated Oligonucleotides

1. Biotinylated oligonucleotide-50 was immobilized on streptavidin-coated Sepharose beads (Amersham Biosciences). Fifty microliters of binding buffer (Pyrosequencing AB) was added to 2 or 0.75 pmol of the oligonucleotides.

2. Then 3 μL of streptavidin-coated Sepharose beads were added and the mixture was vigorously mixed at room temperature for 10 min. The beads and oligonucleotide mixture were transferred to a filter column (Amersham Biosciences) and the binding buffer removed by vacuum [27]. The biotinylated oligonucleotide attached to the beads was denatured in 50 μL denaturation buffer (Pyrosequencing AB) for 1 min.

3. The denaturation buffer was removed by vacuum and oligonucleotide immobilized on the beads was washed twice in 150 μL wash buffer (Pyrosequencing AB). The beads attached oligonucleotides were resuspended in 50 μL of annealing buffer (Pyrosequencing AB) for pyrosequencing [14].

3.7 Degradation of Endogenous Pyrophosphate in dNTPs

Fifty microliters of 10 mM dNTPs containing 25 mM magnesium acetate and 5 mM Tris, pH 7.7, was incubated with 0.4 units of PPase for 30 min at room temperature to degrade the pyrophosphates in monomers [28].

3.8 Pyrosequencing

1. The pyrosequencing apparatus consists of a reaction module with a reaction chamber and four dNTP reservoirs, a side-on photomultiplier tube (PMT, R6355, Hamamatsu Photonics K. K., Shizuoka, Japan), a power supply (Matsusada Precision, Japan), and a computer for collecting data [28].

2. After the ssDNA template immobilized on the gel spots hybridized with the sequencing primer, those gel spots were incubated in 100 μL of pyrosequencing reaction mixture (*see* **Note 4**) containing 0.1 M Tris-acetate (pH 7.7), 2 mM EDTA, 10 mM magnesium acetate, 0.2 % BSA, 10 mM DTT, 10 μM APS, 0.4 mg/mL PVP, 4 mM D-luciferin, 2 U/mL ATP sulfurylase, luciferase in an amount determined to give appropriate sensitivity, 2 U of apyrase VII, and 1–2 U of DNA polymerase I Klenow fragment (exo–).

3. Sequencing reactions were started by sequentially adding dATPαS, dCTP, dTTP, and dGTP. Pyrosequencing was performed at room temperature and the pyrosequencing reaction module was vibrated continuously. The same process was carried out for pyrosequencing ssDNA attached to Sepharose beads.

4   Method Validation

4.1 Influence of Polyacrylamide Gel on Pyrosequencing

Two key points must be addressed regarding the use of attached ssDNA template for pyrosequencing: the immobilization capacity and accessibility of the gel-immobilized templates.

1. First, we investigated whether the polyacrylamide gel can capture enough ssDNA templates to generate detectable pyrosequencing

signals. Figure 2 shows the programs obtained by using the nonimmobilized oligonucleotide template with standard liquid pyrosequencing (Fig. 2a), and the acrylamide-modified oligonucleotide template immobilized on the polyacrylamide gel system (Fig. 2b). The results show that the immobilized oligonucleotides (Fig. 2b) approximate the same signals obtained from nonimmobilized oligonucleotides (Fig. 2a). The height and shape of the peaks in these two pyrograms are nearly identical except that the peak heights from polyacrylamide gel-immobilized oligonucleotides are 36 % of those from nonimmobilized oligonucleotide (only one-quarter high peaks compared to those from nonimmobilized oligonucleotides were obtained when the content of oligonucleotides used in polymerization is 0.5 mM; figures are not shown), suggesting that the polyacrylamide gel is suitable for pyrosequencing, but the immobilization efficiency of different acrylamide-modified oligonucleotide concentrations used was different even when the contents of the gel were same. For comparison, Sepharose bead-based pyrosequencing was also carried out; 0.75 and 2 pmol of biotin oligonucleotides were fixed on 3 mL of streptavidin-Sepharose beads, respectively. As shown in Fig. 2c and d, the signal intensities from 0.75 and 2 pmol of immobilized oligonucleotides were 37 and 20 % of the corresponding amount of nonimmobilized oligonucleotides. As the immobilization efficiency depends on the ratio of DNA molecules to the surface area of supports used for immobilizing the DNA, it is difficult to make a direct comparison of the immobilization efficiency between the two methods. The polymerization method described here costs 0.1 USD *per* purification. In comparison, streptavidin bead-based purification costs about 0.3 USD.

In Fig. 2, the intensity ratios of the peaks are not always proportional to the number of the incorporated nucleotides; this may result from decreasing enzyme activity (due to dilution and reaction duration) and the accumulation of the nonperfect (<100 %) extension in each step. In our pyrosequencing system, more than 20 bases may be accurately called; this is sufficient for most applications, such as SNP genotyping, STR marker analysis, and the identification of short DNA sequences for bacterial typing. In addition, the gel-immobilized templates must be accessible to the primer, enzymes, and dNTPs in order to generate correct sequence signals. Therefore, these pyrosequencing reagents should diffuse quickly to the reaction site through the gel matrix. Otherwise the unextended fragments at each cycle may decrease signal intensities and introduce false extension signal during the next cycle, causing a "frame shift" and limiting the read length. Polyacrylamide is a neutral and hydrophilic polymer that has been widely used by

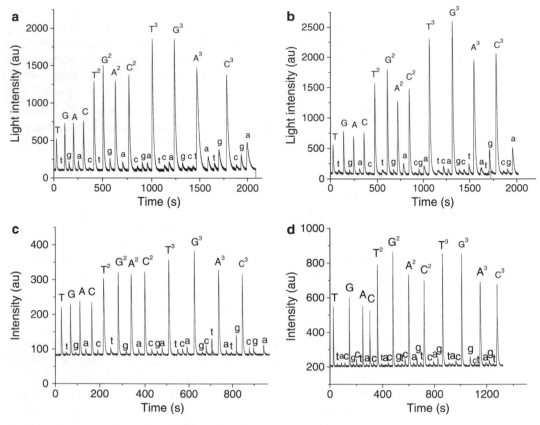

Fig. 2 Pyrograms obtained from 50 base oligonucleotide templates: (**a**) nonimmobilized acrylamide oligonucleotide (0.75 pmol) in solution, (**b**) acrylamide oligonucleotide (2 pmol) immobilized onto 8×1 μL gel spots,(c) oligonucleotides (0.75 pmol) immobilized onto 3 μL of streptavidin-Sepharose beads, and (**d**) biotinylated oligonucleotide (2 pmol) immobilized onto 3 μL of streptavidin-Sepharose beads. *Capital letters* represent signals from dNTP extension; *lower case letters* represent background signals

biologists and chemists. A 7.5 % gel can be used to separate protein up to 56,105 Da or nucleic acid fragments up to 16,105 Da [29]. Recently, a number of chemical and enzymatic reactions have been carried out in polyacrylamide gel films or gel pads [30–32]. Dubiley et al. [33] used T4 polynucleotide kinase and T4 DNA ligase to improve sequencing by hybridization. Mitra and Dubiley showed that the oligonucleotide-immobilized gel support provided a more homogeneous environment for DNA polymerase (90 kDa) in minisequencing than solid glass slides [34, 35]. Our previous experiments showed [26] that the porous sizes of the gel matrix increased with decrease in the acrylamide monomer concentration, allowing unbounded compounds to diffuse in and out of the gel matrix. For the experiment addressed in this paper, a low concentration of acrylamide monomer (3 % w/w) was employed as the immobilization matrix.

2. To investigate the accessibility of the gel-immobilized templates, four samples containing 4 pmol of oligonucleotides and the same volume of gel were divided into different sizes (e.g., eight spots each with 1 μL of gel, four spots each with 2 μL of gel, two spots each with 4 μL of gel, and one spot with 8 μL of gel). These were then used to compare signal intensities and reaction rate. All four dNTPs simultaneously added to the reaction chamber allow multiple, dNTP incorporations and enhance sensitivity. Light intensities versus time are shown in Fig. 3. Four samples showed similar light intensities and reaction rates, indicating that the size of the gel spot does not obviously change the pyrosequencing results. However, the time to reach maximum intensity was about 50 s, longer than the 30 s [11] required for templates immobilized on streptavidin-coated magnetic beads, and 10 s for DNA templates free in solution. It is obvious that the gel matrix limited the diffusion of the pyrosequencing reagents, but the immobilized ssDNA templates were fully accessible in a relatively short diffusion time. Moreover, in Fig. 2, three uncomplementary dNTPs, followed by a complementary dNTP, were sequentially added to the reaction chamber to identify/quantify any false-positive signal. If the gel matrix slows down the diffusion of the pyrosequencing reagents, false-positive signals from the incorporation of added uncomplementary dNTPs would appear. The pyrograms in Fig. 2 demonstrate that no obvious false-positive light signals were detected during the first few cycles. The false-positive light signals increased as the sequencing reaction progressed. Moreover, this was not caused by the gel matrix as the same false-positive signals were also observed in the pyrogram from free templates (Fig. 2a). Though we observed slow diffusion for gel-immobilized templates as shown in Fig. 3, a good pyrogram with no false signal could be still obtained by employing long incubation of the pyrosequencing reaction mixture and an excess amount of the reagents.

4.2 Electrophoresis for Removing the Interfering Components in the Gel Spots

In gel immobilization of PCR products, PCR remnants such as PPi, excess primers, and nucleotides enter into the gel during polymerization. These impurities should be removed prior to pyrosequencing. Two approaches were used to remove these interfering components. The first was the washing approach, in which the gel-attached PCR products were incubated in a 95 °C water bath for 10 min. The other was the electrophoresis approach, in which the gel was subjected to 1× TBE at room temperature at 40 V/cm for 10 min. Figure 4 shows the degree to which interfering components in the gels were degraded after treatment with the above approaches. Curves were recorded from the fifth second after the gel was added in pyrosequencing reaction mixture. In Fig. 4, curve C was obtained from 95 °C water-treated gels, in which PCR

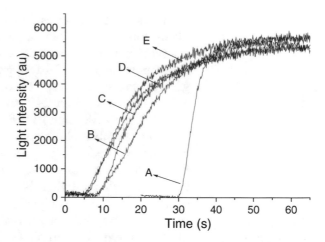

Fig. 3 Bioluminescence profile upon addition of all the four nucleotides (dTTP, dGTP, dCTP, and dATPαS) to the pyrosequencing reaction mixture. (**a**) Nonimmobilized oligonucleotide (1 pmol); (**b**)–(**e**) 4 pmol of oligonucleotide was copolymerized in a total volume of 8 μL of prepolymer: (**b**) one spot with 8 μL of gel; (**c**) two spots each with 4 μL of gel; (**d**) four spots each with 2 μL of gel; (**e**) eight spots each with 1 μL of gel

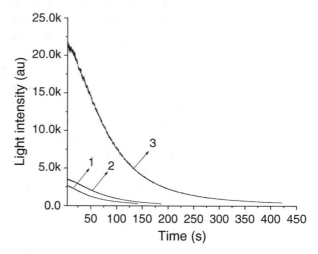

Fig. 4 Bioluminescence from gel-immobilized ssDNA templates (16 μL PCR products) prepared under alkali polymerization conditions and electrophoresis (curve **a**), hot water incubation and electrophoresis (curve **b**), and only hot water incubation (curve **c**), respectively

products were purified by ethanol precipitation and concentrated four times for polymerization; the highest value of the light intensity is 2.2×10^4 AU. It required 400 s for the signals to decrease to 400 au, indicating that not all the interfering components were removed in the 95 °C water process. However, the highest light intensity decreased to 3.2×10^3 from 2.2×10^4 au when electrophoresis was used to remove the impurities (*see* curve B in Fig. 4), suggesting that electrophoresis could effectively eliminate the

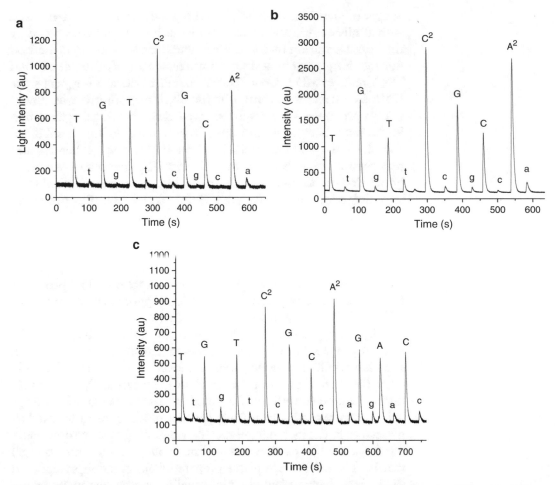

Fig. 5 Sequencing pyrograms of PCR products (DNA135) that were gel-immobilized under different conditions. (**a**) Purified PCR product polymerized under neutral condition; (**b**) purified PCR product polymerized under alkali condition; (**c**) crude PCR products polymerized under alkali condition. The *capital letters* in the pyrograms represent signals from nucleotide extension; *lower case letters* represent background signals

interfering components. An alternative method for preparing ssDNA is to denature dsDNA with alkali condition. The gel polymerization was directly performed in 0.1 M NaOH solution, and then the gel was subjected for electrophoresis treatment. As shown in curve A, background signal due to impurities was much lower than for the other conditions. Therefore electrophoresis is a very efficient method to prepare sufficiently pure ssDNA template for pyrosequencing.

4.3 Preparing ssDNA Templates from PCR Products Using Different Gel Immobilization Conditions

The DNA templates (2.15 pmol) and polyacrylamide prepolymer were copolymerized under different conditions as described. Figure 5 shows the pyrograms of gel-immobilized templates prepared under neutral (a) and alkali conditions (b), respectively. The peaks were well defined and the S/Ns were sufficiently high for correct base calling. The results agreed with those obtained by

Sanger sequencing. Peak heights from ssDNA templates denatured with alkali condition were about twice as high as those prepared by the heat denaturing method. Heat denaturation is a simple method not requiring reagent addition, but reassociation of the denatured DNA reduces ssDNA concentration. Alkali denaturing keeps the DNA in a denatured state, but the alkali may interfere in downstream processes. Our results showed that heat denaturation in a 95 °C water bath could not effectively remove the unimmobilized complementary strands, which might stay in the gel matrix and may reassociate with the immobilized ssDNA templates. An additional electrophoresis step was ineffective to separate the dsDNA, so polymerization in alkali condition was better for preparing ssDNA templates, as our experiments indicate that the PCR products can still be effectively immobilized and remain in the denatured state during copolymerization and electrophoresis. Moreover, electrophoresis effectively removes OH^- ions, which might interfere with the subsequent pyrosequencing reactions. The processes of denaturing, copolymerizing, and electrophoresis in the presence of NaOH were simple, fast, and convenient.

From the pyrograms in Fig. 5a, b, we estimate that the diffusion effect would not influence pyrosequencing. Nonimmobilized strands of PCR amplicons were removed much more efficiently from the surface of the gel spot than from inside the gel matrix during heat denaturation. It is possible that the increased light signals from the alkali denaturing process result from more ssDNA molecules in the internal gel matrix, suggesting that pyrosequencing reagents such as enzymes and nucleotides could enter the gel matrix. The ssDNA templates prepared from ethanol-precipitated PCR fragments yielded high-quality pyrosequencing data. However, the precipitation step was labor and time intensive especially for many samples. So we investigated the feasibility of preparing ssDNA templates directly from crude PCR products. Raw PCR products (1.075 pmol) were denatured, copolymerized, and subjected to electrophoresis in alkali condition. The obtained pyrogram is shown in Fig. 5c and the result was confirmed by ABI Prism 377 DNA sequencer. The immobilization percentages of the PCR products in Fig. 5b, c were almost the same, including that ssDNA templates could be successfully prepared from the crude PCR products. This improvement greatly reduced preparation time and reagent costs; most importantly, the risk of cross contamination was decreased when many different PCR products were processed.

4.4 ssDNA Templates for SNP Genotyping

In SNP genotyping, one of the three possible genotypes (homozygote, heterozygote, and homozygote) needs to be assigned to a specific sample. For homozygous samples, a single peak will be generated by pyrosequencing for a bp at a given variant site. For heterozygous samples, two peaks with half the intensity of the homozygous single

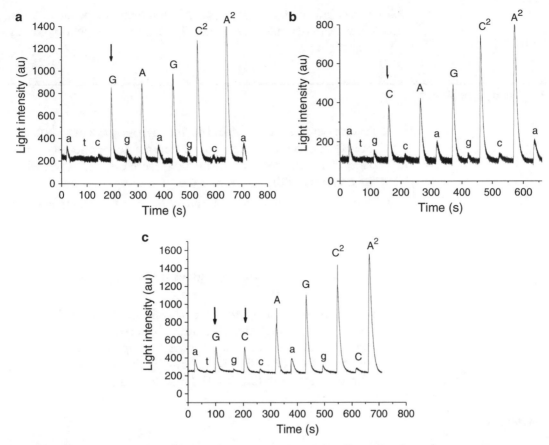

Fig. 6 Pyrograms obtained from three SNP genotyping samples: (**a**) Homozygous sample 14417G/G; (**b**) homozygous sample 14417C/C; and (**c**) heterozygous sample 14417C/G

peak will be observed at the SNP position. To evaluate the template preparation method developed above, three samples selected from volunteers in our laboratory with an OLR-1 gene SNP(C14417G) were used for pyrosequencing. The genotypes of these samples were determined with an ABI Prism 377 DNA sequencer in advance. In this experiment, the sequences of ssDNA templates were known and the sequencing primer was specially designed to extend starting at the SNP locus. Therefore, a single pyrosequencing analysis was enough to determine the genotype of a sample [5, 36]. The correct genotyping results of the two homozygotes, 14417C/C (Fig. 6a) and 14417G/G (Fig. 6b), and the heterozygote 14417C/G (Fig. 6c) were obtained. As for the heterozygote, C and G both occur at the site of a single nucleotide, so the height of each of the two peaks (Fig. 6c) is only the half of that from a homozygous sample. In order to evaluate background signals and fidelity of pyrosequencing results, uncomplementary dNTPs were intentionally added before adding complementary dNTPs. Although dATPαS showed slightly higher background signals, correct dATPαS extension signals could be clearly discriminated. Therefore, ssDNA templates prepared with the described method could be successfully used for SNP genotyping by pyrosequencing.

5 Technical Notes

1. Polyacrylamide gel is suitable for pyrosequencing, but the immobilization efficiency of different acrylamide-modified oligonucleotide concentrations used were different even when the contents of the gel were same.

2. The porous sizes of the gel matrix increased with decrease in the acrylamide monomer concentration, allowing unbounded compounds to diffuse in and out of the gel matrix.

3. Peak heights from ssDNA templates denatured with alkali condition were about twice as high as those prepared by the heat denaturing method.

4. These pyrosequencing reagents should diffuse quickly to the reaction site through the gel matrix. Otherwise the unextended fragments at each cycle may decrease signal intensities and introduce false extension signal during the next cycle, causing a "frame shift" and limiting the read length.

References

1. Ronaghi M, Uhlen M, Nyren P (1998) A sequencing method based on real-time pyrophosphate. Science 281:363–365

2. Nyren P, Karamohamed S, Ronaghi M (1997) Detection of single-base changes using a bioluminometric primer extension assay. Anal Biochem 244:367–373

3. Ronaghi M, Karamohamed S, Pettersson B, Uhlen M, Nyren P (1996) Real-time DNA sequencing using detection of pyrophosphate release. Anal Biochem 242:84–89

4. Nyren P (1994) Apyrase immobilized on paramagnetic beads used to improve detection limits in bioluminometric ATP monitoring. J Biolumin Chemilumin 9:29–34

5. Alderborn A, Kristofferson A, Hammerling U (2000) Determination of single-nucleotide polymorphisms by real-time pyrophosphate DNA sequencing. Genome Res 10:1249–1258

6. Nourizad N, Gharizadeh B, Nyren P (2003) Method for clone checking. Electrophoresis 24:1712–1715

7. Gharizadeh B, Ohlin A, Molling P, Backman A et al (2003) Multiple group-specific sequencing primers for reliable and rapid DNA sequencing. Mol Cell Probes 17:203–210

8. Margulies M, Egholm M, Altman WE, Attiya S et al (2005) Genome sequencing in microfabricated high-density picolitre reactors. Nature 437:376–380

9. Nordstrom T, Nourizad K, Ronaghi M, Nyren P (2000) Method enabling pyrosequencing on double-stranded DNA. Anal Biochem 282:186–193

10. Pacey-Miller T, Henry R (2003) Single-nucleotide polymorphism detection in plants using a single-stranded pyrosequencing protocol with a universal biotinylated primer. Anal Biochem 317:166–170

11. Russom A, Tooke N, Andersson H, Stemme G (2003) Single nucleotide polymorphism analysis by allele-specific primer extension with real-time bioluminescence detection in a microfluidic device. J Chromatogr A 1014:37–45

12. Pettersson M, Bylund M, Alderborn A (2003) Molecular haplotype determination using allele-specific PCR and pyrosequencing technology. Genomics 82:390–396

13. Verri A, Focher F, Tettamanti G, Grazioli V (2005) Two-step genetic screening of thrombophilia by pyrosequencing. Clin Chem 51:1282–1284

14. Palmieri O, Toth S, Ferraris A, Andriulli A et al (2003) CARD15 genotyping in inflammatory bowel disease patients by multiplex pyrosequencing. Clin Chem 49:1675–1679

15. Syed AA, Irving JA, Redfern CP, Hall AG et al (2004) Low prevalence of the N363S polymorphism of the glucocorticoid receptor in South Asians living in the United Kingdom. J Clin Endocrinol Metab 89:232–235

16. Sinclair A, Arnold C, Woodford N (2003) Rapid detection and estimation by pyrosequencing of 23S rRNA genes with a single nucleotide polymorphism conferring linezolid resistance in Enterococci. Antimicrob Agents Chemother 47:3620–3622

17. Holmberg K, Persson ML, Uhlen M, Odeberg J (2005) Pyrosequencing analysis of thrombosis-associated risk markers Clin Chem 51:1549–1552

18. Holmberg A, Blomstergren A, Nord O, Lukacs M et al (2005) The biotin-streptavidin interaction can be reversibly broken using water at elevated temperatures. Electrophoresis 26:501–510

19. Ji M, Hou P, Li S, He N, Lu Z (2004) Microarray-based method for genotyping of functional single nucleotide polymorphisms using dual-color fluorescence hybridization. Mutat Res 548:97–105

20. Ronaghi M (2001) Pyrosequencing sheds light on DNA sequencing. Genome Res 11:3–11

21. Wang H, Li J, Liu H, Liu Q et al (2002) Label-free hybridization detection of a single nucleotide mismatch by immobilization of molecular beacons on an agarose film. Nucleic Acids Res 30, e61

22. Afanassiev V, Hanemann V, Wolfl S (2000) Preparation of DNA and protein micro arrays on glass slides coated with an agarose film. Nucleic Acids Res 28, E66

23. Wang Y, Wang H, Gao L, Liu H et al (2005) Polyacrylamide gel film immobilized molecular beacon array for single nucleotide mismatch detection. J Nanosci Nanotechnol 5:653–658

24. Rubina AY, Pan'kov SV, Dementieva EI, Pen'kov DN et al (2004) Hydrogel drop microchips with immobilized DNA: properties and methods for large-scale production. Anal Biochem 325:92–106

25. Rehman FN, Audeh M, Abrams ES, Hammond PW et al (1999) Immobilization of acrylamide-modified oligonucleotides by co-polymerization. Nucleic Acids Res 27:649–655

26. Xiao PF, Cheng L, Wan Y, Sun BL et al (2006) An improved gel-based DNA microarray method for detecting single nucleotide mismatch. Electrophoresis 27:3904–3915

27. Dunker J, Larsson U, Petersson D, Forsell J et al (2003) Parallel DNA template preparation using a vacuum filtration sample transfer device. Biotechniques 34(862–866):868

28. Zhou G, Kamahori M, Okano K, Harada K, Kambara H (2001) Miniaturized pyrosequencer for DNA analysis with capillaries to deliver deoxynucleotides. Electrophoresis 22:3497–3504

29. Sambrook J, Russell DW (2003) Molecular cloning: a laboratory manual (III). Cold Spring Harbor Laboratory Press, ColdSpring Harbor, Chapters 5 and 10

30. Yershov G, Barsky V, Belgovskiy A, Kirillov E et al (1996) DNA analysis and diagnostics on oligonucleotide microchips. Proc Natl Acad Sci U S A 93:4913–4918

31. Dyukova VI, Dementieva EI, Zubtsov DA, Galanina OE et al (2005) Hydrogel glycan microarrays. Anal Biochem 347:94–105

32. Mitra RD, Church GM (1999) In situ localized amplification and contact replication of many individual DNA molecules. Nucleic Acids Res 27, e34

33. Dubiley S, Kirillov E, Lysov Y, Mirzabekov A (1997) Fractionation, phosphorylation and ligation on oligonucleotide microchips to enhance sequencing by hybridization. Nucleic Acids Res 25:2259–2265

34. Mitra RD, Shendure J, Olejnik J, Edyta Krzymanska O, Church GM (2003) Fluorescent in situ sequencing on polymerase colonies. Anal Biochem 320:55–65

35. Dubiley S, Kirillov E, Mirzabekov A (1999) Polymorphism analysis and gene detection by minisequencing on an array of gel-immobilized primers. Nucleic Acids Res 27, e19

36. Ahmadian A, Gharizadeh B, Gustafsson AC, Sterky F et al (2000) Single-nucleotide polymorphism analysis by pyrosequencing. Anal Biochem 280:103–110

Chapter 7

Multiplex PCR Based on a Universal Biotinylated Primer to Generate Templates for Pyrosequencing

Zhiyao Chen, Yunlong Liu, Hui Ye, Haiping Wu, Jinheng Li, Bingjie Zou, Qinxin Song, and Guohua Zhou

Abstract

Pyrosequencing is a powerful tool widely used in genetic analysis, however template preparation prior to pyrosequencing is still costly and time-consuming. To achieve an inexpensive and labor-saving template preparation for pyrosequencing, we have successfully developed a single-tube multiplex PCR including a pre-amplification and a universal amplification. In the process of pre-amplification, a low concentration of target-specific primers tagged with universal ends introduced universal priming regions into amplicons. In the process of universal amplification, a high concentration of universal primers was used for yielding amplicons with various SNPs of interest. As only a universal biotinylated primer and one step of single-stranded DNA preparation were required for typing multiple SNPs located on different sequences, pyrosequencing-based genotyping became time-saving, labor-saving, sample-saving, and cost-saving. By a simple optimization of multiplex PCR condition, only a 4-plex and a 3-plex PCR were required for typing 7 SNPs related to tamoxifen metabolism. Further study showed that pyrosequencing coupled with an improved multiplex PCR protocol allowed around 30 % decrease of either typing cost or typing labor. Considering the biotinylated primer and the optimized condition of the multiplex PCR are independent of SNP locus, it is easy to use the same condition and the identical biotinylated primer for typing other SNPs. The preliminary typing results of the 7 SNPs in 11 samples demonstrated that multiplex PCR-based pyrosequencing could be promising in personalized medicine at a low cost.

Key words Pyrosequencing, Multiplex polymerase chain reaction, Universal biotinylated primer, Single nucleotide polymorphism

1 Introduction

Pyrosequencing is a gel-free DNA sequencing technique depending on the real-time quantification of pyrophosphates (PPis) released during primer extension reactions [1]. Compared to gel-based Sanger sequencing and other methods for SNP detection, it is much more quantitative, thus peak intensities in a pyrogram can be used to quantify the extended templates [2–16]. In addition to SNP typing and pathogen identification, pyrosequencing is an

Guohua Zhou and Qinxin Song (eds.), *Advances and Clinical Practice in Pyrosequencing*, Springer Protocols Handbooks, DOI 10.1007/978-1-4939-3308-2_7, © Springer Science+Business Media New York 2016

accurate tool for analyzing methylated DNA and mutant DNA in a clinical sample [17–20].

Although an automatic pyrosequencer has helped to increase sequencing throughput, template preparation prior to pyrosequencing is still costly and time-consuming. Conventionally, each pyrosequencing needs the step of PCR with a biotinylated primer and the step of single-stranded DNA (ssDNA) preparation with streptavidin-coated beads. As biotinylated primers and beads are expensive, it should be much costly if multiple targets are pyrosequenced at a time. On the other hand, it is still time-consuming and laborious to perform PCR and ssDNA preparation for each template although an automatic ssDNA preparation device can be employed.

To avoid ssDNA preparation prior to pyrosequencing, Linear-After-The-Exponential (LATE)-PCR, an efficient asymmetric amplification method to directly generate ssDNA amplicons, has been used to provide templates for pyrosequencing [21, 22]. Due to no need for ssDNA preparation, the total process for pyrosequencing is simplified; however, the strict conditions for designing qualified LATE-PCR primers greatly limit the wide application of LATE-PCR [23]. Moreover, as for targets with AT-rich or GC-rich sequences, it is difficult to yield ssDNA adequate enough for pyrosequencing. Most importantly, the ssDNA generated via LATE-PCR contains a lot of unwanted components, such as PPi, excess primers, dNTPs; hence, an additional template processing step is still required to achieve a pyrogram of high quality before pyrosequencing.

To achieve a method capable of inexpensive template preparation, simple PCR set-up, and more efficient use of DNA samples, multiplex PCR is conventionally used to simultaneously amplify multiple targets of interest within a single reaction [24]. However, every target needs a biotinylated primer to allow the following ssDNA preparation, in addition to common shortcomings such as complex manipulation, low sensitivity, and primer–primer interactions in multiplex PCR. Although multiplex PCR based on the ligation of a universal adapter with fragmented targets is efficient for the amplification of multiple targets, specific fragmentation of targets of interest is difficult [25]. An alternate way is to use a primer consisted of a target-specific sequence and a tagged sequence to introduce a universal priming site. Hence, two steps of amplification are needed: a target-specific PCR to generate a small amount of templates with universal ends, and a PCR using a pair of universal primers to amplify all templates with the universal ends [26]. As only a pair of universal primers is employed, all targets have similar amplification efficiency even though the target sequences are different (Fig. 1). Most importantly, this protocol is cost-effective to supply pyrosequencing templates because only a universal

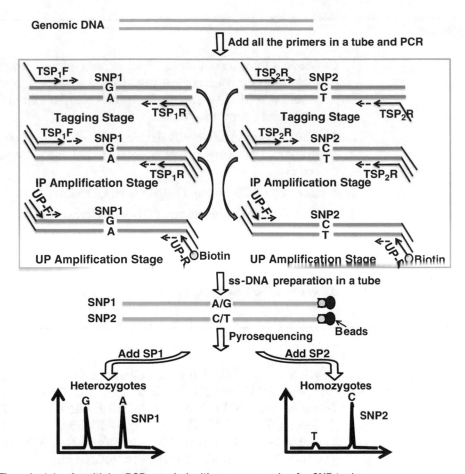

Fig. 1 The principle of multiplex PCR coupled with pyrosequencing for SNP typing

biotinylated primer is required for amplifying any target of interest. Therefore, we used this multiplex PCR approach based on a universal biotinylated primer for typing multiple SNPs in a single PCR. As a single PCR and a single step of ssDNA preparation are performed for multiple targets, the whole process for multiplex SNP typing becomes time-saving, labor-saving, sample-saving, and cost-saving.

As an example, 6 SNPs in cytochrome P450 2D6 (CYP2D6) gene and 1 SNP in sulfotransferase 1A1 (SULT1A1) gene were employed for investigation. Many studies have shown that these SNPs are related to the metabolism of tamoxifen, which is used for the treatment of hormone receptor-positive breast cancer [27, 28]. By a simple optimization of multiplex PCR condition, only a 4-plex and a 3-plex PCR are required for typing the 7 SNPs with pyrosequencing, indicating that pyrosequencing coupled with an improved multiplex PCR protocol allows personalized medicine at a low cost [29–30].

2   Materials

1. Genomic DNA was isolated from whole blood samples by phenol-chloroform extraction protocol. All of the blood samples were provided by Jinling Hospital (Nanjing, China) with the informed consent form.

2. The DNA concentration was determined by a UV–Vis spectrophotometer (Naka Instruments, Japan), and stored at −20 °C before use.

3. Mastercycler PCR system (Eppendorf, Germany).

4. *HotStarTaq* DNA polymerase (Qiagen, Germany).

5. Streptavidin Sepharose™ High Performance Beads (GE Healthcare Bio-Sciences AB, Sweden).

6. Portable bioluminescence analyzer (HITACHI, Ltd., Central Research Laboratory, Japan).

3   Methods

3.1   Primer Design

1. Seven SNPs in CYP2D6 gene (GenBank ID: NG_008376.1) and SULT1A1 gene (GenBank ID: NC_000016.9) were investigated: CYP2D6*3 (rs35742686), CYP2D6*4 (rs3892097), CYP2D6*6 (rs5030655), CYP2D6*9 (rs5030656), CYP2D6*10 (rs1065852), CYP2D6*41 (rs28371725), and SULT1A1*2 (rs9282861).

2. A pair of primers (each consists of a target-specific sequence region and a universal sequence region) was designed for analyzing SNPs of interests.

3.2   Multiplex PCR

1. PCR amplifications were performed on Mastercycler PCR system. A 50 μL of PCR contained 5 μL of 10× PCR buffer, 4.0 mM $MgCl_2$, 0.8 mM each dNTP, 0.5 mM betaine, 3 % DMSO, 0.08 μM each of target-specific primers, 2 μM each of universal primers, 150 ng genomic DNA, 2.5 U of HotStarTaq DNA polymerase (Qiagen, Germany), and H_2O was added up to 50 μL.

2. The PCR program was as follows: 94 °C for 15 min, followed by 10 cycles of 94 °C for 30 s, 55 °C for 90 s, 72 °C for 60 s; then 10 cycles of 94 °C for 30 s, 72 °C for 90 s; 35 cycles of 94 °C for 20 s, 60 °C for 20 s, 72 °C for 20 s, and a final extension at 72 °C for 3 min.

3.3   Template Preparation for Pyrosequencing

1. The biotinylated multiplex PCR products were immobilized onto Streptavidin Sepharose™ High Performance Beads. DNA strands were denatured by 0.1 M NaOH, then washed by 1×

annealing buffer (4 mM Tris–HCl [pH 7.5], 2 mM $MgCl_2$, 5 mM NaCl).

2. The immobilized strands were divided into aliquots, then annealed to different sequencing primer, respectively, at 94 °C for 30 s and 55 °C for 3 min.

3.4 Pyrosequencing

1. We used a portable bioluminescence analyzer for pyrosequencing [14, 15] (*see* **Note 1**).

2. Pyrosequencing was carried out by the reported method. The reaction volume was 40 µL, containing 0.1 M Tris–acetate (pH 7.7), 2 mM EDTA, 10 mM magnesium acetate, 0.1 % BSA, 1 mM dithiothreitol, 2 µM adenosine 5′-phosphosulfate, 0.4 mg/mL PVP, 0.4 mM D-luciferin, 2 µM ATP sulfurylase, 5.7×10^8 RLU QuantiLum recombinant luciferase, 18 U/mL Exo⁻ Klenow Fragment, and 1.6 U/mL apyrase.

4 Method Validation

4.1 Typing 7 SNPs Related to Tamoxifen Metabolism

It is well-known that the efficiency and specificity of multiplex PCR was affected by various conditions, such as the concentrations of dNTPs, Mg^{2+}, DNA polymerase, primers TSPs and UPs. After pretesting the concentration range of each component, we investigated the interactions among these five factors by L16 (3^5) orthogonal test designed by SPSS (Statistical Package for the Social Science). The results showed that the optimized concentration of dNTPs, Mg^{2+}, DNA polymerase, TSPs, and UPs was 0.8 mM, 4.0 mM $MgCl_2$, 2.5 U/50 µL, 0.08 µM, and 2 µM, respectively.

As reported, betaine and DMSO could improve the yield of PCR amplification [16, 17]; thus, different concentrations of these additives were added into our multiplex PCR system to improve amplification efficiency. The results showed that the optimum concentration of betaine and DMSO was 0.5 M and 3 %.

The melting temperature (T_m) of a TSP, consisted of target-specific sequence and a universal priming sequence, was around 87 °C, while the T_m of its target-specific sequence was around 57 °C; thus, the annealing temperature at a tagging stage should be around 55 °C. The amount of amplicons from different PCR cycles at the tagging stage indicated that the tagging step was necessary to the success of multiplex PCR, and ten cycles were sufficient for generating enough amplicons (Fig. 2).

Pyrosequencing on ssDNA amplicons from PCR with different plexing numbers was performed. The results showed that pyrograms of good quality were obtained when pyrosequencing templates were from 1-plex, 2-plex, 3-plex, and 4-plex PCR. However, noisy peaks appeared in pyrograms when the plexing number was more than 4. Although genotypes can still be unambiguously

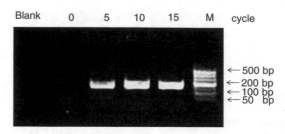

Fig. 2 Influence of different PCR cycles at the tagging stage on the amplicons yield of a 3-plex PCR

identified, the pyrogram quality became poor considering the peak intensities were disproportional to the expected base numbers. Therefore, the selected 7 SNPs were grouped into a 4-plex and a 3-plex PCR amplification. After two multiplex PCRs in individual tubes, ssDNA was prepared for pyrosequencing. The typical pyrograms of a sample were successfully obtained from typing the 7 SNPs (see Panel B and D in Fig. 3 for details). To verify the accuracy of the proposed method, single-plex PCR was performed for all 7 SNPs individually. As shown in the Panel A and C in Fig. 3, no obvious difference in pyrogram quality was observed between multiplex-PCR and single-plex PCR, indicating that a multiplex PCR assay using a universal biotinylated primer can be used to simultaneously generate multiple templates for pyrosequencing efficiently [31–33].

To further illustrate the clinical application of our method, 11 clinical samples (whole blood) were selected. After a 4-plex and a 3-plex PCR on the genomic DNA from blood samples, 7 SNPs were genotyped by pyrosequencing. Typing results were shown in Fig. 4 and Table 1. After statistical analysis, the inactive genotype CYP2D6 (*3, *4, *5, *6, *9) with the phenotype of poor metabolizers (PM) was not detected among 11 samples, indicating that the frequency of PM was quite low in Chinese population. Also, the frequency of reduced active genotype CYP2D6*41 and SULT1A1*2 with the phenotype of intermediate metabolizers (IM) was very low in Chinese population. However, the frequency of CYP2D6*10 with the phenotype of intermediate metabolizers (IM) was as high as 63.1 % in Chinese population.

5 Technical Notes

1. This apparatus has a portable size of 140 mm (W) × 158 mm (H) × 250 mm (D), which uses an array of eight photodiodes (Hamamatsu Photonics K.K., Japan) to detect photo signals, and employs four separate capillaries for dispensing small amounts of dNTPs into the reaction chamber.

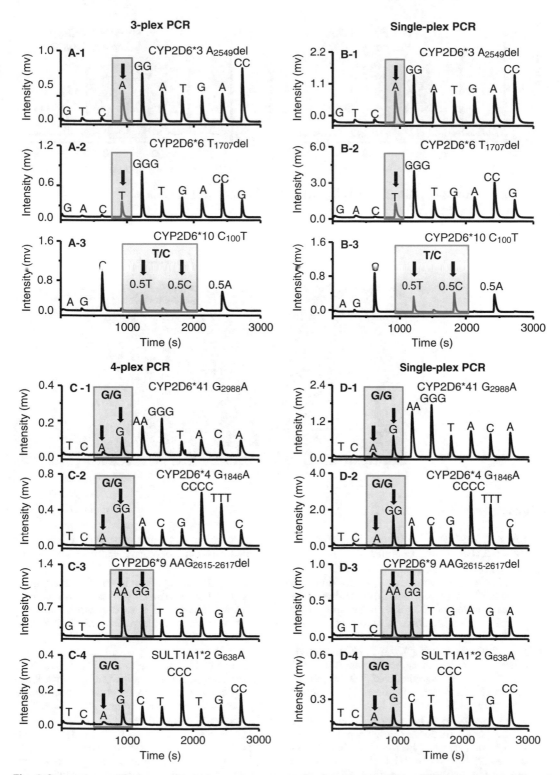

Fig. 3 Comparison of typing results between pyrosequencing based on multiplex PCR (panels A and C) and single-plex PCR (panels B and D)

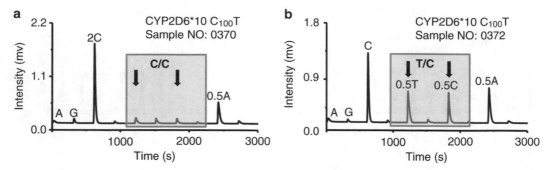

Fig. 4 Typical pyrograms of CYP2D6*10 typing results in different clinical samples

Table 1
Genotyping results of 7 SNPs in 11 clinical samples by the proposed method

Genes	Alleles/position	Number of homozygote	Number of heterozygote	Phenotype
CYP2D6 ($n=11$)	*3/A_{2549}del	11	0	PM
	*4/G_{1846}A	11	0	PM
	*6/T_{1707}del	11	0	PM
	*9/$AAG_{2615-2617}$ del	11	0	PM
	*10/C_{100}T	4	7	IM
	*41/G_{2988}A	11	0	IM
SULT1A1 ($n=11$)	*2/G_{638}A	11	0	IM

References

1. Ronaghi M (2001) Pyrosequencing sheds light on DNA sequencing. Genome 11:3
2. Bai Y, Han Q, Lin D, Luo J, Tu J, Ge Q, Lu Z (2012) Structure-function relationships of three kinds of immobilized DNA probes in the discrimination abilities of single nucleotide variation. J Nanosci Nanotechnol 12:1748–1753
3. Xiao P, Chen J, Tang J, Lu Z (2011) Single nucleotide variation detection on 3D DNA microarray by ligation of two-terminal-modified universal probes. J Nanosci Nanotechnol 11:7627–7634
4. Xia G, Gao W, Ji K, Liu S, Wan B, Luo J, Bai Y (2011) Single nucleotide polymorphisms analysis of noise-induced hearing loss using three-dimensional polyacrylamide gel-based microarray method. J Nanosci Nanotechnol 7:807–812
5. Li Y, Tang J, Pan Z, Xiao P, Zhou D, Jin L, Pan M, Lu Z (2011) Single nucleotide polymorphism genotyping and point mutation detection by ligation on microarrays. J Nanosci Nanotechnol 11:994–1003
6. Cheng L, Ge Q, Sun B, Yu P, Ke X, Lu Z (2009) Polyacrylamide gel-based microarray: a novel method applied to the association study between the polymorphisms of BDNF gene and autism. J Nanosci Nanotechnol 5:542–550
7. Li S, Liu H, Tian L, Liu L, He N (2010) A novel single nucleotide polymorphisms detection sensors based on magnetic nanoparticles array and dual-color single base extension. J Nanosci Nanotechnol 10:5311–5315
8. Li S, Liu H, Jia Y, Deng Y, Zhang L, Lu Z, He N (2012) A novel SNPs detection method based on gold magnetic nanoparticles array and single base extension. Theranostics 2:967–975
9. Li S, Liu H, Liu L, Tian L, He N (2010) A novel automated assay with dual-color hybrid-

ization for single-nucleotide polymorphisms genotyping on gold magnetic nanoparticle array. Anal Biochem 405:141–143

10. Xiao L, Zhang J, Sirois P, He N, Li K (2011) A new strategy for next generation sequencing: merging the Sanger's method and the sequencing by synthesis through replacing extension. J Nanosci Nanotechnol 7:568–571

11. Liu H, Li S, Liu L, Tian L, He N (2010) An integrated and sensitive detection platform for biosensing application based on Fe@Au magnetic nanoparticles as bead array carries. Biosens Bioelectron 26:1442–1448

12. Bai Y, Lin D, Han Q, Jia Y, Tu J, Luo J, Ge Q, Zhang D, Lu Z (2011) Discrimination of single nucleotide mutation by using a new class of immobilized shared-stem double-stranded DNA probes. J Nanosci Nanotechnol 7:640–647

13. Fang Wang CM, Zeng X, Li C, Deng Y, He N (2012) Chemiluminescence molecular detection of sequence-specific HBV-DNA using magnetic nanoparticles. J Biomed Nanotechnol 8:786–790

14. Tian L, Li S, Liu H, Wang Z, He N (2009) An automated MagStation for high-throughput single nucleotide polymorphism genotyping and the dual-color hybridization. J Biomed Nanotechnol 5:511–515

15. Zhao H, Ma X, Li M, Zhou D, Xiao P, Lu Z (2011) Analysis of CpG island methylation using rolling Circle amplification (RCA) product microarray. J Biomed Nanotechnol 7:292–299

16. Tu J, Bai Y, Ge Q, Yang Q, Lu Z (2011) 2-color encoding solid phase minisequencing. J Nanosci Nanotechnol 11:2305–2307

17. Quillien V, Lavenu A, Karayan-Tapon L, Carpentier C, Labussiere M, Lesimple T, Chinot O, Wager M, Honnorat J, Saikali S, Fina F, Sanson M, Figarella-Branger D (2012) Comparative assessment of 5 methods (methylation-specific polymerase chain reaction, MethyLight, pyrosequencing, methylation-sensitive high-resolution melting, and immunohistochemistry) to analyze O6-methylguanine-DNA-methyltranferase in a series of 100 glioblastoma patients. Cancer 118:4201–4211

18. Garcia-Gonzalez C, Garcia-Bujalance S, Ruiz-Carrascoso G, Arribas JR, Gonzalez-Garcia J, Bernardino JI, Pascual-Pareja JF, Martinez-Prats L, Delgado R, Mingorance J (2012) Detection and quantification of the K103N mutation in HIV reverse transcriptase by pyrosequencing. Diagn Microbiol Infect Dis 72:90–96

19. van Schaik W, Top J, Riley DR, Boekhorst J, Vrijenhoek JE, Schapendonk CM, Hendrickx AP, Nijman IJ, Bonten MJ, Tettelin H, Willems RJ (2010) Pyrosequencing-based comparative genome analysis of the nosocomial pathogen *Enterococcus faecium* and identification of a large transferable pathogenicity island. BMC Genomics 11:239

20. Satkoski JA, Malhi R, Kanthaswamy S, Tito R, Malladi V, Smith D (2008) Pyrosequencing as a method for SNP identification in the rhesus macaque (*Macaca mulatta*). BMC Genomics 9:256

21. Salk JJ, Sanchez JA, Pierce KE, Rice JE, Soares KC, Wangh LJ (2006) Direct amplification of single-stranded DNA for pyrosequencing using linear-after-the-exponential (LATE)-PCR. Anal Biochem 353:124–132

22. Sanchez JA, Pierce KE, Rice JE, Wangh LJ (2004) Linear-after-the-exponential (LATE)-PCR: an advanced method of asymmetric PCR and its uses in quantitative real-time analysis. Proc Natl Acad Sci U S A 101:1933–1938

23. Pierce KE, Sanchez JA, Rice JE, Wangh LJ (2005) Linear-After-The-Exponential (LATE)-PCR: primer design criteria for high yields of specific single-stranded DNA and improved real-time detection. Proc Natl Acad Sci U S A 102:8609–8614

24. Aquilante CL, Langaee TY, Anderson PL, Zineh I, Fletcher CV (2006) Multiplex PCR-pyrosequencing assay for genotyping CYP3A5 polymorphisms. Clin Chim Acta 372:195–198

25. Wang WP, Ni KY, Zhou GH (2006) Multiplex single nucleotide polymorphism genotyping by adapter ligation-mediated allele-specific amplification. Anal Biochem 355:240–248

26. Krjutskov K, Andreson R, Magi R, Nikopensius T, Khrunin A, Mihailov E, Tammekivi V, Sork H, Remm M, Metspalu A (2008) Development of a single tube 640-plex genotyping method for detection of nucleic acid variations on microarrays. Nucleic Acids Res 36, e75

27. Gjerde J, Hauglid M, Breilid H, Lundgren S, Varhaug JE, Kisanga ER, Mellgren G, Steen VM, Lien EA (2008) Effects of CYP2D6 and SULT1A1 genotypes including SULT1A1 gene copy number on tamoxifen metabolism. Ann Oncol 19:56–61

28. Irvin WJ Jr, Walko CM, Weck KE, Ibrahim JG, Chiu WK, Dees EC, Moore SG, Olajide OA, Graham ML, Canale ST, Raab RE, Corso SW, Peppercorn JM, Anderson SM, Friedman KJ, Ogburn ET, Desta Z, Flockhart DA, McLeod HL, Evans JP, Carey LA (2011) Genotype-guided tamoxifen dosing increases active metabolite exposure in women with reduced CYP2D6 metabolism: a multicenter study. J Clin Oncol 29:3232–3239

29. Wu H, Wu W, Chen Z, Wang W, Zhou G, Kajiyama T, Kambara H (2011) Highly sensitive pyrosequencing based on the capture of free adenosine 5′ phosphosulfate with adenosine triphosphate sulfurylase. Anal Chem 83:3600–3605

30. Chen Z, Fu X, Zhang X, Liu X, Zou B, Wu H, Song Q, Li J, Kajiyama T, Kambara H, Zhou G (2012) Pyrosequencing-based barcodes for a dye-free multiplex bioassay. Chem Commun 48:2445–2447

31. Henke W, Herdel K, Jung K, Schnorr D, Loening SA (1997) Betaine improves the PCR amplification of GC-rich DNA sequences. Nucleic Acids Res 25:3957–3958

32. Winship PR (1989) An improved method for directly sequencing PCR amplified material using dimethyl sulphoxide. Nucleic Acids Res 17:1266

33. Xu Y, Sun Y, Yao L, Shi L, Wu Y, Ouyang T, Li J, Wang T, Fan Z, Fan T, Lin B, He L, Li P, Xie Y (2008) Association between CYP2D6*10 genotype and survival of breast cancer patients receiving tamoxifen treatment. Ann Oncol 19:1423–1429

Part II

Template Innovation

Chapter 8

A Novel Pyrosequencing Principle Based on AMP–PPDK Reaction for Improving the Detection Limit

Guohua Zhou, Tomoharu Kajiyama, Mari Gotou, Akihiko Kishimoto, Shigeya Suzuki, and Hideki Kambara

Abstract

Highly sensitive real-time pyrosequencing seems promising for constructing an inexpensive and small DNA sequencer with a low running cost. A DNA sample of a picomole level is usually used in the conventional pyrosequencing based on a luciferase assay coupled with an APS–ATP sulfurylase reaction for producing ATP from pyrophosphate (PPi). Although the luminescence intensity could be increased by increasing the amount of luciferase, it was impossible to reduce the target DNA amount because of a large background luminescence due to the luciferase–APS reaction. In this report, a novel approach using a new conversion reaction of PPi to ATP is proposed. This method has a very low background and can produce high signals in the presence of a large amount of luciferase; thus, the sample amount required for sequencing is significantly reduced. The ATP production from PPi is catalyzed with pyruvate orthophosphate dikinase (PPDK) using AMP and phosphoenolpyruvate as the substrates, which are inactive for the luciferase-catalyzed reaction. All of the components in the AMP–PPDK-based pyrosequencing system are suitable for highly sensitive DNA sequencing in one tube. Real-time DNA sequencing with a readable length up to 70 bases was successfully demonstrated by using this system. By increasing the amount of luciferase, as low as 2.5 fmol of DNA templates was accurately sequenced by the proposed method with a novel simple and inexpensive DNA sequencer having a photodiode array as a sensor instead of a PMT or CCD camera. A sample amount as low as two orders of magnitude smaller than that used in the conventional pyrosequencer can be used.

Key words Pyrosequencing, Pyruvate orthophosphate dikinase (PPDK), DNA sequencing, High sensitivity, Luminometric assay, Luciferase, Pyrophosphate (PPi), Photodiode, Sequencer

1 Introduction

The robust and high-throughput DNA-sequencing method based on Sanger's principle hastened the sequencing of the whole human genome [1]. As the human genome sequencing has been completed, the sequencing of short fragments is becoming more important for identifying microbial types, SNP typing, and gene expression analysis in the post genome era. Various new attempts [2, 3] along this line, such as sequencing by hybridization [4, 5],

Guohua Zhou and Qinxin Song (eds.), *Advances and Clinical Practice in Pyrosequencing*, Springer Protocols Handbooks, DOI 10.1007/978-1-4939-3308-2_8, © Springer Science+Business Media New York 2016

sequencing by synthesis [6–8], and sequencing by exonuclease digestion [9–12], have been proposed. Pyrosequencing is a newly developed sequencing-by-synthesis method based on the bioluminometric detection of inorganic pyrophosphates (PPi) coupled with four enzymatic reactions [13].

In the conventional pyrosequencing method, four enzymes are employed. They are DNA polymerase for extending DNA strands, ATP sulfurylase for converting PPi to ATP in the presence of adenosine 5' phosphosulfate (APS), luciferase for producing visible light by consuming ATP to convert luciferin to oxyluciferin, and apyrase for degrading ATP and unincorporated dNTPs into AMP and dNMPs. When the added dNTP is complementary to the base in a template strand hybridized with a sequencing primer, a strand extension reaction occurs. It is followed by ATP production and luciferase reaction. A light signal is detected as a peak in a pyrogram. The relative intensity of each peak is proportional to the number of incorporated nucleotides. Consequently, the nucleotide sequence is determined from the incorporated nucleotide species and the peak heights in the pyrogram. Pyrosequencing has several advantages over other new sequencing methods in terms of base-calling accuracy, system flexibility, and automating the whole sequencing process. It is thus becoming popular for SNP typing [14], microbial typing [15, 16], and resequencing [17].

Although pyrosequencing is based on a sensitive bioluminometric assay, it still requires DNA templates at a picomole level. In many cases, the reduction of template DNA amount as well as the reagent amount is preferable for reducing the sequencing cost, and a highly sensitive ATP detection is therefore required. However, in the conventional pyrosequencing method, a large background signal due to a side reaction of APS with luciferase makes a highly sensitive assay impossible as the concentration of luciferase cannot be much higher. In this report, we describe a novel method enabling pyrosequencing with a very small amount of template DNA by reducing the background due to the side reaction. It uses pyruvate orthophosphate dikinase (PPDK) [18, 19] instead of ATP sulfurylase to convert PPi into ATP in the presence of AMP. This system successfully demonstrated the long-read sequencing of up to 70 bases. Since the method is sensitive enough to sequence several femtomoles of DNA, a novel small and inexpensive DNA sequencer with a photodiode array as a sensor instead of a PMT or CCD camera can be constructed.

The detection of small amount of PPi produced during nucleotide incorporation reactions is very difficult in a luciferase assay with APS as a substrate because a large background is produced. Another way of producing ATP from PPi is to use PPDK and AMP. The enzymatic cycle reactions are shown in Eqs. (1) and (2), where AMP produced in Eq. (1) is converted to ATP again by PPDK in the presence of PPi and phosphoenolpyruvate (PEP). As neither AMP nor PEP is a substrate for the luciferase reaction, a highly sensitive ATP detection is possible by increasing the luciferase amount in the reaction mixture. The cycle reaction continues for a long time by consuming PEP (Eq. (1)) and luciferin (Eq. (1)). A constant signal intensity, which enables the use of a large amount of luciferase to realize long-time signal integration for highly sensitive detection, is therefore observed. By optimizing the conditions of these reactions, ATP as low as 0.4 amol could be detected [18].

$$AMP + PPi + PEP \xrightarrow{\text{PPDK,Mg}^{2+}} ATP + \text{Pyruvate} + Pi \qquad (1)$$

$$ATP + \text{Luciferin} + O_2 \xrightarrow{\text{Luciferase,Mg}^{2+}} AMP + \text{Oxyluciferase} + CO_2 + PPi + \text{Light} \qquad (2)$$

The detection target in pyrosequencing is PPi, and the principle of the proposed pyrosequencing is shown schematically in Fig. 1. All reactions including DNA strand extension, ATP production from PPi, luminometric reaction, and degradation of dNTP by apyrase are carried out in one tube. The reaction mixture contains all of the substrates and enzymes together. After hybridizing a sequencing primer to a single-stranded DNA template, the primer extension starts by the addition of dNTP only when the added dNTP is complementary to the base of the template. The dNTP incorporation reaction produces PPi, which reacts with AMP to produce ATP in the presence of PPDK. The ATP is used to convert luciferin to oxyluciferin with the release of visible light. The luminescence is proportional to the number of nucleotides incorporated. The base sequence can then be determined from the luminescence intensity and the iterative base addition sequence.

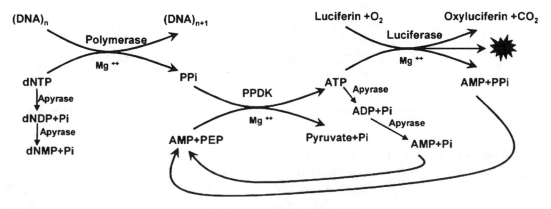

Fig. 1 Principle of pyrosequencing using PPDK for converting PPi to ATP

2   Materials

1. Thermostable PPDK (8.6 U/mg of protein, 24 mg of protein/mL) and thermostable luciferase (1.4×10^{11} RLU/mg of protein, 18 mg of protein/mL) were supplied by Kikkoman (Chiba, Japan).

2. D-Luciferin, luciferase *Photinus pyralis* (firefly), phosphoenolpyruvate trisodium (PEP), pyrophosphate decahydrate (PPi), ATP sulfurylase, apyrase-VI, bovine serum albumin (BSA), and APS were purchased from Sigma (St. Louis, MO).

3. 2′-deoxyadenosine-5′-O-(1-thiotriphosphate), Sp isomer (Sp-dATP-α-S) was from Biolog Life Science Institute (Bremen, Germany).

4. Single-stranded DNA binding protein (SSB), deoxynucleotide (dNTPs) were purchased from Amersham Biosciences (Piscataway, NJ).

5. Exo-Klenow was purchased from Ambion (Austin, TX).

6. Inorganic pyrophosphatase (40 U/mL) was obtained from USB Corp. (Cleveland, OH).

7. Platinum Taq DNA polymerase was purchased from Invitrogen (Carlsbad, CA).

8. Poly(vinylpyrrolidone) (PVP), dNTPs, and QuantiLum recombinant luciferase were purchased from Promega (Madison, WI).

9. Sodium DynabeadsM-280 streptavidin (2.8-μm i.d.) was purchased from Dynal A. C. (Oslo, Norway).

10. ATP and AMP were obtained from Oriental Yeast (Osaka, Japan).

11. The oligonucleotides were purchased from Sigma Genosys (Hokkaido, Japan). PCR primers were 5′-tgttgaagtaccagcatgcac-3′ (TF) and 5′-biotin-aaaattacttaccatttgcgatca-3′ (TRb) for amplifying TPMT gene (NCBI accession no. AB045146), and 5′-biotin-cagcagaggggacatgaa-at-3′ (UFb) and 5′-caaaaacattatgcccgagac-3′ (UR) for amplifying UGT1A1 gene (NCBI accession no. NM_000463).

3   Methods

3.1 Template DNA Preparation

1. Genomic DNAs were extracted from the blood of volunteers in our laboratory with Dnazol reagent (Invitrogen). The template DNA was obtained by PCR reactions with primer pairs of TF and TRb from human genomic DNA to get 181-bp fragments of TPMT gene, and with primers of UF band UR to get 151-bp fragments of UGT1A1 gene.

2. Fifty microliters of each PCR reaction mixture contained 1.5 mM $MgCl_2$, 0.2 mM of each dNTP, 1.25 U of Platinum Taq polymerase, 20 pmol of biotinylated primer, and 40 pmol of another primer.

3. Amplification was performed on a PTC-200 thermocycler PCR system (MJ Research, Inc.) according to the following protocol: denaturing at 94 °C for 2 min, followed by 35 thermal reaction cycling (94 °C for 30 s; 56 °C for 60 s; 72 °C for 60 s). After the thermal cycle reaction, the product was incubated at 72 °C for 7 min to ensure the complete extension of the amplified DNA.

4. Super-paramagnetic beads were used to immobilize biotinylated PCR products. The immobilization was performed by incubating the mixture of DNA and beads at room temperature for 10 min. Single-stranded DNAs were obtained by incubating the immobilized double-stranded DNAs in 0.1 M NaOH for 5 min. The supernatant fluid was neutralized by 1 M HCl, and the immobilized DNA strand was washed according to the manufacturer's instructions.

5. Annealing of a primer with the single-stranded template was carried out in the buffer of 50 mM tris–acetate (pH 7.8) and 20 mM magnesium acetate at 92 °C for 30 s, 65 °C for 3 min, and room temperature for 5 min.

3.2 Preparation of AMP–PPDK-Based Sequencing Solution

One milliliter of the AMP–PPDK-based sequencing mixture (*see* **Note 1**) contained the following components: 60 mM Tricine (pH 7.8), 2 mM EDTA, 20 mM magnesium acetate, 0.2 mM dithiothreitol, 0.4 mM D-luciferin, 0.08 mM PEP (*see* **Note 2**), 0.4 mM AMP, 0.1 % BSA, 50 U of Exo-Klenow, 15 U of PPDK, 2 U of apyrase (*see* **Note 3**), and an appropriate amount of luciferase (*see* **Note 4**).

3.3 Preparation of the Conventional APS–ATP Sulfurylase-Based Sequencing Solution

For comparison, the buffer condition for the APS–ATP sulfurylase system [20, 21] (*see* **Note 5**) was the same as that for the AMP–PPDK system. One milliliter of solution contained the following components: 60 mM Tricine (pH 7.8) (*see* **Note 6**), 2 mM EDTA, 20 mM magnesium acetate, 0.2 mM dithiothreitol, 0.4 mM D-luciferin, 0.1 % BSA, 5 μM APS, 200 mU of ATP sulfurylase, 50 U of Exo-Klenow, 2 U of apyrase and an appropriate amount of luciferase.

3.4 Gel-Based DNA Sequencing

1. The PCR products obtained with primers of TF and TRb and primers of UFb and UR were sequenced by conventional Sanger's method on an ABI Prism 310Genetical Analyzer. The purified PCR products were sequenced with a Thermo Sequenase sequencing kit (RPN2440, Amersham) using the primers described above.

2. The sequencing reaction was carried out on a PTC200 instrument at 96 °C for 2 min, followed by 25 thermal reaction cycles (96 °C for 10 s; 50 °C for 5 s; 60 °C for 4 min). The products were recovered by ethanol precipitation.

3.5 Apparatus for Pyrosequencing

1. We used two types of instruments for pyrosequencing. One was an in-house pyrosequencer, which employed capillaries for dispensing small amounts of dNTPs into the reaction chamber, for evaluation as previously reported [21]. A side-on photo-multiplier tube (PMT, R6355, Hamamatsu Phonics K. K., Shizuoka, Japan), an amplifier (AMP, NF Corp., Yokohama, Japan), a power supply (C3830, Hamamatsu Phonics K. K.), and a computer for collecting data were used. The diameter of the capillary used for connecting dNTP reservoirs to the reaction chamber was 50 μm. The whole system was packed into a small box and vibrated by a Votex mixer.

2. The other was a small prototype pyrosequencer developed in our laboratory. It used an array of photodiodes (S1133; Hamamatsu Photonics K.K.) to detect photo signals instead of PMT. The array of photodiodes was placed on a base plate having in-house-produced amplifiers [22]. A resistor for converting a photocurrent to a voltage was 10^{10} Ω, and the gain of a buffer amplifier was 17.85. Transmission efficiency at the detector surface is 92 %. To vibrate the reaction chamber, a cell phone motor fixed on the base support was employed. A plate holding the reaction chambers was vibrated with the motor.

4 Method Validation

4.1 The Optimum pH of the Pyrosequencing

The optimum pH values for PPDK, Exo-Klenow, luciferase, and apyrase reactions are 7.0, 8.0, 7.8, and 6.0, respectively (according to the protocols by the manufacturers). As all of the enzymatic reactions are carried out in a single tube, the pH value should be optimized. The peak intensities obtained at various pHs of tricine-HAc buffer in a range of pH 7.2–8.2 are shown in Fig. 2. They are in good proportion to the number of incorporated nucleotides in a pH range higher than 7.4, although the signal intensities obtained at pH 7.2 are not in good proportion to the number of incorporated nucleotides. The pyrograms also indicate that peak intensities decrease gradually with the increase of buffer pH while the activity of luciferase increases with the increase of the buffer pH [23]. On the other hand, the activity of apyrase is reduced at pH higher than 6.0; the signal should thus be increased at the high pH region. Therefore, the reduction of signal intensities with the increase of the pH value in Fig. 2 does not originate in the activity changes of luciferase or apyrase, but is likely due to the activity change of PPDK because PPDK is significantly deactivated at a

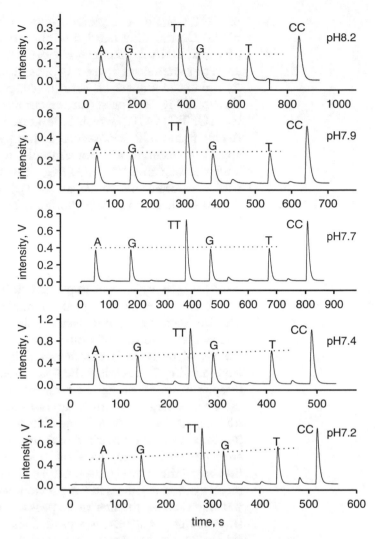

Fig. 2 pH dependence of DNA sequencing patterns determined from AMP–PPDK-based pyrosequencing reactions. The pH of the buffer is indicated in the right side of each sequencing profile. The buffer was 60 mM tricine, and HAc was used to adjust the pH. The DNA template was single-stranded PCR products of UGT1A gene. The cyclic dNTP dispensing order was A → T → G → C → A. The base species on the top of each peak indicated the sequence complementary to the template. The detection was carried out by PMT at 800 V

high pH region [23]. Considering that the optimum pH for Klenow or luciferase is about pH 8, we determined the pH value of the sequencing reaction buffer to be 7.8.

4.2 Selection of an Appropriate Concentration of Apyrase

In pyrosequencing, it is very important to select an appropriate concentration of apyrase. This is because insufficient apyrase will cause a plus frame shift of a sequencing profile, where some of the extended DNA strands are longer than expected as the degradation of dNTP is not completed before dispensing the subsequent dNTP. On the other hand, a minus frame shift, where some of the extended DNA fragments are shorter than expected, occurs when an excess amount of apyrase is present in the sequencing mixture. Pyrograms obtained at various concentrations of apyrase are shown in Fig. 3. The sequence complementary to the template is "AGTTGTCCT," which is indicated at the top of each peak. A plus frame shift is observed in the pyrograms obtained at low apyrase concentrations. For example, when dCTP was dispensed after the sequence of "AGTTG," the undesired signals marked with the dotted line circles at "c" appeared in Fig. 3e, d. These signals are due to the incorporation of two bases "CC" into the T-terminated undesired fragments (AGTTGT) produced by small amounts of undegraded dTTP at the preceding dGTP dispension. Since a part of the fragments were already incorporated with dCTP at an early stage, the peak CC marked with a short dash-dotted cycle (Fig. 3d, e) is lower than the height of a two-base extension. For the same reason, the peaks T marked with dotted rectangles are also lower than the expected height, but they have the signal intensity close to that of a one-base incorporation. This is because the signal decrease is compensated by the undesired extension from another T following the CC sequence. The plus frame shift disappears by increasing the concentration of apyrase (Fig. 3a–c). However, a large amount of apyrase causes a rapid degradation of dNTPs, so that a minus frame shift appears in the pyrograms, as indicated by a and g marked with arrows in Fig. 3. Peaks G and T after peak TT are higher than peaks G and A before peak TT because of the extra signals produced by the incomplete nucleotide incorporation reactions in the previous steps. No minus frame shift was observed for the first three peaks A, G, and TT even though a large amount of apyrase was used. This is because the minus frame shift only occurs when the same base is present in the upward sequence. The minus frame shift can be reduced by decreasing the apyrase concentration in the sequencing solution (Fig. 3c). Although a low apyrase concentration is effective for removing the minus frame shift, it requires a long time to degrade the dispensed dNTP; therefore, a long sequencing time is required. We overcame this difficulty by using a rather high apyrase concentration (2 U/mL) coupled with a double-dispensing method, where the same dNTP species was dispensed repeatedly in a short period of time.

4.3 Base Calling in the Homopolymeric Stretch

The determination of base numbers in homopolymeric stretches is very important. It is carried out by the quantitative detection of peak heights in pyrosequencing because peak intensities should be in proportion to the base numbers incorporated at a time. To investigate the relation between peak heights and the number of incorporated bases, different template DNAs prepared from TPMT and UGT1A1 genes were investigated. The pyrograms are shown

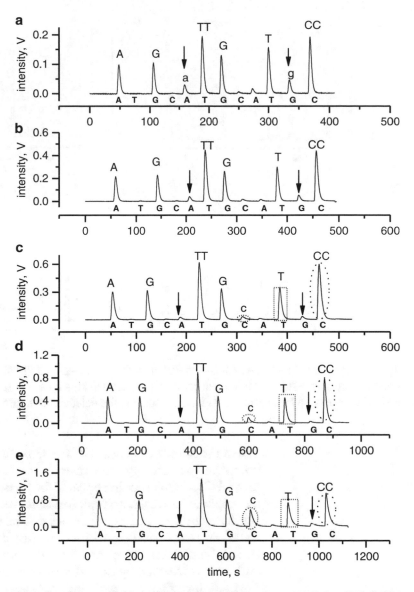

Fig. 3 Pyrograms obtained with various amounts of apyrase in an AMP–PPDK-based system. Programs (**a–e**) were obtained with the apyrase concentrations of 6.7 mU/μL, 3.3 mU/μL, 2.2 mU/μL, 1.1 mU/μL, and 0.6 mU/μL, respectively. The DNA template was a single-stranded PCR product of UGT1A gene. The dNTP dispensing order was A → T → G → C → A. The base species on the top of each peak indicated the sequence complementary to the template. The detection was carried out by PMT at 800 V

in Fig. 4, which clearly shows a linear relationship between the peak heights and the number of incorporated bases up to four identical nucleotides in a homopolymeric stretch. In Fig. 4c, the peak intensity of G (marked by an arrow) was not in proportion to five Gs, although it was a little higher than that for four Gs.

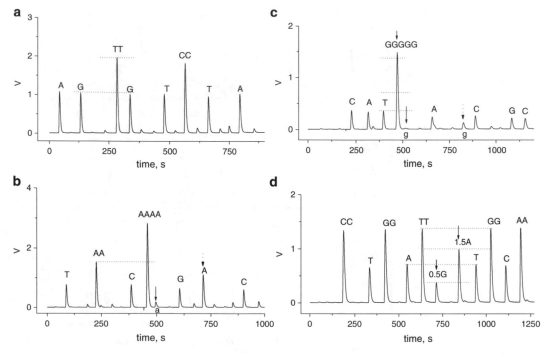

Fig. 4 Pyrograms for templates containing various kinds of nucleotides in homopolymeric stretches. The templates are single-stranded PCR products of UGT1A1 gene in (**a**) a liquid phase and (**b**) a solid surface and of TPMT gene in (**c**) a liquid phase and (**d**) a solid surface. The detection was carried out by PMT at 800 V

When the double dispension of the same dGTP was carried out to complete the incorporation reaction of base G, a peak after the second dispension should appear if the incorporation of base G was incomplete. However, no peak was observed. This might be due to the formation of secondary structures in the template. We also found an unexpected signal increase just behind a homogeneous stretch (containing more than four identical bases) such as peak A and peak G (marked by dotted arrows in Fig. 4b, c, respectively). Further investigation will be necessary to understand this phenomenon.

4.4 Comparison between the Present System and the Conventional Pyrosequencing System with APS–ATP Sulfurylase Reaction

To compare the two systems at the same conditions, all of the components including pH and buffer species in the reaction mixtures were kept identical except for the use of APS and ATP sulfurylase in APS–ATP sulfurylase-based mixture and AMP, PEP, and PPDK in the AMP–PPDK-based mixture. The details of each mixture were described in the experimental section. Almost the same photoemission profiles were obtained by the addition of ATP and PPi or by the nucleotide incorporation reactions in both systems. There was no large difference in the photo emission between the two systems as far as the same reaction conditions, such as luciferase and reaction buffers, were used. Good pyrograms for UGT1A1

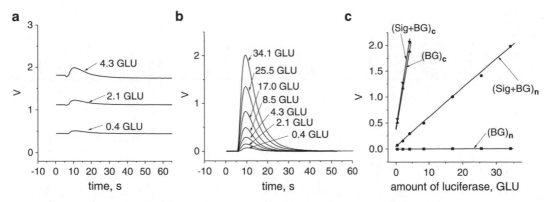

Fig. 5 Comparison of the present system based on AMP–PPDK reaction with the conventional system based on APS–ATP sulfurylase reaction. The signal intensities obtained with 18 fmol of PPi in 40 μL of reaction mixture at various amounts of luciferase (Kikkoman) were obtained. *Graph A* shows the baselines and the signals of 10 fmol of PPi in APS–ATP sulfurylase-based system at various amounts of luciferase. APS concentration was 5 μM. (**b**) Shows the signal profiles of 18 fmol of PPi by AMP–PPDK-based mixture at various concentration of luciferase. The amount of luciferase is indicated beside each trace. (**c**) Is the linear relationship between the signal intensities and the amount of luciferase. Lines $(BG)_c$ and $(Sig + BG)_c$ are the backgrounds and signals plus backgrounds in (**a**), respectively. Lines $(BG)_n$ and $(Sig + BG)_n$ are the backgrounds and signals plus backgrounds in (**b**), respectively. GLU means 10^9 luciferase units. The detection was carried out by a PD array

genes were obtained in both systems. However, a high background signal due to APS was observed in the conventional pyrosequencing. Although the signal intensities increase with the amount of luciferase, a large luciferase amount could not be used in the conventional system because of the high background signal. Consequently, the detection sensitivity in the conventional system is significantly limited. On the contrary, almost no background signal appeared in a pyrogram obtained with the present system based on the AMP–PPDK system. A highly sensitive detection of PPi as small as 18 fmol could be realized as shown in Fig. 5. The signal intensity increased with the amount of luciferase, as shown in Fig. 6b and the line $(Sig + BG)_n$ in Fig. 5c, while the background stayed constant even at a high concentration of luciferase, as shown by line $(BG)_n$ in Fig. 5c. While, the background signal increased due to the APS reaction with luciferase as well in the conventional system as shown in Fig. 5a and line $(BG)_c$ in Fig. 5c. The large background prevented the highly sensitive detection of PPi by conventional pyrosequencing reactions, as shown in Fig. 5a and lines $(BG)_c$ and $(Sig + BG)_c$ in Fig. 5. Consequently, the present system based on the AMP–PPDK reaction allows the detection or sequencing of trace DNAs by increasing the amount of luciferase.

4.5 Long-Read DNA Sequencing

Long-base reading is of great importance in applying pyrosequencing to microbial typing as well as mutation screening and resequencing. Base reading up to 100 bases was reported by the conventional pyrosequencing system with APS–ATP sulfurylase

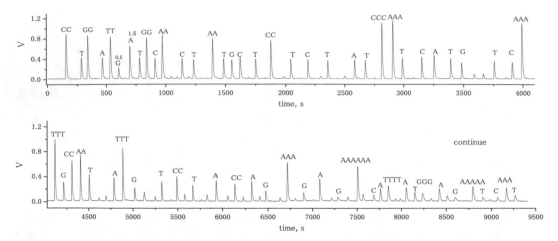

Fig. 6 Long-base read pyrogram obtained using single-stranded DNA-binding protein (SSB). The sequencing was performed on the liquid phase of the single-stranded 181-bp PCR products of TPMT gene. The dNTP dispensing order was A → T → G → C → A. A double dispensation of the same dNTP was carried out when a peak occurred. The base species on the top of each peak indicated the sequence complementary to the template. The detection was carried out by PMT at 800 V

and dATPαS [24]. The performance of the present AMP–PPDK system for long-base reading was investigated. To improve the accuracy of base calling, single-stranded DNA-binding protein (SSB) was used [25, 26]. As shown in Fig. 6, DNA sequencing up to 70 bases was successfully carried out, although the proportion of the peak intensities to the incorporated base number was worse in a long-base region. More than 100 bases could be identified; while the sequence data of the last 30 bases were not good enough for sequencing accurately. The readable base length was limited mainly by the undesired peaks due to secondary structures of a template, misannealing of a sequencing primer to the target, and frame shifts due to incomplete extension reactions. Besides the addition of SSB for improving the sequencing quality, the double dispension of each dNTP was effective to minimize minus frame shifts that accumulate incomplete extension products.

4.6 Inexpensive Detector for Pyrosequencing and the Detection Limit

The present sequencing system gave a high detection sensitivity because of the low background signal. As a large amount of luciferase could be employed without producing a large background, a small amount of DNA could be sequenced by a simple and inexpensive DNA sequencing system with an inexpensive photodiode (PD) array instead of a PMT or CCD camera. Although the sensitivity of the constructed device was one order of magnitude lower than that with a PMT, it was sensitive enough for pyrosequencing based on the proposed AMP–PPDK system. To demonstrate the sequencing capability of the prototype instrument with a PD array, a 181-bp single-stranded PCR fragment of TPMT

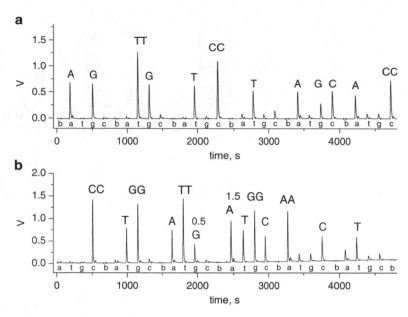

Fig. 7 Pyrograms obtained by using an inexpensive photodiode array as the detector. The sequencing detection was performed on 250 fmol of the liquid phase of single-stranded PCR products of UGT1A1 gene (**a**) and TPMT gene (**b**) simultaneously. The dNTP dispensing order was A→T→G→C→b (blank). A double dispensing of dNTP was used, and the interval was 35 s. The time interval between two different dNTP dispensations was 120 s. The base species on the top of each peak indicated the sequence complementary to the template. The detection was carried out by a PD array

gene and a 151-bp single-stranded PCR fragment of UGT1A1 gene were sequenced by AMP–PPDK-based reactions (Fig. 7). It showed that the inexpensive sequencer works well.

5 Technical Notes

1. Pyrograms at various amounts of AMP indicated a suitable AMP concentration of 0.1–0.4 mM for sequencing reactions. It was found that a high concentration of AMP inhibits the luciferase-catalyzed reaction; large amounts of AMP are therefore not preferable for pyrosequencing. Consequently, 0.4 mM AMP was employed for a routine pyrosequencing.

2. We did not observe any significant change in signal intensities in a range from 80 to 320 μM PEP, so 80 μM of PEP was used for a routine sequencing.

3. Considering that the optimum pH for Klenow or luciferase is about pH 8, we determined the pH value of the sequencing reaction buffer to be 7.8.

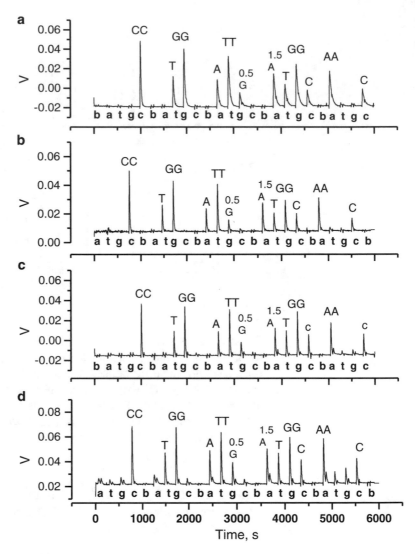

Fig. 8 Sensitivities in pyrosequencing with various amounts of luciferase obtained by using an inexpensive photodiode array as the detector. The measurements were performed with 500 fmol (**a**), 125 fmol (**b**), 12.5 fmol (**c**), and 2.5 fmol (**d**) of the liquid phase of single-stranded PCR products of TPMT gene, respectively. The concentration of luciferase was 0.1 GLU/25 μL, 0.4 GLU/25 μL, 4 GLU/25 μL, and 20 GLU/25 μL for pyrogram **a**, **b**, **c**, and **d**, respectively. The concentration of apyrase was the half of that described in the experiment section. The concentration of dATPαS was 100 μM, 100 μM, 40 μM, and 10 μM for pyrogram **a**, **b**, **c**, and **d**, respectively, and the concentration of other three dNTPs was the half of dATPαS. The dNTP dispensing order was A → T → G → C → b (blank). The base species on the top of each peak indicated the sequence complementary to the template. The detection was carried out by a PD array

4. DNA sequencing at various concentrations of luciferase is shown in Fig. 8. A small amount of DNA could be sequenced with a large amount of luciferase even if a photodiode detector was used. While as small as 2.5 fmol of DNA was successfully

sequenced by increasing the luciferase amount to 20 GLU/25 μL (Fig. 8d). This amount was at least two orders of magnitude lower than that consumed in a conventional pyrosequencing system.

5. All of the enzymatic reactions used in the conventional pyrosequencing based on the APS–ATP sulfurylase system were concordant at room temperature. However, the optimum temperature for PPDK-catalyzed reaction was rather high, i.e., 55–60 °C, and the activity went down to 20 % of the maximum value at room temperature [23]. To compensate the low activity of PPDK at room temperature, a large amount of PPDK, i.e., 15 U/mL, was used. And it was clarified from the experiment that ~83 % of PPi was converted into ATP at room temperature.

6. A large amount of apyrase causes a rapid degradation of dNTPs while a low apyrase concentration is effective for removing the minus frame shift, it requires a long time to degrade the dispensed dNTP; therefore, a long sequencing time is required. We overcame this difficulty by using a rather high apyrase concentration (2 U/mL) coupled with a double-dispensing method, where the same dNTP species was dispensed repeatedly in a short period of time.

References

1. Zubritsky E (2002) How analytical chemists saved the human genome project...or at least gave it a helping hand. Anal Chem 74: 23A–26A

2. Shendure J, Mitra RD, Varma C, Church GM (2004) Advanced sequencing technologies: methods and goals. Nat Rev Genet 5:335–344

3. Chan EY (2005) Advances in sequencing technology. Mutat Res 573:13–40

4. Drmanac R, Drmanac S, Strezoska Z, Paunesku T, Labat I, Zeremski M, Snoddy J, Funkhouser WK, Koop B, Hood L et al (1993) DNA sequence determination by hybridization: a strategy for efficient large-scale sequencing. Science 260:1649–1652

5. Broude NE, Sano T, Smith CL, Cantor CR (1994) Enhanced DNA sequencing by hybridization. Proc Natl Acad Sci U S A 91: 3072–3076

6. Ronaghi M, Uhlen M, Nyren P (1998) A sequencing method based on real-time pyrophosphate. Science 281(363):365

7. Elahi E, Ronaghi M (2004) Pyrosequencing: a tool for DNA sequencing analysis. Methods Mol Biol 255:211–219

8. Seo TS, Bai X, Kim DH, Meng Q, Shi S, Ruparel H, Li Z, Turro NJ, Ju J (2005) Four-color DNA sequencing by synthesis on a chip using photocleavable fluorescent nucleotides. Proc Natl Acad Sci U S A 102:5926–5931

9. Jett JH, Keller RA, Martin JC, Marronc BL, Moyzis RK, Ratliff RL, Seitzinger NK, Shera EB, Stewart CC (1989) High-speed DNA sequencing: an approach based upon fluorescence detection of single molecules. J Biomol Struct Dyn 7:301–309

10. Sauer M, Angerer B, Ankenbauer W, Foldes-Papp Z, Gobel F, Han KT, Rigler R, Schulz A, Wolfrum J, Zander C (2001) Single molecule DNA sequencing in submicrometer channels: state of the art and future prospects. J Biotechnol 86:181–201

11. Werner JH, Cai H, Jett JH, Reha-Krantz L, Keller RA, Goodwin PM (2003) Progress towards single-molecule DNA sequencing: a one color demonstration. J Biotechnol 102:1–14

12. Brakmann S (2004) High-density labeling of DNA for single molecule sequencing. Methods Mol Biol 283:137–144

13. Ronaghi M (2001) Pyrosequencing sheds light on DNA sequencing. Genome Res 11:3–11

14. Ahmadian A, Gharizadeh B, Gustafsson AC, Sterky F, Nyren P, Uhlen M, Lundeberg J (2000) Single-nucleotide polymorphism analysis by pyrosequencing. Anal Biochem 280:103–110

15. Ronaghi M, Elahi E (2002) Pyrosequencing for microbial typing. J Chromatogr B Analyt Technol Biomed Life Sci 782:67–72

16. Pourmand N, Elahi E, Davis RW, Ronaghi M (2002) Multiplex pyrosequencing. Nucleic Acids Res 30, e31

17. Nourizad N, Gharizadeh B, Nyren P (2003) Method for clone checking. Electrophoresis 24:1712–1715

18. Sakakibara T, Murakami S, Eisaki N, Nakajima M, Imai K (1999) An enzymatic cycling method using pyruvate orthophosphate dikinase and firefly luciferase for the simultaneous determination of ATP and AMP (RNA). Anal Biochem 268:94–101

19. Zhou G, Gotou M, Kajiyama T, Kambara H (2005) Multiplex SNP typing by bioluminometric assay coupled with terminator incorporation (BATI). Nucleic Acids Res 33:e133

20. Ronaghi M, Nygren M, Lundeberg J, Nyren P (1999) Analyses of secondary structures in DNA by pyrosequencing. Anal Biochem 267:65–71

21. Zhou G, Kamahori M, Okano K, Harada K, Kambara H (2001) Miniaturized pyrosequencer for DNA analysis with capillaries to deliver deoxynucleotides. Electrophoresis 22:3497–3504

22. Kamahori M, Harada K, Kambara H (2002) A phase III randomized trial of 5-fluorouracil, doxorubicin, and mitomycin C versus 5-fluorouracil and mitomycin C versus 5-fluorouracil alone in curatively resected gastric cancer. Meas Sci Technol 13:1779–1785

23. Eisaki N, Tatsumi H, Murakami S, Horiuchi T (1999) Pyruvate phosphate dikinase from a thermophilic actinomyces *Microbispora rosea* subsp. aerata: purification, characterization and molecular cloning of the gene. Biochim Biophys Acta 1431:363–373

24. Gharizadeh B, Nordstrom T, Ahmadian A, Ronaghi M, Nyren P (2002) Long-read pyrosequencing using pure 2′-deoxyadenosine-5′-O′-(1-thiotriphosphate) Sp-isomer. Anal Biochem 301:82–90

25. Ronaghi M (2000) Improved performance of pyrosequencing using single-stranded DNA-binding protein. Anal Biochem 286:282–288

26. Ehn M, Ahmadian A, Nilsson P, Lundeberg J, Hober S (2002) Escherichia coli single-stranded DNA-binding protein, a molecular tool for improved sequence quality in pyrosequencing. Electrophoresis 23:3289–3299

Chapter 9

Pyrosequencing Chemistry Coupled with Modified Primer Extension Reactions for Quantitative Detection of Allele Frequency in a Pooled Sample

Guohua Zhou, Masao Kamahori, Kazunori Okano, Gao Chuan, Kunio Harada, and Hideki Kambara

Abstract

A new method for SNP analysis based on the detection of pyrophosphate (PPi) is demonstrated, which is capable of detecting small allele frequency differences between two DNA pools for genetic association studies other than SNP typing. The method is based on specific primer extension reactions coupled with PPi detection. As the specificity of the primer-directed extension is not enough for quantitative SNP analysis, artificial mismatched bases are introduced into the 3′-terminal regions of the specific primers as a way of improving the switching characteristics of the primer extension reactions. The best position in the primer for such artificial mismatched bases is the third position from the primer 3′-terminus. Contamination with endogenous PPi, which produces a large background signal level in SNP analysis, was removed using PPase to degrade the PPi during the sample preparation process. It is possible to accurately and quantitatively analyze SNPs using a set of primers that correspond to the wild-type and mutant DNA segments. The termini of these primers are at the mutation positions. Various types of SNPs were successfully analyzed. It was possible to very accurately determine SNPs with frequencies as low as 0.02. It is very reproducible and the allele frequency difference can be determined. It is accurate enough to detect meaningful genetic differences among pooled DNA samples. The method is sensitive enough to detect 14 amol ssM13 DNA. The proposed method seems very promising in terms of realizing a cost-effective, large-scale human genetic testing system.

Key words SNP, Bioluminometric assay, Specific primer extension reactions

1 Introduction

Single nucleotide polymorphisms (SNPs) are the most frequent form of sequence variation among individuals and may be responsible for a number of heritable diseases. As approximately one nucleotide in every 1000 bases is estimated to differ between any two copies in the human chromosome, more than 3,000,000 SNPs may be present in the whole human genome [1]. Some of these

Guohua Zhou and Qinxin Song (eds.), *Advances and Clinical Practice in Pyrosequencing*, Springer Protocols Handbooks, DOI 10.1007/978-1-4939-3308-2_9, © Springer Science+Business Media New York 2016

may be the causative factors of serious diseases. It is necessary to analyze a tremendous number of individual DNA samples at various loci to clarify the relationships between SNPs and diseases. Consequently, an extremely efficient technology for screening large numbers of SNPs in samples from many patients and with high throughput, relative ease, low cost, and high accuracy will be required for both basic research and routine diagnostic testing. Many methods have been developed as attempts to achieve these goals, including electrophoresis [2, 3], amplification refractory mutation system (ARMS) [4], Invader [5, 6], 5′-nuclease TaqMan [7, 8], dynamic allele-specific hybridization (DASH) [9], molecular beacon probes [10], mass spectrometry [11, 12], pyrosequencing [13–15], DNA chips [3, 16], electric field-controlled nucleic acid hybridization [17, 18], electrocatalysis [19], and bead technology [20, 21]. Each method has its advantages and disadvantages, and these have been covered in several reviews [22–25]. Most of these methods are for typing one SNP or multiple SNPs for one individual at a time. To associate SNPs with diseases, we have to analyze multiple SNPs for large numbers of patient samples and control samples. This will be a time-consuming and laborious task. An alternative method is to quantitatively investigate pooled DNA samples [16, 26].

When the frequency of a given allele within the population is very low, such as ≤1 %, this will represent a rare case and should be considered individually. Here, targets should be those that appear more frequently. An allele that appears with a frequency of <5 % is likely, in most circumstances, to be of very minor importance in its effect on a population. Therefore, polymorphisms that occur with a frequency of at least 5 % in normal individuals are usually considered for further analysis when searching for SNPs in genes that might have meaningful associations with diseases [27]. To determine this small frequency value in DNA pools with a high degree of accuracy, an approach with a high specificity and reproducibility is necessary.

We propose a method which provides the required accuracy in determining allele frequencies. The method uses specific primer extension reactions coupled with detection of inorganic pyrophosphate (PPi) by a bioluminometric method in which luciferin and luciferase are employed. The primer extension produces a long strand of complementary DNA as well as a lot of PPi which can be easily detected by bioluminometric methods. The key points in the technology are how to improve the specificity of primer extension (switching of extension reactions according to allele species) and to reduce background signals caused by contaminant PPi in the reagents and by thermal decomposition of dNTPs at high extension temperatures. A specific primer extension can be controlled by a match or mismatch at the 3′-terminus of the primer which is hybridized to the target. This technique is frequently used to distinguish a variant from the wild type. Switching of the primer extension reaction by nucleotide variations must be accurately controlled for SNP typing. The switching characteristics are improved by repeated extension reactions (ARMS; [4]) or by modifying the primer sequences. We have successfully used DNA primers that contain mismatched bases near their 3'-termini to reduce false-positive signals in selective primer extension reactions [28]. In the work presented here, we use this technology to increase the switching characteristics of primer extension. Bioluminescence assay, which is based on detecting the PPi released during incorporation of dNTP into the template, has been used successfully in pyrosequencing [13] as well as in a form of antibody assay in which a dendritic DNA is used as the label [29]. However, endogenous contaminant PPi in reagents must be removed to obtain high sensitivity.

After artificially introducing a mismatched base into the 3'-terminal region of the primer and optimizing the conditions of reaction for PPi assay, the method becomes applicable to highly accurate determination of allele frequency. Here, we report on the characteristics of the method and the experimental conditions for determination of allele frequency.

The principle of allele frequency determination is shown in Fig. 1, where two specific primers are used to discriminate wild-type and mutant DNA. In the first step, genomic DNA gathered from multiple patients (or from control subjects) is equally mixed prior to preparation of the DNA samples. The mixed DNA is then amplified by PCR (Polymerase Chain Reaction) followed by single-strand DNA separation, for which a bead technology is used. Finally, the sample is divided into two equal aliquots, and one of the two primers is then added. After a primer-directed polymerase extension with all four deoxynucleotides, PPi is produced if the 3'-terminus of the specific primer is complementary to the base in the template. The released PPi can be converted to ATP with adenosine 5'-phosphosulfate (APS) and ATP sulfurylase. A luciferin and luciferase assay can then be used to detect the ATP. When there is a mismatch in the primer–template duplex at the 3'-terminus of the primer, either no PPi or a very small amount of PPi is released. The match or mismatch at the 3'-terminus of the primer–DNA duplex thus acts as a switch in DNA strand extension. The signal intensities obtained from the two aliquots can be used to determine the frequency of the alleles. However, the switching characteristics of the primer for starting the extension reaction are not perfect; mismatched primer extension frequently occurs. Such reactions make it difficult to correctly determine frequencies of alleles. To minimize the occurrence of false-positive signals, a mismatched nucleotide is artificially introduced into the 3'-terminal region of each specific primer employed in the strand extension, as shown in Fig. 2. In order to prevent mismatch extension, the

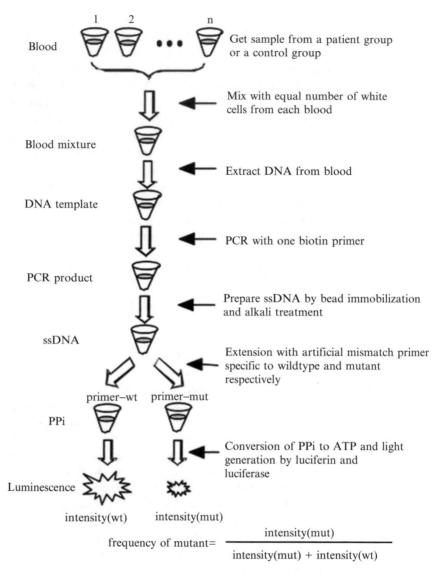

Fig. 1 The principles of allele frequency assay using PPi detection coupled with strand extension of two primers specific to the allele. Only matched primers can be extended to produce PPi. The PPi is then used to emit bioluminescence

artificial mismatched nucleotide in the primer is designed so that it is the same as the nucleotide at the corresponding position of the template. Since a single potential mutation site exists on both strands, the accuracy of the allele frequency at a site can be improved by analyzing the two complementary strands. As strand extension proceeds by several hundred steps at a time, the amount of PPi produced is more than two orders of magnitude greater than that produced in pyrosequencing. A small amount of DNA can thus be used for the analysis of SNPs.

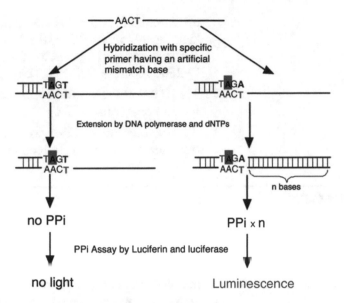

Fig. 2 A mismatch base artificially introduced into primers at the third position from the 3′-terminus improved the switching characteristics of primer extension reactions. To detect the mutant or wild-type DNAs, two extension reactions are carried out, and the emissions were compared to determine the heterozygosity or allele frequency

This approach is called bioluminometric assay using a modified primer extension reaction (BAMPER).

2 Materials

1. Platinum *Taq* DNA polymerase was purchased from Gibco BRL Life Technologies (Grand Island, NY).

2. Polyvinylpyrrolidone (PVP), dNTPs, and QuantiLum recombinant luciferase (95 %) were purchased from Promega (Madison, WI).

3. Sodium pyrophosphate decahydrate (PPi), ATP sulfurylase, apyrase VI, bovine serum albumin (BSA), D-luciferin, inorganic pyrophosphatase (PPase), and APS were purchased from Sigma (St. Louis, MO).

4. Dynabeads M-280 Streptavidin (2.8 μm i.d.) was from Dynal (Oslo, Norway).

5. Sodium 2′-deoxyadenosine 5′-O-(1-triphosphate) (dATPαS) was from Amersham Pharmacia Biotech.

6. The intensity of bioluminescence was measured using a luminometer made in our laboratory consisting of a side-on

photomultiplier tube (R6355; Hamamatsu Photonics, Shizuoka-ken, Japan), an amplifier (AMP; NF Corp., Yokohama, Japan), a power supply (Matsusada Precision, Japan), and a Hitachi D-2500 recorder (Hitachi, Tokyo, Japan).

7. The data was acquired with LabVIEW software (National Instruments, Austin, TX).

8. All the oligonucleotides were synthesized and purified by Amersham Pharmacia Biotech (Hokkaido, Japan).

3   Methods

3.1   Degradation of Endogenous PPi Contamination in Reagents

1. Reagents such as dNTPs and ATP sulfurylase generally contain a lot of endogenous PPi. To obtain high sensitivity, PPase was used to degrade endogenous PPi before the nucleotide incorporation reaction (*see* **Note 1**).

2. To remove PPi in dNTPs, 50 μL of 10 mM dNTPs containing 25 mM magnesium acetate tetrahydrate and 5 mM Tris–acetate, pH 7.7, was incubated with 0.4 U PPase for 30 min at room temperature.

3. Excess PPase was removed by ultrafiltration through a centrifugal filter tube with a nominal molecular weight cutoff of 10,000 (Millipore, Japan). To remove PPi in the PPi detection mixture, PPase was directly added to the solution before adding APS, and the solution was incubated for 30 min at room temperature (*see* **Note 2**).

3.2   Primer and Target Sequences

1. A partial sequence of the P53 gene (exon 8) was synthesized and used as a model target, called P53-A. The sequence was 5′-CTTTCTTGCGGAGATTCTCTTCCTCTGTGCGC CGGTCTCTCCCAGGACAGGCACAAACACGCAC CTCAAAGCTGTTCCGTCCCAGTAGATTACCA-3′.

2. To investigate the primer extension characteristics, we prepared four target DNAs which were denoted P53-C, P53-T, P53-G, and P53-A. Their sequences were identical except for the base species at the polymorphic site position 55 (underlined). As P53-T is the mutant of P53-A, they are termed P53Mut and P53Wt, respectively, here. The primers specific to each template described above were 5′-AACAGCTTTGAGGTGCGTGTTN-3′ (N = A, C, T, or G).

3. To optimize the position of the artificially mismatched base in each primer (*see* **Note 3**), primer extension reactions were carried out with various primers having an artificial mismatched base in a different position from the 3′-terminus, whose sequences were the same as the primers described above except for the artificial mismatched base.

4. For determining the allele frequency of a site, the complementary strand of P53Wt was also analyzed; the specific primer for this strand was 5′-GGTCTCTCCCAGGACAGGCTCN-3′ (N = T or A). M13mp18 single-strand DNA (0.2 μg/μL), purchased from Takara (Shiga, Japan), was used as the template DNA to evaluate the sensitivity. The extension primer for M13 was 5′-TGTAAAACGACGGCGAG-3′.

3.3 Real Sample Preparation by PCR

1. Genome DNA was extracted from the blood (supplied by volunteers in our laboratory) using DNAzol reagent (Gibco BRL, Life Technologies). DNA fragments used for SNP detection were amplified from the genomic DNA by PCR with a PTC-225 thermocycler system (MJ Research, MA) according to the following procedure: denaturation at 94 °C for 2 min, followed by 35 cycles of 94 °C for 30 s, 57 °C for 60 s, and 72 °C for 1 min, with a final incubation at 72 °C for 5 min.

2. The primers for amplifying the P53 exon 8 fragment were 5′-biotin-gtcctgcttgcttac-ctcgcttagt-3′ and 5′-acctgatttccttact-gcctcttgc-3′. The PCR products were purified using a QIAquick PCR purification kit (Qiagen, Hilden, Germany).

3. After purification and quantification, the single-strand DNA was trapped on streptavidin-coated magnetic Dynabeads M-280 and then recovered using 0.1 M NaOH.

3.4 Allele-Specific Extension Reactions

1. A thermostable DNA polymerase without exonuclease activity was used for the allele-specific extension reaction. The reaction mixtures contained 50 mM KCl, 20 mM Tris–HCl pH 8.4, 1.5 mM $MgCl_2$, 50 μM dNTPs (*see* **Note 4**), 50 nM SNP primers, 0.05 U/μL Platinum *Taq* DNA polymerase, and synthetic oligonucleotides or PCR products.

2. Each reaction mixture of 10 μL was incubated at 95 °C for 30 s, 57 °C for 30 s, and 72 °C for 1 min in a PTC-225 thermocycler (MJ Research). Finally, the product was kept on ice before the PPi assay.

3.5 PPi Detection

The detection of PPi produced in the DNA polymerase reaction was carried out by a method similar to that reported by Ronaghi et al. except for the use of apyrase [13]. The reaction   v o l u m e was 75 μL, containing 0.1 M Tris–acetate pH 7.7, 2 mM EDTA, 10 mM magnesium acetate, 0.1 % BSA, 1 mM dithiothreitol, 2 μM APS (*see* **Note 5**), 0.4 mg/mL PVP, 0.4 mM D-luciferin, 200 mU/mL ATP sulfurylase, and 3 μg/mL luciferase. As described above, endogenous PPi was removed by incubating the mixture with PPase for 30 min before adding APS.

4   Method Validation

4.1   Modification of Primers and Their Switching Characteristics

To improve the switching characteristics of specific primers, a single base of each primer was modified to create an artificial mismatch in the primer–DNA duplex in the 3′-terminal region of the primer. This modification of the primers improved the switching characteristics of primer extension according to the match or mismatch at the 3′-terminus. The switching characteristics in terms of primer extension reactions were evaluated with a template DNA containing a partial sequence of the human P53 gene (exon 8). The base type at the polymorphic site is A for wild-type DNA and T for mutant DNA. These are referred to as P53Wt and P53Mut, respectively. Four groups of primers were prepared. Each group contained four primers with the four possible terminal bases. Their 3′-termini are at the nucleotide position where a mutation can be observed. The first group had no modification in the terminal region. The other three groups contained a modification to cause an artificial mismatch in the primer–DNA duplexes at the second, third, and fourth nucleotide positions from the 3′-termini of the primers, respectively.

Whether or not mismatch primer extension occurs depends on the DNA polymerase as well as on the annealing temperature used in the extension step. In general, higher temperatures are preferred, as they prevent mismatch primer extension. However, mismatch extension frequently occurs even at a high temperature such as 55 °C. The artificial mismatch which we introduced at the third position from the 3′-terminus of the primer prevents mismatch primer extension. As shown in Fig. 3, mismatch primer extension, which otherwise produced a signal as strong as several tenths of the matched signal, was decreased to a few percent of the matched signal by the artificial introduction of a mismatched base into the third position from the 3′-terminus of the primer. Only the matched primers produced large signals resulting from strand extension. The primer extension reactions can thus be controlled by the match or mismatch, at the 3′-terminus of the primer, with the template DNA. This switching characteristic in strand extension reactions is very accurate and is reliable enough to distinguish between wild-type and mutant DNAs. The ratios of mismatch extension products to match extension products were 0.66 % for primer A, which matched with P53Mut, and 1.4 % for primer T, which matched with P53Wt, as shown in Fig. 3c. This technique is thus successful as an accurate way of determining the frequencies of alleles.

To confirm the switching characteristics of primers in DNA strand extension reactions, the results for all four possible bases at the polymorphic site were investigated using synthesized P53 gene fragments. We refer to these as P53-A, P53-C, P53-T, and P53-G, respectively, according to the base in the allele. It was possible to

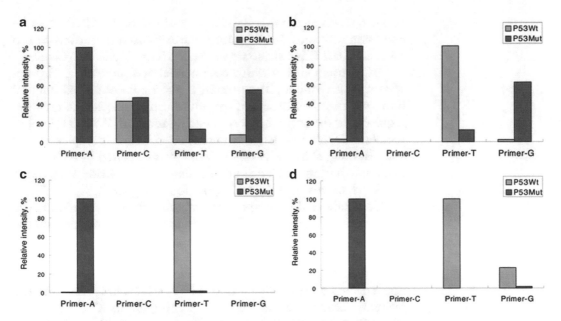

Fig. 3 Comparison of primer extensions for wild-type and mutant targets. In (**a**) there is no artificial mismatch base in the primer; while in (**b–d**) an artificial mismatch base has been placed at the second, third, and fourth positions from the 3′-terminus of the primer, respectively. The sequences of primers A, C, T, and G were the same except for the base at the 3′-terminus. The concentrations of template, primers, and each dNTP were 25 nM, 50 nM, and 50 μM, respectively. The injection volume of the sample was 1 μL, which includes 25 fmol template. The intensities shown were normalized so that the maximum value in each figure is 100

perfectly control all primer extension reactions by the terminal base match or mismatch, as long as specific primers with an artificial mismatched base at the third position from the 3′-terminus were used. As a small amount of strand extension from mismatched primers occurred, a calibration curve should be used to obtain an exact allele frequency. More recently, it has been reported that extension from a mismatched primer can be minimized by adding single-stranded DNA-binding protein (SSB) to the extension solution [30].

4.2 Factors Determining Levels of Background Signals and the Sensitivity of Detection

If, in the present experiment, it were possible to use an ATP-degrading enzyme such as apyrase (as used in pyrosequencing), any endogenous PPi would be effectively degraded in the presence of APS and ATP sulfurylase, which would make highly sensitive detection of newly produced PPi possible. Unfortunately, this approach is not applicable to the present system because having the degradation of PPi proceeding in competition with the PPi assay reaction would affect quantitative SNP determination. However, a reduction in the amount of endogenous PPi remains very important in the realization of accurate allele frequency measurements. There are several possible sources of background signals. The reagents include a lot of PPi as a contaminant. Exogenous PPi is also produced by the thermal decomposition of dNTPs during the extension reactions. Furthermore, the APS used to convert PPi to ATP, and dATP, is a substrate of the luciferin–luciferase reaction.

In pyrosequencing with a commercial pyrosequencer, ~1 pmol of sample is required. The present experiment consumed only 10 fmol, which is two orders of magnitude smaller than the quantity required for the current pyrosequencing method. When 10 fmol of template DNA was used to produce 55 base complementary strands, a signal intensity of ~100 mV was obtained in the present detection system. Background signals could be made very much smaller than this value by taking the following steps.

To analyze the components which affect bioluminometric measurement, various reagents were added to the bioluminometric detection system in a step-by-step fashion. The base solution contained luciferin, luciferase, template DNAs, and polymerase. Even without adding other reagents such as ATP sulfurylase, the solution emitted a photo signal of 1.5 mV, which indicated that the reagents contained small amounts of endogenous ATP. By adding APS and ATP sulfurylase to the above solution, the background signal produced by endogenous PPi was evaluated as 146 mV, which included the contribution from the APS. As well as the contaminants in these reagents, solutions of dNTPs were found to contain a lot of endogenous PPi. As APS is an analog of ATP, it also reacts directly with luciferin to emit a photon, as has been reported previously [31]. Although dATP was a strong background source by reacting directly with luciferin to emit a photon, this was overcome by using dATPαS instead of dATP in BAMPER, a step that has previously been reported in work on pyrosequencing [13, 32].

In general, DNAs produced by a PCR process include a lot of PPi as well as unreacted dATP. This leads to a large background signal in a subsequent luminometric assay. PPi is produced by PCR and thermal decomposition of dNTPs in the process of producing template DNA. This PPi and the dNTPs were removed by taking the following steps. The template DNA was initially purified using a QIAquick PCR purification kit. Single-stranded DNA was then prepared by a bead technology. Both endogenous PPi and residual dATP in PCR products were efficiently removed by the purification and bead washing procedures. As commercially available dNTP solutions contain large amounts of endogenous PPi, this PPi should be degraded using PPase, as described in Materials and Methods. Exogenous PPi is also produced by thermal decomposition of dNTPs. As such thermal decomposition will occur in the BAMPER process, we investigated this problem by heating a dNTP mixture to different temperatures for 2 min as shown in Fig. 4. Little decomposition of the dNTPs was seen below 70 °C, but this decomposition increased at higher temperatures. The use

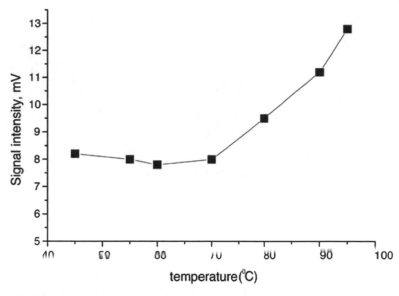

Fig. 4 Signal intensity change from decomposition of dNTPs for 2 min at various temperatures. The concentration of each dNTP was 20 nM

of a thermostable DNA polymerase requires a hot start where the reaction mixture is heated to 95 °C. As decomposition of dNTPs is unavoidable in this case, reductions in the reaction time at high temperature and in the amounts of dNTPs present were both necessary as ways of reducing the amount of dNTP decomposition products and thus the levels of background signals. Therefore, a short reaction time of 30 s at 95 °C and a reduced amount of dNTPs were used. To optimize this reduced amount of dNTPs, an experiment was carried out to determine the relationship between the amount of dNTPs and the bioluminescence signal intensity produced by DNA extension reactions with 50 nM P53Wt, as shown in Fig. 5. This indicated that the amount of PPi produced with 50 nM template DNA was unchanged with a dNTP concentration >35 μM. So 50 μM of each of the dNTPs was a suitable concentration in this case. Since the amount of dNTPs was dependent on the amount of template used and the extension base length, we were able to adjust the amount of template on the basis of its extension base length. A concentration of 10–50 nM template P53Wt with an extension base length of 54 was appropriate for routine analysis, so 50 μM each dNTP with 50 nM template, P53Wt, was enough in most cases. This was about one-quarter of the amount of dNTPs used in the normal PCR protocol. The blank signal was decreased from 95 to 10 mV by this optimization. The background of the solution for detecting PPi was reduced to 6.5 mV by using PPase to degrade the PPi. This value was small enough to allow the detection of 10 fmol target DNA.

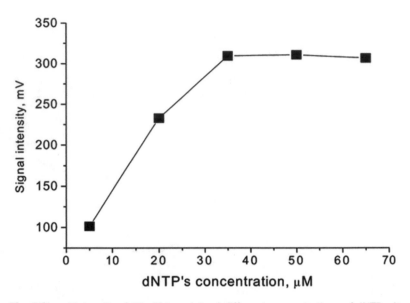

Fig. 5 Signal intensity of 50 nM template at different concentrations of dNTPs. In the extension step, the concentrations of template (P53Wt) and of primer were 50 and 100 nM, respectively. One microliter was injected for the determination. The concentration of each dNTP was the same

In BAMPER, the addition of PPase to the reaction solution as an agent for degrading endogenous PPi is very important for reducing the background level. To prevent PPase degrading the PPi produced by the extension reaction, only a small amount of PPase was added. The amount of PPase was so small that the reaction solution had to be incubated for ~30 min to remove all of the endogenous PPi before adding APS to the solution. In this case, it is not necessary to worry about the side effects of PPase on PPi detection, because the PPi produced by the polymerase reaction was instantly and completely converted into ATP by ATP sulfurylase and APS before its degradation by the PPase present in the reaction mixture. This addition of PPase had no effect on the signal intensity produced by ATP but significantly reduced the background level that arises from contaminant PPi in the reagents.

The background level produced by APS was linearly proportional to its concentration. Therefore, a small concentration of APS was preferable in terms of decreasing the level of the background signal. When a sufficient amount of luciferin was present in the reaction mixture, the signal intensity stayed constant at APS concentrations >1.5 μM. In the present experiment, 2 μM APS was used in the SNP assay, and this produced a background signal level of 2.5 mV. With a fixed amount of APS, this background signal was stable during detection, and it was thus easy to subtract it from the observed signals to obtain a reliable signal from the extension reaction.

The reduction in the amount of residual PPi and optimization of the reaction conditions allowed us to obtain a high degree of sensitivity of detection. For extension of a 54 base strand, the lower detection limit was 0.27 ± 0.02 fmol, and the quantitative limit was 0.83 ± 0.05 fmol. This indicated that 10 fmol of a short strand of DNA, such as 200 bases, would be enough for routine SNP analysis. When a long DNA was used as template, the sensitivity of detection was improved. For example, for ssM13, with an extension length of 6289 bp, the lower detection limit was 14 amol. This is the most important advantage of BAMPER. It is impossible to detect 0.5 fmol ssM13 by pyrosequencing, while the signal produced with the same amount of ssM13 template in BAMPER was very strong. This is shown in Fig. 6, where the same instrument was used for both forms of measurement. Although the intensity of the signal did not increase in linear proportion to base length, it did increase quite a lot. For a long strand of DNA, the extension reaction might be incomplete, which is not good for quantitative determination. However, applying primer extension to a long strand of DNA is still useful in terms of highly sensitive detection of SNPs.

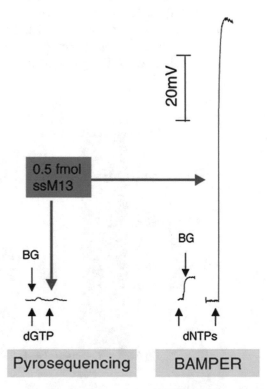

Fig. 6 Comparison of signal intensities obtained with the prototype instrument in two different modes, pyrosequencing and BAMPER. The experimental conditions were the same, except that apyrase was not used in BAMPER. The sample was 0.5 fmol ssM13. BG indicates the background signal level

4.3 A Simple Instrument for BAMPER

The instrument for use in BAMPER may be very simple because it does not require iterative addition of four different dNTPs. While we have made a small device coupled to a photomultiplier for BAMPER, a commercially available bioluminometer would also be suitable. Precise control of reagent injection is not necessary in BAMPER because a one-shot injection is enough to add the detection solution. The reaction volume was 10–40 μL for SNP typing, with both the prototype BAMPER device and a commercial bioluminometer. The amount of sample required for SNP typing can be decreased by reducing the reaction volume. For example, 10 fmol PPi, which corresponds to <100 amol target DNA (when, for example, the extension length is 100 bases), was successfully detected in a 500 nl solution with a good signal-to-noise ratio by BAMPER.

4.4 SNP Typing and Allele Frequency Analysis

SNP typing and allele frequency analysis were carried out with genomic DNA from our colleagues and with synthesized DNA. Typing one SNP for a homozygous or a heterozygous sample is the simplest case of allele frequency analysis. To start with, samples containing P53Wt, P53Mut, and an equimolar mixture of P53Wt and P53Mut were analyzed, and the results are shown in Fig. 7. The bioluminescence intensities obtained with the two specific primers were normalized to the total intensity. The results were almost as expected, which indicates that the method is applicable to SNP typing of a small amount of sample. In order to

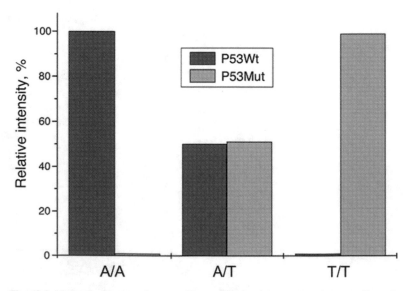

Fig. 7 A bioluminescence assay with modified primer extension reactions for genotyping. Targets containing A (P53Wt) and T (P53Mut) at the polymorphic site were used. For homo-templates, it was only possible to extend one primer. However, both primers extended for a hetero-template

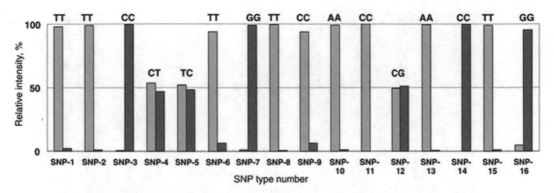

Fig. 8 Results of using BAMPER to type 16 SNPs. The intensity was normalized to the total intensity. The details of each SNP, including the corresponding gene name, mutation point, and specific primers, are given in Table 1

confirm the applicability of BAMPER to various SNPs, 16 polymorphic sites in human genomic DNA extracted from the blood were investigated. As shown in Fig. 8, all of the SNPs were accurately typed. The results are listed in Table 1 and coincide with the sequencing results obtained by gel-based electrophoresis. Although some of the priming regions contained GC-rich sequences, these tests showed that BAMPER was effective for typing all the SNPs analyzed in this study. In some cases, mismatch extension still occurred, but the relative proportion was <10 % of the matched extensions, proving the usefulness of artificial introduction of a mismatched base into the primer. For example, the proportion of mismatch extensions for SNP16 was ~40 % when such an artificial mismatched base was not introduced. The reproducibility of BAMPER analysis results was very good. For SNP-13 the whole SNP typing process, including PCR, preparation of single-stranded DNA, the bead washing process and BAMPER detection, was repeated eight times in parallel, and the relative standard deviation was 3.8 % ($n=8$).

As it would have been difficult to obtain real samples for an allele frequency study, synthetic wild-type and mutant P53 DNAs mixed in various ratios were used. Reactions with the two primers were carried out for each sample. The allele frequencies of P53Mut (T allele) in the artificially prepared samples were 0.02, 0.05, 0.1, and 0.7. The wild-type allele was A. The correlation between the estimated allele frequencies and those observed for the artificially prepared DNA was very high, at $r^2 = 0.9999$. The measurements were repeated four times, and the results were highly reproducible. The largest uncertainty in frequency determination was estimated to be 0.9 % for a frequency <10 %. This is enough to distinguish differences between the allele frequencies of two groups in terms of medical characteristics. There may be some difficulty with accuracy in applying the method to determining allele frequencies of <5 %.

Table 1
SNPs used for the evaluation and typing analyses

SNP code	Gene name	SNP	Specific primer sequence[a]	Typing by BAMPER	Typing by GE[b]
SNP-1	Angiotensin II type 1 receptor	A1166C	aattctgaaaagtagctTaT/G (30)	T/T	T/T
SNP-2	Aldosterone synthase	Lys173Arg	gttctgcagcacttctAcT/C (50)	T/T	T/T
SNP-3	Paraoxonase1	Arg192Gln	caatacatctccaggTtT/C (40)	C/C	C/C
SNP-4	Methylenetetrahydrofolate reductase	C677T	gagaaggtgtctgcgggTgC/T (65)	C/T	C/T
SNP-5	Methionine synthase	D919G	cttgagagactcataatCgT/C (40)	T/C	T/C
SNP-6	Cholesteryl ester transfer protein	Ile405Val	gaaacagtctttggtgtTaT/C (35)	T/T	T/T
SNP-7	Peroxisome proliferator-activated receptor γ	Pro12Ala	ctgatcccaagttggtCgC/G (55)	G/G	G/G
SNP-8	Glutathione S-transferase P1	Ile105Val	ttggtgtagatgagggaCaT/C (45)	T/T	T/T
SNP-9	Angiotensinogen	G−6A	caacggcagcttcttccGcC/T (60)	C/C	C/C
SNP-10	eNOS	T−786C	ggctgaggcagggtcagGcA/G (75)	A/A	A/A
SNP-11	Prothrombin	G20210A	cactgggagcattgaggGtC/T (60)	C/C	C/C
SNP-12	8-Oxyguanin DNA glycosylase	Ser326Cys	agtgccgacctgcgccaTtC/G (65)	C/G	C/G
SNP-13	P53 gene (exon 8)	Cys275Ser	aacagctttgaggtgcgtgAtA/T (45)	A/A	A/A
SNP-14	P53 gene (exon 8)	Pro278His	aggtgcgtgtttgtgcctgAcA/C (59)	C/C	C/C
SNP-15	P53 gene (exon 8)	Arg282Trp	tgtgcctgtctgggagagTcT/C (64)	T/T	T/T
SNP-16	P53 gene (exon 8)	Arg283His	gcctgtcctgggagaccgCcA/G (74)	G/G	G/G

[a]The two capital letters at the 3′-terminus of the primer are the specific bases of the SNP type, while the third capital letter is the artificially mismatched base. The number in parentheses represents the GC content in the probe. The sequences of PCR primers are available on request
[b]GE is SNP typing by gel-based electrophoresis

Table 2

Comparison of calculated and observed allele frequencies for synthesized pooled DNA samples (four independent measurements were carried out to estimate the error rates _n_= 4)

Known allele frequency[a]	0.020	0.050	0.100	0.700
Allele frequency observed using strand one[b]	0.021 ± 0.001	0.045 ± 0.008	0.095 ± 0.009	0.691 + 0.010
Allele frequency observed using strand two[b]	0.017 ± 0.003	0.057 ± 0.004	0.098 ± 0.006	0.698 ± 0.009
Average allele frequency[c]	0.019 ± 0.003	0.051 ± 0.008	0.096 ± 0.002	0.694 ± 0.005

The artificial pools were constructed by mixing different ratios of synthesized wild-type and mutant P53 DNA in one tube directly

[a]Frequency = concentration of P53Mut/(concentration of P53Mut + concentration of P53Wt)

[b]Frequency = intensity produced by primer A complementary to P53Mut/(intensity produced by primer A + intensity produced by primer T complementary to P53Wt). Frequency was obtained by calibration with samples having known frequencies of 0, 0.30, 0.50, 0.90, and 1.0. Calibration was carried out using a regression line, and the allele frequency was obtained by the regression equation. Strands one and two are complementary

[c]The average frequencies were obtained from strands one and two

However, those frequencies that are <5 % are likely to be of very minor importance and are usually not considered for further analysis, as has been discussed by Nigel Spurr [27].

The complementary strand was also analyzed using two other specific primers to obtain a reliable frequency value. The observed allele frequencies in pooled DNA samples for both P53 strands were compared with estimated values and are listed in Table 2. The observed allele frequencies were consistent for both strands, which indicated that the results obtained were reliable and that frequency analysis of one strand would be enough to determine the allele frequency in practical applications.

For allele frequency analysis, the accuracy of pipetting operations as well as the number of samples in a pool must be carefully considered. The expected sampling error can be expressed as $\sqrt{[f(1-f)/2n]}$, where f is the allele frequency of one of the two alleles and n is the sample size [33]. The calculated errors due to sampling (sampling error) at different allele frequencies for $n=100$ and $n=1000$ are shown as the black and purple lines in Fig. 9, respectively. It was found that when the sample size is smaller than 1000, the sampling error is greater than the standard deviation of the measurement (measurement error) at each allele frequency, as shown in Fig. 9. On the other hand, the measurement error, which is small and independent of the number of samples, becomes dominant in allele frequency determination for large sample sizes such as $n>1000$. To obtain a reliable allele frequency, a large sample size (n) is necessary.

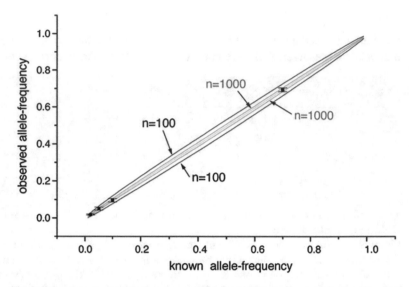

Fig. 9 Comparison of sampling errors (*black* and *purple lines*) and measurement errors (error bars) at different allele frequencies. Sample sizes were 100 for the black line and 1000 for the *purple line*, respectively. The *green line* was drawn by the regression equation obtained using the observed allele frequency and the known allele frequency. The error bar represents the measurement error (color figure online)

5 Technical Notes

1. Before PPi detection, a reduction in endogenous PPi in reagents was necessary in BAMPER because apyrase, which is used to degrade dNTPs and ATP in pyrosequencing, was not included in the reaction mixture for BAMPER.

2. To prevent PPase degrading the PPi produced by the extension reaction, only a small amount of PPase was added. The amount of PPase was so small that the reaction solution had to be incubated for ~30 min to remove all of the endogenous PPi before adding APS to the solution.

3. To prevent mismatch primer extension, an artificial mismatched base was introduced into the terminal region of each primer.

4. The amount of PPi produced with 50 nM template DNA was unchanged with a dNTP concentration >35 μM. So 50 μM of each of the dNTPs was a suitable concentration in this case. Since the amount of dNTPs was dependent on the amount of template used and the extension base length, we were able to adjust the amount of template on the basis of its extension base length. A concentration of 10–50 nM template P53Wt with an extension base length of 54 was appropriate for routine analy-

sis, so 50 μM each dNTP with 50 nM template, P53Wt, was enough in most cases.

5. The background level produced by APS was linearly proportional to its concentration. Therefore, a small concentration of APS was preferable in terms of decreasing the level of the background signal.

References

1. Wang DG, Fan JB, Siao CJ, Berno A, Young P, Sapolsky R, Ghandour G, Perkins N, Winchester E, Spencer J et al (1998) Large-scale identification, mapping, and genotyping of single-nucleotide polymorphisms in the human genome. Science 280:1077–1082

2. See D, Kanazin V, Talbert H, Blake T (2000) Electrophoretic detection of single-nucleotide polymorphisms. Biotechniques 28(710):714, 716

3. Schmalzing D, Belenky A, Novotny MA, Koutny L, Salas-Solano O, El-Difrawy S, Adourian A, Matsudaira P, Ehrlich D (2000) Microchip electrophoresis: a method for high-speed SNP detection. Nucleic Acids Res 28:e43

4. Newton CR, Graham A, Heptinstall LE, Powell SJ, Summers C, Kalsheker N, Smith JC, Markham AF (1998) Analysis of any point mutation in DNA. The amplification refractory mutation system (ARMS). Nucleic Acids Res 17:2503–2516

5. Lyamichev V, Mast AL, Hall JG, Prudent JR, Kaiser MW, Takova T, Kwiatkowski RW, Sander TJ, de Arruda M, Arco DA, Neri BP, Brow MA (1998) Polymorphism identification and quantitative detection of genomic DNA by invasive cleavage of oligonucleotide probes. Nat Biotechnol 17:292–296

6. Hall JG, Eis PS, Law SM, Reynaldo LP, Prudent JR, Marshall DJ, Allawi HT, Mast AL, Dahlberg JE, Kwiatkowski RW, de Arruda M, Neri BP, Lyamichev VI (2000) Sensitive detection of DNA polymorphisms by the serial invasive signal amplification reaction. Proc Natl Acad Sci U S A 97:8272–8277

7. Jeffreys AJ, MacLeod A, Tamaki K, Neil DL, Monckton DG (1991) Minisatellite repeat coding as a digital approach to DNA typing. Nature 354:204–209

8. Whitcombe D, Brownie J, Gillard HL, McKechnie D, Theaker J, Newton CR, Little S (1998) A homogeneous fluorescence assay for PCR amplicons: its application to real-time, single-tube genotyping. Clin Chem 44:918–923

9. Howell WM, Jobs M, Gyllensten U, Brookes AJ (1999) Dynamic allele-specific hybridization. A new method for scoring single nucleotide polymorphisms. Nat Biotechnol 17:87–88

10. Tyagi S, Bratu DP, Kramer FR (1998) Multicolor molecular beacons for allele discrimination. Nat Biotechnol 16:49–53

11. Sauer S, Lechner D, Berlin K, Lehrach H, Escary JL, Fox N, Gut IG (2000) A novel procedure for efficient genotyping of single nucleotide polymorphisms. Nucleic Acids Res 28:e13

12. Fei Z, Smith LM (2000) Analysis of single nucleotide polymorphisms by primer extension and matrix-assisted laser desorption/ionization time-of-flight mass spectrometry. Rapid Commun Mass Spectrom 14:950–959

13. Ronaghi M, Uhlen M, Nyren P (1998) A sequencing method based on real time pyrophosphate. Science 281:363–365

14. Nyren P, Karamohamed S, Ronaghi M (1997) Detection of single-base changes using a bioluminometric primer extension assay. Anal Biochem 244:367–373

15. Ahmadian A, Gharizadeh B, Gustafsson AC, Sterky F, Nyren P, Uhlen MA, Lundeberg J (2000) Single- nucleotide polymorphism analysis by pyrosequencing. Anal Biochem 280:103–110

16. Fan JB, Chen X, Halushka MK, Berno A, Huang X, Ryder T, Lipshutz RJ, Lockhart DJ, Chakravarti A (2000) Parallel genotyping of human SNPs using generic high-density oligonucleotide tag arrays. Genome Res 10:853–860

17. Gilles PN, Wu DJ, Foster CB, Dillon PJ, Chanock SJ (1999) Single nucleotide polymorphic discrimination by an electronic dot blot assay on semiconductor microchips. Nat Biotechnol 17:365–370

18. Sosnowski RG, Tu E, Butler WF, O'Connell JP, Heller MJ (1997) Rapid determination of single base mismatch mutations in DNA hybrids by direct electric field control. Proc Natl Acad Sci U S A 94:1119–1123

19. Boon EM, Ceres DM, Drummond TG, Hill MG, Barton JK (2000) Mutation detection by electrocatalysis at DNA-modified electrodes. Nat Biotechnol 18:1096–1100

20. Chen J, Iannone MA, Li MS, Taylor JD, Rivers P, Nelsen AJ, Slentz-Kesler KA, Roses A, Weiner MP (2000) A microsphere-based assay for multiplexed single nucleotide polymorphism analysis using single base chain extension. Genome Res 10:549–557

21. Lannone MA, Taylor JD, Chen J, Li MS, Rivers P, Slentz-Kesler KA, Weiner MP (2000) Multiplexed single nucleotide polymorphism genotyping by oligonucleotide ligation and flow cytometry. Cytometry 39:131–140

22. Syvanen AC (1999) From gels to chips: "minisequencing" primer extension for analysis of point mutations and single nucleotide polymorphisms. Hum Mutat 13:1–10

23. Landegren U, Nilsson M, Kwok PY (1998) Reading bits of genetic information: methods for single-nucleotide polymorphism analysis. Genome Res 8:769–776

24. Nollau P, Wagener C (1997) Methods for detection of point mutations: performance and quality assessment. IFCC Scientific Division, Committee on Molecular Biology Techniques. Clin Chem 43:1114–1128

25. Whitcombe D, Newton CR, Little S (1998) Advances in approaches to DNA-based diagnostics. Curr Opin Biotechnol 9:602–608

26. Breen G, Harold D, Ralston S, Shaw D, St Clair D (2000) Determining SNP allele frequencies in DNA pools. Biotechniques 28:464–466, 468, 470

27. Campbell DA, Valdes A, Spurr N (2000) Making drug discovery a SN(i)P. Drug Discov 5:388–396

28. Okano K, Uematsu C, Matsunaga H, Kambara H (1998) Characteristics of selective polymerase chain reaction (PCR) using two-base anchored primers and improvement of its specificity. Electrophoresis 19:3071–3078

29. Capaldi S, Getts RC, Jayasena SD (2000) Signal amplification through nucleotide extension and excision on a dendritic DNA platform. Nucleic Acids Res 28:e21

30. Ronaghi M (2000) Improved performance of pyrosequencing using single-stranded DNA-binding protein. Anal Biochem 286:282–288

31. Hyman ED (1998) A new method of sequencing DNA. Anal Biochem 174:423–436

32. Ronaghi M, Karamohamed S, Pettersson B, Uhlen M, Nyren P (1996) Real-time DNA sequencing using detection of pyrophosphate release. Anal Biochem 242:84–89

33. Germer S, Holland MJ, Higuchi R (2000) High-throughput SNP allele-frequency determination in pooled DNA samples by kinetic PCR. Genome Res 10:258–266

Chapter 10

A Gel-Free SNP Genotyping Method Based on Pyrosequencing Chemistry Coupled with Modified Primer Extension Reactions Directly from Double-Stranded PCR Products

Guohua Zhou, Hiromi Shirakura, Masao Kamahori, Kazunori Okano, Keiichi Nagai, and Hideki Kambara

Abstract

Inexpensive, high-throughput genotyping methods are needed for analyzing human genetic variations. We have successfully applied the regular bioluminometric assay coupled with modified primer extension reactions (BAMPER) method to single-nucleotide polymorphism (SNP) typing as well as the allele frequency determination for various SNPs. This method includes the production of single-strand target DNA from a genome and a primer extension reaction coupled with inorganic pyrophosphate (PPi) detection by a bioluminometric assay. It is an efficient way to get accurate allele frequencies for various SNPs, while single-strand DNA preparation is labor-intensive. The procedure can be simplified in the typing of SNPs. We demonstrate that a modified BAMPER method in which we need not prepare a single-strand DNA can be carried out in one tube. A PCR product is directly used as a template for SNP typing in the new BAMPER method. Generally, tremendous amounts of PPi are produced in a PCR process, as well as many residual dNTPs, and residual PCR primers remain in the PCR products, which cause a large background signal in a bioluminometric assay. Here, shrimp alkaline phosphatase (SAP) and *E. coli* exonuclease I were used to degrade these components prior to BAMPER detection. The specific primer extension reactions in BAMPER were carried out under thermocycle conditions. The primers were extended to produce large amounts of PPi only when their bases at 30-termini were complementary to the target. The extension products, PPis, were converted to ATP to be analyzed using the luciferin–luciferase detection system. We successfully demonstrated that PCR products can be directly genotyped by BAMPER in one tube for SNPs with various GC contents. As all reactions can be carried out in a single tube, the method will be useful for realizing a fully automated genotyping system.

Key words SNP, Genotyping, BAMPER, Bioluminometric assay, Mutation detection

Guohua Zhou and Qinxin Song (eds.), *Advances and Clinical Practice in Pyrosequencing*, Springer Protocols Handbooks, DOI 10.1007/978-1-4939-3308-2_10, © Springer Science+Business Media New York 2016

1   Introduction

The completion of the human genome sequence [1, 2], as well as an initial map of human genome sequence variation [3], will help enable the provision, of medical care to patients based on each individual's specific genotype. Although the map identifies and localizes 1.42 million single nucleotide polymorphisms (SNPs) in the genome, the relationships between diseases and SNPs have not being clarified. To associate genetic variations with a variety of diseases, a large amount of SNPs need to be analyzed. Consequently, an automated and high-throughput SNP typing method is required. Previously, various SNP genotyping approaches have been developed to identify genetic alterations, including electro-phoresis [4], denaturing liquid chromatography [5], mass spec-trometry [6], flow-cytometry with color beads containing DNA probes [7], DNA chips coupled with electric field-controlled DNA hybridization [8], minisequencing [9, 10], dynamic allele specific hybridization (DASH) [11], enzymatic cleavage methods such as Invader [12] and 50-nuclease TaqMan [13], pyrosequenc-ing [14, 15], amplification refractory mutation system (ARMS) [16], molecular beacon probes [17], METPOC [18], and other high-throughput technologies [19, 20]. From the viewpoint of practical testing, however, an easy-to-use genotyping system that is also inexpensive with respect to both instruments and reagents is still needed.

We have recently reported a new gel-free genotyping approach for allele frequency analysis [21]. It is based on bioluminometric assay coupled with modified primer extension reactions (BAMPER) (*see* **Note 1**), in which an inexpensive and simple luminometer can be used. In BAMPER, primers with artificially mismatched bases near the 30-termini hybridize on the targets to extend their strands when the terminal bases match the expected alleles in the targets. The artificially introduced mismatch bases are used to reduce false-positive signals due to the mismatch primer extension reactions (*see* **Note 2**). The primer extension reactions produce large amounts of inorganic pyrophosphate (PPi), which are detected by a luminometric method. Therefore, the key point of the assay is how to remove the residual PPi in the reagents, as well as to avoid the nonspecific primer extension reaction. In the reported BAMPER assay, template DNAs were prepared as single-strand DNAs through a time-consuming and labor-intensive process.

Here, we demonstrate a simplified procedure for BAMPER detection in which all the reactions necessary for sample prepara-tion and genotyping are carried out in one tube. We also demon-strate that this simplified BAMPER is a reliable method for SNP

Table 1

SNP code	Gene symbol	Accession number	SNP identifier[a]	PCR primer sequences[b]	Specific primer sequences[c]	Typing by BAMPER	Typing by GE[d]
SNP-1	AGT	AF424741.1	g.1218A>G	FW: 5′-aagaggtccagcgtgag RV: 5′-ccccggcttaccttc	5′-aacggcagcttcttccGcC/T (60)	C/C	C/C
SNP-2	AGTR1	AY436325.1	g.47009A>C	FW: 5′-caaaatgagcacgctttc RV: 5′-cagccgtcatctgtctaatg	5′-atttctgaaagtagctTaT/G (30)	T/T	T/T
SNP-3	NOS3	AF519768.1	g.1132T>C	FW: 5′-gaccagatgcccagctagtg RV: 5′-cagtgacgcacgcttcc	5′-ggctgaggcagggtcagGcA/G (75)	A/A	A/A
SNP-4	F2	AF493953.1	g.322G>A	FW: 5′-caaatgggcatcgtctca RV: 5′-ggactaccagcgtgcacc	5′-cactgggagcattgaggGtC/T (60)	C/C	C/C
SNP-5	PON1	AF539592.1	g.18152A>G	FW: 5′-catgggtatacagaaagcctaa RV: 5′-ccatataatcgcattcatcaat	5′-aacccaaatacatctcccaggTtT/C	C/C	C/C
SNP-6	MTHFR	AF105980.1	g.129C>T	FW: 5′-cagtccctgtggtcttca RV: 5′-gaactcagcgaactcagcac	5′-ggaaggtgtctgcgggTgC/T (65)	C/T	C/T
SNP-7	MTR	U73338.1	c.2756A>G	FW: 5′-tgatccaaagcctttacact RV: 5′-aagggagagaaatgaagtraag	5′-ctgagagactcataatCgT/C (40)	T/C	T/C
SNP-8	CYBA	NT_010542.14	g.271036A>G	FW: 5′-cctcgatttggagtggat RV: 5′-ccttggtgcttgtgggta	5′-ccccagggacagaTgT/C (70)	C/C	C/C
SNP-9	CETP	AY008270.1	g.493A>G	FW: 5′-gcaaatctcaaggaatagc RV: 5′-ggttgcctgatttcctttag	5′-aacagtctttggtgtTaT/C (35)	T/T	T/T
SNP-10	NPPA	NM_006172.1	c.94G>A	FW: 5′-ctttcctgccctacctt RV: 5′-ataaaagagggcggcact	5′-ataggtctgcgttggaGaC/T (55)	T/T	T/T
SNP-11	OGG1	AF521807.1	g.9184C>G	FW: 5′-actcttccacctccaacac RV: 5′-tagccgctgtctccctcaata	5′-agccgactggccaTtC/G (65)	C/G	C/G

(continued)

Table 1
(continued)

SNP code	Gene symbol	Accession number	SNP identifier[a]	PCR primer sequences[b]	Specific primer sequences[c]	Typing by BAMPER	Typing by GE[d]
SNP-12	ABCA1	AF275948.1	g.105057A>G	FW: 5′-aggatgtgtcaaggaggaaat RV: 5′-gagccaagacaacaaagaaa	5′-cctggttccaaccagaagagaTtA/G (50)	A/A	A/A
SNP-13	PPARG	AY157024.1	g.28910C>G	FW: 5′-gggtgacttccttctatcata RV: 5′-gttcttgtgaatggaatgtctt	5′-ctgatcccaagttggtCgC/G (55)	G/G	G/G
SNP-14	ITGB3	M32672.1	g.1498T>C	FW: 5′-tccccttttcgtacaacgg RV: 5′-aagagtccagcctacct	5′-gtcttacaggccctgccAcT/C (65)	C/C	C/C
SNP-15	ITGA2	AF035968.2	g.2719T>C	FW: 5′-atattgaattgctccgaatgt RV: 5′-gaagtgatgccttaagctacc	5′-ttctttggtttatatgttcaagAtA/G (46)	G/G	G/G
SNP-16	PON1	NM_000446.3	c.163T>A	FW: 5′-catgggtatacagaaagcctaa RV: 5′-ccatataatcgcattcatcaat	5′-ccattaggcagtatctcGaA/T ((45)	A/A	A/A
SNP-17	GP1BA	AF395009.1	g.2217C>T	FW: 5′-cctggatctatcccacatc RV: 5′-aaaaagccctttggtattgtata	5′-cttctccagcttgggtgtggCcA/G (65)	G/G	G/G
SNP-18	PON2	NM_000305.1	c.932G>C	FW: 5′-gtggtataagtgcctatgagc RV: 5′-ggtaactgctattttcaacagc	5′-aaactgtagtcactgtaggcttctGaG/C (44)	G/G	G/G
SNP-19	CD14	U00699.1	g.210T>C	FW: 5′-ttggtgccaacagatgaggttcac RV: 5′-ttctttcctacacagcggcaccc	5′-accaccagagaaggcttagCcT/C (65)	T/T	T/T
SNP-20	LPL	NM_000237.1	c.106G>A	FW: 5′-aatagcatcagcggtggtt RV: 5′-ggccagtcaggatactca	5′-ctttcagaaagaagagatttaAcG/A (35)	G/G	G/G
SNP-21	LPL	AC107964.4	g.2394A>C	FW: 5′-taagcgacaggagcctaac RV: 5′-aagaggggggaatcgagtct	5′-ctcaaacgtttagaagtgaatttaCgT/G (37)	T/T	T/T
SNP-22	UCP1	U28479.1	g.292A>G	FW: 5′-cagtggtggctaatgagagaat RV: 5′-gaagaagcagagggtaaaga	5′-gatttctgattgaccacagtttgaAcA/G (41)	A/A	A/A

SNP	Gene	Accession	Variant	Primer	Probe			
SNP-23	GSTP1	NM_000852.1	c.313A>G	FW: 5′-tgtgttggcagtcttcatcc RV: 5′-gtgcaggttgtgtcttgtcc	5′- atag⬛tggtgtgtagatgagggaCaT/C (⬛8)	T/T	T/T	T/T
SNP-24	KL	AB009666.1	g.1686A>G	FW: 5′-cggccagtccctaattg RV: 5′-gagccgtgcaggacgtt	5′-⬛gaaa⬛ggcgccgaccaactArT/C (⬛8)	C/C	C/C	C/C
SNP-25	NOS3	AF519768.1	g.7164G>T	FW: 5′-tgaggagggcatgaggc RV: 5′-tggggtgtgggatcagc	5′-⬛ctg⬛gcaggcccagatCaG/T (⬛5)	G/G	G/G	G/G
SNP-26	LEPR	NM_002303.1	c.668A>G	FW: 5′-tctagaagcactcttaataccc RV: 5′-tcaataggcctgaagtgttag	5′-t⬛acat⬛tggtggagtaattttGcA/G (⬛4)	G/G	G/G	G/G
SNP-27	EDN1	NM_001955.2	c.594T>G	FW: 5′-ggggcaggctttattta RV: 5′-caggaaccagcagaggatg	5′-t⬛acat-acgctctctggagCgC/A (57)	C/C	C/C	C/C

Note: [a]The nucleotide residue 1 is located at the start of the reference sequence for "g." numbers, and at the A of the A⬛G translation initiation start site for "c." numbers
[b]FW and RV represent forward and reverse primer, respectively
[c]The two capital letters in the 3-terminus of the primer represent the specific base to the SNP type, and the third capital letter represents the artificially mismatched base. The number in the brackets represents the GC content in a probe
[d]GE means SNP typing by gel-based electrophoresis

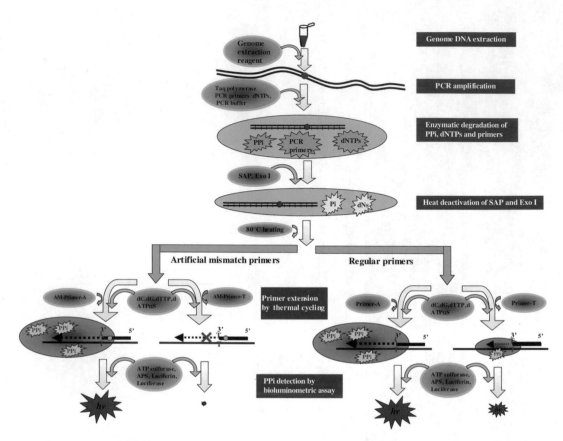

Fig. 1 Schematics of BAMPER using double-stranded PCR products for SNP typing. *Pi* phosphate, *dNs* deoxynucleosides, *SAP* shrimp alkaline phosphatase, *Exo I* exonuclease I, *APS* adenosine phosphosulfate. AM-Primer: artificial mismatch primers

typing using multiplex PCR products directly (*see* Fig. 1). The method is shown to be applicable for typing many SNPs with various GC contents in different genome samples.

2   Materials

1. Platinum Taq DNA polymerase was purchased from Gibco-BRL Life Technologies (Grand Island, NY).

2. Polyvinylpyrrolidone (PVP), deoxynucleotide (dNTPs), and QuantiLum™ recombinant luciferase (95 %) were purchased from Promega (Madison, WI; www.promega.com).

3. Sodium pyrophosphate decahydrate (PPi), ATP sulfurylase, apyrase-VI, bovine serum albumin (BSA), D-luciferin, inorganic pyrophosphatase (PPase), and adenosine 5′-phosphosulfate (APS) were purchased from Sigma (St. Louis, 30-termini MO).

4. Dynabeads M-280 Streptavidin (2.8 μm inner diameter [ID]) was purchased from Dynal A.C. (Oslo, Norway).

5. All solutions were prepared in deionized and sterilized water.

6. Sodium 2′-deoxyadenosine 5′-O-(1-triphosphate) (dATPaS) was purchased from Amersham Biosciences (Piscataway, NJ).

7. Other chemicals were of a commercially extra-pure grade.

8. The bioluminescence was measured with a LUMINOUS CT-9000D luminometer (DIA-IATRON, Tokyo, Japan).

3 Methods

3.1 Degradation of Endogenous PPi Contaminated in Reagents

1. A total of 50 μL of 10 mM dNTPs containing 25 mM magnesium acetate tetrahydrate (Mg(Ac)$_2$) and 5 mM Tris–HAc, pH 7.7, were incubated with 0.4 U PPase for 30 min at room temperature.

2. The residual PPase was removed by ultrafiltration with a centrifugal filter-tube having the nominal molecular weight cut off of 10,000 (Millipore, Japan; www.millipore.com).

3. To remove PPi in the PPi detection mixture, 0.1 U PPase was directly added to 50 mL PPi detection solution before adding APS, and the solution was incubated for 30 min at room temperature.

3.2 Primer and Target Sequences

1. Pairs of genotyping probes (primers) were designed so as to hybridize in the target-specific regions. As there were two choices for selecting the target DNA strand, two sets of genotyping primers could be designed.

3.3 PCR Amplification and Enzymatic Cleanup

1. DNA fragments used for SNP testing were amplified from the genome DNA with a PTC-225 thermocycler PCR System according to the following protocol: denatured at 94 °C for 2 min, followed by 35 thermal reaction cycles (94 °C for 30 s; 57 °C for 60 s; 72 °C for 1 min) (see **Note 1**).

2. After the cycle reaction, the product was incubated at 72 °C for 5 min and held at 4 °C.

3. In the case of multiplex PCR, 10 mL of the amplification was carried out in a 384-well plate. The concentration of each primer used in single-PCR or multiplex-PCR was identical, 0.2 pmol/mL (see **Note 2**).

4. Residual components, such as PCR primers, dNTPs, and PPis produced in the PCR step, produce a large background signal. These components were degraded by adding 1 U of shrimp alkaline phosphatase (SAP) and 2 U of exonuclease I to 5 μL of the PCR product.

5. The mixture was thoroughly mixed and incubated at 37 °C for 40 min, and then heated at 80 °C for 10 min to inactivate the enzymes (see **Note 3**).

3.4 Allele-Specific Extension Reactions

1. Thermostable DNA polymerase without exonuclease activity was used for allele-specific primer extension reactions. A pair of extension reactions for one template species with two typing primers, corresponding to wild-type and mutant, respectively, was carried out under the same conditions.

2. The reaction mixtures contained 50 mM KCl, 20 mM Tris–HCl (pH 8.4), 1.5 mM magnesium chloride, 125 mM of deoxy-CTP (dCTP), 125 mM of deoxy-TTP (dTTP), 125 mM of deoxy-GTP (dGTP), 125 mM of deoxyadenosine triphosphate-αS (dATPαS), 1.25 mM of genotyping primers, 0.05 U/mL of Platinum Taq DNA polymerase, and 1 μL of PCR products.

3. Each 4 μL reaction mixture was incubated at 94 °C for 30 s. This was followed by five thermal cycles (94 °C for 10 s; 55 °C for 10 s; 72 °C for 20 s) in a PTC-225 thermocycler.

4. Finally, the product was kept on ice before the PPi assay (*see* **Note 4**).

3.5 PPi Detection

1. The detection of PPi produced in the genotyping primer extension reactions was performed by a method similar to one previously reported [21]. The PPi detection solution contained the following components: 0.1 M Tris–acetate (pH 7.7), 2 mM EDTA, 10 mM magnesium acetate, 0.1 % BSA, 1 mM dithiothreitol, 2 mM APS, 0.4 mg/mL PVP, 0.4 mM D-luciferin, 200 mU/mL ATP sulfurylase, and 3 mg/mL luciferase.

2. We also added 40 mL of PPi detection solution to each well containing extension solution.

4 Method Validation

4.1 Typing Many SNPs with Various GC Contents in Different Genome Samples

To evaluate the primer extension characteristics, we used an SNP, I823M in the ABCA1 gene, as a test target. Three samples including two homo-samples (AA or GG) and a hetero-sample (A/G) were analyzed. A pair of primers containing the artificial mismatch bases in the third positions from the 3′ ends was designed to distinguish the wild and mutant types. Also, a pair of genotyping primers without an artificial mismatch base at the 3′ terminus region was used for the control experiment. The results (Fig. 2) indicate that the introduction of the artificial mismatch base was an effective way to decrease the false-positive signals. For example, the false-positive signal for the homo-G case was decreased to several percents from 36 %.

We used thermosensitive enzymes for the degradation at first and followed this with heating-inactivation of the enzymes. Here, Exonuclease I was used for degrading PCR primers and Shrimp

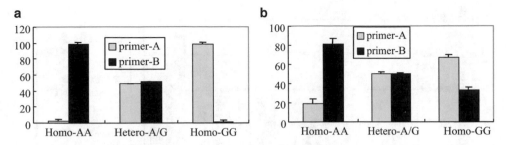

Fig. 2 SNP typing of I823M in the ABCA1 gene using artificial mismatch primers (**a**) and regular primers (**b**) in cycle extension reactions for BAMPER. Three samples with different SNP types were analyzed: homo-AA, hetero-AG, and homo-GG. Primer-A and primer-B represent the specific primer for typing homo-A and homo-G, respectively

Alkaline Phosphatase (SAP) was used for degrading dATP and PPi. Both of these were inactivated by high-temperature incubation. This treatment had no observed effect on the subsequent SNP detection. As a result, one-tube cleanup of the PCR products was realized by simply adding a small amount of SAP and Exonuclease I. The optimum concentrations of SAP and Exonuclease I were 0.5–2 U and 1–4 U, respectively, for 10 μl of PCR products. If a large background signal is still observed after the enzyme treatment, a single-strand DNA binding protein (SSB) can be added to prevent primer dimer production.

The background signal due to the dATP used for the extension reactions was very strong. We reduced this signal to a level corresponding to about one-fiftieth of the normal positive signal observed in BAMPER by using the analog, dATPαS. The thermal decomposition of dNTPs was the main background source in BAMPER using the thermal-cycling procedure, and this was minimized by decreasing the dNTP concentration and shortening the high-temperature incubation time. However, the signal intensity from the cycle extension reaction is affected by the amount of dNTPs. Therefore, a balance must be struck between the background and the positive signal.

As shown in Fig. 3a, the positive signal intensities became stronger with an increasing dNTP concentration as well as with an increased cycling number applied for the extension reaction. However, the background mainly produced by the decomposition of dNTPs also increased in proportion to the cycles, as shown in Fig. 3b. The optimum dNTP concentration for genotyping was obtained from Fig. 3c. When dNTP concentration was more than 0.1 mM, one cycle was enough to get a good signal-to-background ratio. The plural of cycle reactions were needed when the dNTP concentration was less than 0.01 mM. From the viewpoint of rapid analysis with adequate sensitivity, we selected a concentration of 0.125 mM for each dNTP and five cycles for the extension reaction in the simplified BAMPER experiment.

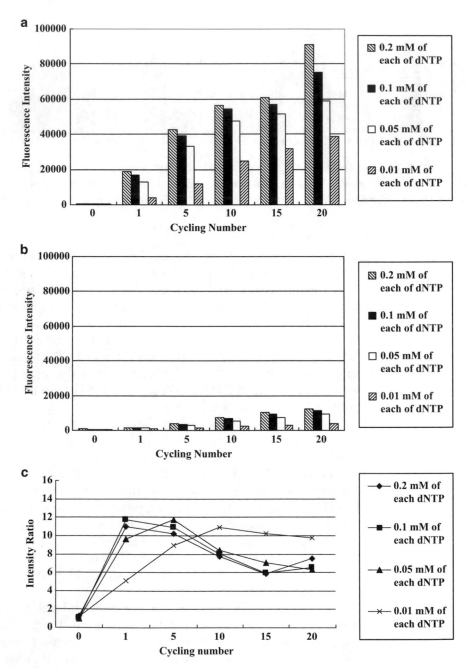

Fig. 3 SNP typing of I823M in the ABCA1 gene by BAMPER using different amounts of dNTPs and different cycling numbers. The extension conditions were 94 °C for 30 s, 50 °C for 30 s, and 72 °C for 30 s, and the cycling number is shown on the *x*-axis. Four kinds of dNTP concentration were used in the extension reactions, as indicated by the bar shades. (**a**) Signal produced by the matched primer extension reaction; (**b**) background in the case of a mismatched primer; (**c**) ratio of the signal intensity for the extension reaction in **a** to the background in **b**

4.2 Genotyping of Various SNPs for Different Genome Samples

Genotyping of 27 individual SNPs in different heart-related genes was carried out with the modified BAMPER. The result was good enough for genotyping of the 27 different SNPs (Fig. 4a). The BAMPER genotyping results coincided with results obtained through DNA sequencing, indicating that BAMPER worked well for genotyping primers containing GC-rich sequences, such as eNOS-786T/C.

To investigate the sample-to-sample instability of typing results in BAMPER, we analyzed ten different SNPs for various genomic samples. All the results coincided with those obtained by DNA sequencing. Part of the genotyping results for 23 genomic samples are shown in Fig. 4b. These results show that the simplified BAMPER method is applicable to different kinds of genome samples, and is accurate enough to type either allele of an SNP.

We attempted 2-plex, 3-plex, 4-plex, and 5-plex PCR for SNP typing by BAMPER. For comparison, we also carried out regular PCRs for all five SNPs. As shown in Fig. 5, BAMPER could be

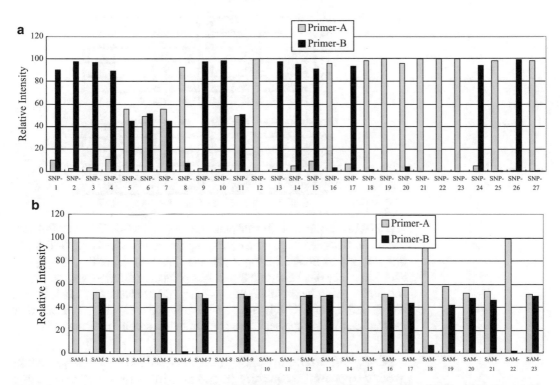

Fig. 4 Genotyping results from the simplified BAMPER using double-stranded DNAs directly. (**a**) Typing various SNPs in a genome sample. The information on SNP-1 to SNP-27 is listed in Table 1. Primer-A and primer-B correspond to a pair of genotyping primers for strand extension after target hybridization. (**b**) Typing an SNP, G664A in the ANP gene, for 23 different genome samples. Primer-A and primer-B denote the genotyping primers for distinguishing allele C and allele T, respectively. In both figures, the relative intensities were obtained after subtracting the control background (no specific primer) from the observed signals. The intensities with primer-A and primer-B are shown as *grey bars* and *black bars*, respectively

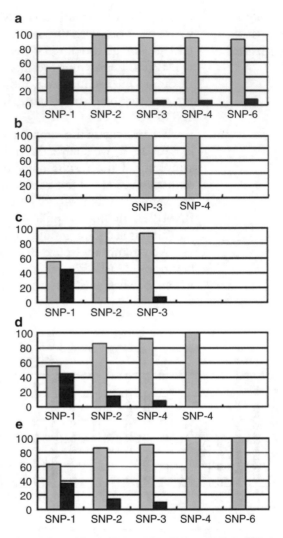

Fig. 5 BAMPER coupled with multiplex PCR. SNP-1, SNP-2, SNP-3, SNP-4, and SNP-6. (**a**) Detection of genotype using regular PC R products. (**b**) SNP-3 and SNP-4 typing by BAMPER using 2-plex PCR products. (**c**) SNP-1, SNP-2, and SNP-3 typing by BAMPER using 3-plex PCR products. (**d**) SNP-1, SNP-2, SNP-3, and SNP-4 typing by BA MPER using 4-plex PCR products. (**e**) SNP-1, SNP-2, SNP-3, SNP-4, and SNP-6 typing by BAMPER using 5-plex PCR products. *Gray bars* and *black bars* represent the signals from two specific extension primers

applied with multiplex PCR products. Although a large background appeared frequently in the multiplex mode, we overcame this problem by adding a single-strand binding protein.

5   Technical Notes

1. Genome DNA for method development was extracted from the blood of volunteers in our laboratory with DNAZOL™ Reagent (Gibco BRL, Life Technologies). Various genome

samples for method validation were obtained from the Department of Cardiovascular Medicine, Graduate School of Medicine, University of Tokyo [22–24].

2. The cycling condition was the same as that described above except for the annealing temperature, which was the average of each primer's T_m.

3. Generally, 3 mL of PCR products were used for each SNP typing: three BAMPER reactions (for wild-type, mutant, and control) were carried out, and each reaction used only 1 µL of PCR products.

4. Because of the small volume of extension solution, mineral oil was added to prevent the evaporation of water.

References

1. Ahmadian A, Gharizadeh B, Gustafsson AC, Sterky F, Nyren P, Uhlen M, Lundeberg J (2000) Single-nucleotide polymorphism analysis by pyrosequencing. Anal Biochem 280:103–110

2. Baner J, Isaksson A, Waldenstrom E, Jarvius J, Landegren U, Nilsson M (2003) Parallel gene analysis with allele-specific padlock probes and tag microarrays. Nucleic Acids Res 31:e103

3. Bray MS, Boerwinkle E, Doris PA (2001) High-throughput multiplex SNP genotyping with MALDI-TOF mass spectrometry: practice, problems and promise. Hum Mutat 17:296–304

4. Cai H, White PS, Torney D, Deshpande A, Wang Z, Marrone B, Nolan JP (2000) Flow cytometry-based minisequencing: a new platform for high-throughput single-nucleotide polymorphism scoring. Genomics 66:135–143

5. Chen J, Iannone MA, Li MS, Taylor JD, Rivers P, Nelsen AJ, Slentz-Kesler KA, Roses A, Weiner MP (2000) A microsphere-based assay for multiplexed single nucleotide polymorphism analysis using single base chain extension. Genome Res 10:549–557

6. Hampe J, Wollstein A, Lu T, Frevel HJ, Will M, Manaster C, Schreiber S (2001) An integrated system for high throughput TaqMan™ based SNP genotyping. Bioinformatics 17:654–655

7. Hardenbol P, Baner J, Jain M, Nilsson M, Namsaraev EA, Karlin-Neumann GA, Fakhrai-Rad H, Ronaghi M, Willis TD, Landegren U, Davis RW (2003) Multiplexed genotyping with sequence-tagged molecular inversion probes. Nat Biotechnol 21:673–678

8. Hsu TM, Law SM, Duan S, Neri BP, Kwok PY (2001) Genotyping single-nucleotide poly-morphisms by the invader assay with dual-color fluorescence polarization detection. Clin Chem 47:1373–1377

9. Li Z, Tsunoda H, Okano K, Nagai K, Kambara H (2003) Microchip electrophoresis of tagged probes incorporated with one-colored ddNTP for analyzing single-nucleotide polymorphisms. Anal Chem 75:3345–3351

10. McPherson JD, Marra M, Hillier L, Waterston RH, Chinwalla A, Wallis J, Sekhon M, Wylie K, Mardis ER, Wilson RK et al (2001) A physical map of the human genome. Nature 409:934–941

11. Medintz I, Wong WW, Berti L, Shiow L, Tom J, Scherer J, Sensabaugh G, Mathies RA (2001) High-performance multiplex SNP analysis of three hemochromatosis-related mutations with capillary array electrophoresis microplates. Genome Res 11:413–421

12. Newton CR, Graham A, Heptinstall LE, Powell SJ, Summers C, Kalsheker N, Smith JC, Markham AF (1989) Analysis of any point mutation in DNA. The amplification refractory mutation system (ARMS). Nucleic Acids Res 17:2503–2516

13. Nordstrom T, Nourizad K, Ronaghi M, Nyren P (2000) Method enabling pyrosequencing on double-stranded DNA. Anal Biochem 282:186–193

14. Nordstrom T, Ronaghi M, Forsberg L, de Faire U, Morgenstern R, Nyren P (2000) Direct analysis of single-nucleotide polymorphism on double-stranded DNA by pyrose-quencing. Biotechnol Appl Biochem 31:107–112

15. Prince JA, Brookes AJ (2001) Towards high-throughput genotyping of SNPs by dynamic

allele-specific hybridization. Expert Rev Mol Diagn 1:352–358

16. Ronaghi M (2000) Improved performance of pyrosequencing using single-stranded DNA-binding protein. Anal Biochem 286:282–288

17. Ronagh M, Uhlen M, Nyren P (1998) A sequencing method based on real-time pyrophosphate. Science 281:363, 365

18. Sachidanandam R, Weissman D, Schmidt SC, Kakol JM, Stein LD, Marth G, Sherry S, Mullikin JC, Mortimore BJ, Willey DL et al (2001) A map of human genome sequence variation containing 1.42 million single nucleotide polymorphisms. Nature 409:928–933

19. Sosnowski RG, Tu E, Butler WF, O'Connell JP, Heller MJ (1997) Rapid determination of single base mismatch mutations in DNA hybrids by direct electric field control. Proc Natl Acad Sci U S A 94:1119–1123

20. Syvanen AC (1999) From gels to chips: "minisequencing" primer extension for analysis of point mutations and single nucleotide polymorphisms. Hum Mutat 13:1–10

21. Taylor JD, Briley D, Nguyen Q, Long K, Iannone MA, Li MS, Ye F, Afshari A, Lai E, Wagner M et al (2001) Flow cytometric platform for high-throughput single nucleotide polymorphism analysis. Biotechniques 30:661–666, 668–669

22. Tyagi S, Bratu DP, Kramer FR (1998) Multicolor molecular beacons for allele discrimination. Nat Biotechnol 16:49–53

23. Venter JC, Adams MD, Myers EW, Li PW, Mural RJ, Sutton GG, Smith HO, Yandell M, Evans CA, Holt RA et al (2001) The sequence of the human genome. Science 291:1304–1351

24. Xiao W, Oefner PJ (2001) Denaturing high-performance liquid chromatography: a review. Hum Mutat 17:439–474

25. Zhou G, Kamahori M, Okano K, Chuan G, Harada K, Kambara H (2001) Quantitative detection of single nucleotide polymorphisms for a pooled sample by a bioluminometric assay coupled with modified primer extension reactions (BAMPER). Nucleic Acids Res 29:e93

Chapter 11

Improvement of Pyrosequencing to Allow Multiplex SNP Typing in a Pyrogram

Guohua Zhou, Mari Gotou, Tomoharu Kajiyama, and Hideki Kambara

Abstract

A multiplex single-nucleotide polymorphism (SNP) typing platform using "bioluminometric assay coupled with terminator (2′,3′-dideoxynucleoside triphosphates [ddNTPs]) incorporation" (named "BATI" for short) was developed. All of the reactions are carried out in a single reaction chamber containing target DNAs, DNA polymerase, reagents necessary for converting PPi into ATP, and reagents for luciferase reaction. Each of the four ddNTPs is dispensed into the reaction chamber in turn. PPi is released by a nucleotide incorporation reaction and is used to produce ATP when the ddNTP dispensed is complementary to the base in a template. The ATP is used in a luciferase reaction to release visible light. Only 1 nt is incorporated into a template at a time because ddNTPs do not have a 3′ hydroxyl group. This feature greatly simplifies a sequencing spectrum. The luminescence is proportional to the amount of template incorporated. Only one peak appears in the spectrum of a homozygote sample, and two peaks at the same intensity appear for a heterozygote sample. In comparison with pyrosequencing using dNTP, the spectrum obtained by BATI is very simple, and it is very easy to determine SNPs accurately from it. As only one base is extended at a time and the extension signals are quantitative, the observed spectrum pattern is uniquely determined even for a sample containing multiplex SNPs. We have successfully used BATI to type various samples containing plural target sequence areas. The measurements can be carried out with an inexpensive and small luminometer using a photodiode array as the detector. It takes only a few minutes to determine multiplex SNPs. These results indicate that this novel multiplexed approach can significantly decrease the cost of SNP typing and increase the typing throughput with an inexpensive and small luminometer.

Key words Multiplex single-nucleotide polymorphism typing, Bioluminometric assay, 2′,3′-dideoxynucleoside triphosphates, Terminator incorporation

1 Introduction

Although extensively characterized set of single-nucleotide polymorphisms (SNPs) covering the human genome are available [1], the role of hereditary traits on clinical consequences has still not been clarified. As there are a huge number of polymorphisms in the human genome, an accurate, high-throughput, and low-cost genotyping method is required [2]. At the moment, many SNP typing methods based on various principles [3], e.g.,

Guohua Zhou and Qinxin Song (eds.), *Advances and Clinical Practice in Pyrosequencing*, Springer Protocols Handbooks, DOI 10.1007/978-1-4939-3308-2_11, © Springer Science+Business Media New York 2016

sequencing-by-synthesis [4, 5], allele-specific hybridization [6–8], allele-specific extension [9, 10], allele-specific ligation [11, 12], and structure-specific cleavage [13] have been developed. In the meantime, many detection platforms have been constructed with various readouts [14], such as fluorescence [15–18], mass spectrometry [19, 20], luminescence [21–23], and electrochemical detection [24]. Minisequencing is a 2′,3′-dideoxynucleoside triphosphates (ddNTP)-based sequencing-by-synthesis method, and it is widely used for SNP typing detected by fluorescence and mass spectrometry. When using fluorescence for the detection, ddNTPs are labeled with different dyes, and the SNP types are based on the signal intensity at each dye-specific emission wavelength. When mass spectrometry is used for SNP detection, modified ddNTPs or a mixture of dNTPs and ddNTP are required in order to enlarge the mass differences between the extension products from each allele [20]. It is expensive to employ dyes, a laser, a modified ddNTP, and a mass spectrometer for a routine SNP typing at a small scale. We have developed a METPOC method that uses chip electrophoresis with a single colored ddNTP for SNP typing as well as allele frequency analysis [25]. However, it still requires two types of primers for each SNP typing and, therefore, is not so convenient. Pyrosequencing is a promising sequence-by-synthesis technology employing bioluminescence detection, which does not need dye labeling, laser excitation, and electrophoresis [26]. And it has been proven to be an efficient method for SNP typing.

Pyrosequencing uses four enzymatic reactions carried out in a single tube [27, 28]. They include a DNA polymerase reaction for extending DNA strands, PPi conversion for producing ATP by the catalysis of ATP sulfurylase in the presence of adenosine 5′-phosphosulfate (APS), light production by a luciferase–luciferin reaction, and a dNTP degradation reaction by apyrase. A peak in a sequencing spectrum is observed when the added dNTP is complementary to the base in a template strand and incorporated into the hybridized sequencing primer. The DNA sequence is determined from the incorporated nucleotide species and the peak intensities in the spectrum. Because of the advantages of pyrosequencing in terms of the base-calling accuracy, the system flexibility and the high quantitative performance, it is widely used for SNP typing. However, it is not necessary to sequence a long DNA for SNP detections. In most cases, two-base sequencing is enough for biallelic genotyping. On the other hand, it is time-consuming to sequence a long DNA for typing a known SNP by pyrosequencing, which in turn limits the sample processing speed and throughput. Moreover, the use of expensive dATPαS instead of dATP for sequencing increases the cost. Multiplex pyrosequencing for SNP typing is one way to reduce the cost [29]; however, if a pyrogram contains peaks disproportional to the incorporated base number or contains a frame shift caused by incomplete extension, reaction or undegraded dNTPs, the accuracy of pyrosequencing for multiplex genotyping would be reduced. To simplify the sequencing spectrum in multiplex SNP typing, we demonstrated a novel SNP-typing platform based on a "bioluminometric assay coupled with terminator (ddNTPs) incorporation" (or "BATI" for short). This platform does not require the use of dATPαS. There are two possible ways to increase the efficiency of SNP detection. One way is to use multiple primers to hybridize a template simultaneously and then detect the sequencing spectrum for the multiplexed SNP typing by adding ddNTPs in turn (*see* **Note 3**). The other way is to successively add a SNP-specific primer to a reaction mixture containing multiple templates at every cycle of four ddNTPs injection.

As ddNTPs are used instead of dNTPs for nucleotide incorporation, only one base is extended at a time. The signal intensity is proportional to the amount of DNA template in the mixture. In the case of a single SNP typing, only one peak appears in a spectrum for a homozygote and two peaks with equal height for a heterozygote. A schematic illustration for multiplex SNP typing is shown in Fig. 1. There are two possible ways of multiplex typing. The first way can be applied to two-plex or three-plex SNP typing, where SNPs are determined by comparing the obtained results

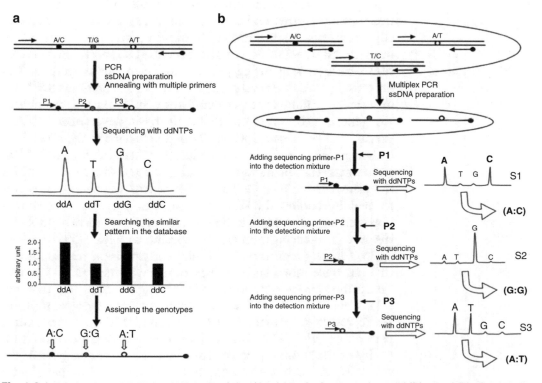

Fig. 1 Schematic view of BATI for SNP typing based on (**a**) a single-step primer addition and (**b**) step-by-step primer additions

with the estimated patterns. The second way can be applied to SNP typing with a multiplex level of more than three by adding different primers in turn. The first case is illustrated in Fig. 1a for typing three SNPs with the alleles A/C, T/G, and A/T on a DNA target. Firstly, a target DNA template is amplified by using a pair of primers with one biotin-primer. After preparing a single-stranded DNA, three sequencing primers with the 3′ ends located just before the SNP points are hybridized with the template simultaneously. A typing spectrum is obtained by carrying out one-base extension reactions by adding ddNTP in turn, and a peak appears in a spectrum if the added ddNTP is complementary to the target at any SNP point. As signal intensities are dependent on the template amounts, the spectral patterns obtained are uniquely determined when the molar concentrations of multiple templates are equal. The result in the case that all three SNPs are on one template is shown in Fig. 1a. It is easy to determine the genotypes of three SNPs by comparing the observed spectral pattern with those estimated from possible combinations of known genotypes. There are 27 different spectral patterns corresponding to three-plex SNP typing. The observed spectrum in Fig. 1a matches the standard pattern for the genotypes AC, GG, and AT.

As shown in Fig. 1b, multiplex SNP typing can also be performed by successive addition of sequencing primers. As the sequencing primers incorporated with ddNTPs cannot extend their strands further and the added ddNTPs are degraded gradually by apyrase in the detection solution, the previously added primers and ddNTPs do not affect the next strand extension reaction with new sequencing primers added in the same tube. The detection procedure is very simple, just like a single-plex SNP typing. At first, multiple target templates containing polymorphisms are generated by multiplex PCR. Next, single-stranded DNA is prepared. A sequencing primer P1 that is specific to the allele A/C is then added into the reaction solution containing the above template mixtures. The mixture is incubated for 3–5 min at 32 °C for the primer hybridization. The one-base extension reaction is performed by adding ddNTPs in turn, and a typing spectrum is obtained as "s1" in Fig. 1b. Following a cyclic addition of ddNTPs, the next sequencing primer, P2, specific to allele T/G is added again. After hybridization for 3 min, the extension reaction is carried out once more, and the spectrum is obtained as "s1" in Fig. 1b. In the same way, a spectrum by adding the sequencing primer P3 is obtained as "s3." The genotypes at all three polymorphisms are therefore determined as A:C, G:G, and A:T from the spectral patterns of "s1", "s2," and "s3", respectively. Because of the simplicity of the spectral patterns (one peak or two equal peaks), the typing is carried out very accurately and rapidly. Compared with the principle described in Fig. 1a, this scheme is not limited to a multiplex level or to the type of alleles at each polymorphism.

2   Materials

1. Thermostable pyruvate orthophosphate dikinase (PPDK) and thermostable luciferase were supplied by Kikkoman (Chiba, Japan).

2. Phosphoenolpyruvate trisodium (PEP), pyrophosphate deca-hydrate (PPi), apyrase-VI, bovine serum albumin (BSA), and D-luciferin were purchased from Sigma (St Louis, MO).

3. 2′-deoxyadenosine-5′-O-(1-thiotriphosphate),   Sp-isomer (Sp-dATP-α-S),   and   2′,3′-dideoxyadenosine-5′-O-(1-thiotriphosphate) (ddATP-α-S) were purchased from Biolog LifeScience Institute (Bremen, Germany).

4. ddNTPs were purchased from Amersham Biosciences (Piscataway, NJ).

5. Exo⁻ Klenow was purchased from Ambion (Austin, TX).

6. Inorganic pyrophosphatase (40 U/mL) and Sequenase version 2.0T7 DNA polymerase (13 U/μL) were obtained from USB Corporation (Cleveland, Ohio).

7. Platinum Taq DNA polymerase was purchased from Invitrogen (Carlsbad, CA).

8. Sodium Dynabeads M-280 Streptavidin (2.8 μm ID) was purchased from Dynal AC (Oslo, Norway).

9. ATP and AMP were obtained from Oriental Yeast (Osaka, Japan).

10. All solutions were prepared in deionized and sterilized water. Other chemicals were of a commercially extra-pure grade.

3   Methods

3.1   Primers and Target Sequences

1. All of the oligonucleotides were purchased from Sigma Genosys (Hokkaido, Japan). The sequences of the PCR primers and SNP-typing primers are listed in Table 1. DNA fragments from TPMT and UGT1A1 genes, respectively, were amplified using the PCR primers listed in Table 1 and employed as templates for SNP typing.

2. SNP-1, SNP-2, SNP-3, and SNP-4 are on the same DNA fragment amplified by the primer pair TF and TR. SNP-5 and SNP-6 are on the same DNA fragment amplified by the primer pair GF and GR.

3. To capture a single-strand DNA with Streptavidin beads, the 5′ ends of primers TR, GR, and PR were modified by biotin. All the oligonucleotides were high-performance liquid chromatography purified.

Table 1

SNPs used for the evaluation and typing analysis

Gene symbol	PCR primer sequences	SNP code	SNP typing primer sequences	SNP identifier
TPMT		SNP-1	5′-ttttctctttctggtaggac	NM_000367:c423A>C
	TF:5′-tgttgaagtaccagcatgcac	SNP-2	5′-tttctggtaggacaaatatt	NM_000367:c.430G>C
	TR:5′-aaaattacttaccatttg cgatca	SNP-3	5′-catgatttgggatagagga	NM_000367:c.460G>A
		SNP-4	5′-agaggagcattagttgccat	NM_000367:c.474C>T
UGTIAI	GF:5′-cagcagaggggacatgaaat	SNP-5	5′-cctcgttgtacatcagagac	NM_000463:c.211G>A
	GR:5′-caaaaacattatgcccgagac	SNP-6	5′-aagacgtaccctgtgcca	NM_000463:c.247T>C
TP53	PFI:5′- gttgaaagtcagggcacaagt	SNP-7	5′-aacagataaagcaactggaa	dbSNPrs2856920:gG>C
	PRI:5′-agcctgggtaacatgat gaaa-biotin	SNP-8	5′-gcagcaaagaaacaaacatg	dbSNPrs2909430:gC>T
		SNP-6	5′-tcttcccacctcagcctcct	dbSNPrs1794287:gA>G
TP53	PF2:5′- agagatcacacattaagtggg	SNP-10	5′-aaaacactgacaggaagcc	dbSNPrs1794286:gA>T
		SNP-11	5′-cagaatgcaagaagcccaga	dbSNPrs11540656:gC>A
	PR2:5′-ctgctcttttcacccat ctac-biotin	SNP-12	5′-tgctggtgcaggggccacg	dbSNPrs1042522:gC>G
		SNP-13	5′-tccattgcttgggacggcaa	dbSNPrs11575998:gG>T

3.2 Template DNA Preparation

1. Genome DNAs were extracted from the blood of volunteers (staff from our laboratory) by using DNAZOL Reagent (Invitrogen) (*see* **Note 1**).

2. Each PCR mixture (50 μL) contained 1.5 mM of $MgCl_2$, 0.2 mM each of dNTPs, 1.25 U of Platinum Taq polymerase, 20 pmol of biotinylated primer, and 40 pmol of another primer.

3. Amplification was performed on a PTC-200 thermocycler PCR system according to the following protocol: denatured at 94 °C for 2 min and followed by 35 thermal reaction cycles (94 °C for 30 s; 56 °C for 1 min; and 72 °C for 1–3 min).

4. After the cycle reaction, the product was incubated at 72 °C for 7 min to ensure the complete extension of the amplified DNA.

5. Super-paramagnetic beads were used to immobilize biotinylated PCR products. The immobilization was performed by incubating the mixture of DNA and beads at room temperature for 15–40 min.

6. Single-stranded DNAs were obtained by incubating the beaded DNAs in 0.1 M NaOH for 5–10 min.

7. The supernatant fluid was neutralized by 1 M HCl, and the immobilized strand was washed by the buffer described in the instructions for the beads (*see* **Note 2**).

8. Annealing of the single-stranded template with sequencing primer was carried out in a buffer of 50 mM Tris–acetate (pH 7.8) and 20 mM magnesium acetate at 92 °C for 30 s, at 65 °C for 3 min, and at room temperature for 5 min.

3.3 PPi Conversion Reaction

1. One milliliter of the AM-PPDK-based reaction mixture contained the following components: 60 mM of Tricine (pH 7.8), 2 mM of EDTA, 20 mM of magnesium acetate, 0.2 mM of DTT, 0.4 mM of D-luciferin, 0.04 mM of PEP, 0.4 mM of AMP, 0.1 % BSA, 65 U of Sequenase 2.0, 10 U of PPDK, 1 U of apyrase, and an appropriate amount of luciferase (*see* **Notes 3** and **4**).

3.4 Degradation of Endogeneous PPi Contained in Reagents

1. One milliliter of 500 mM ddNTPs containing 60 mM of Tricine (pH 7.8), 2 mM of EDTA, and 20 mM of magnesium acetate was incubated with 20 mU of PPase for 10 min at room temperature.

2. The desired concentration of ddNTP solution was diluted directly before the incorporation reaction.

3. For a routine detection, the concentration is 50 μM for ddATP, 100 μM for ddTTP, 100 μM for ddGTP, and 300 μM for ddCTP.

4. The treated AMP is added just before the detection. Usually 40 mU of PPase is enough for degrading the background in 1 mL of detection mixture to a baseline (*see* **Note 5**).

3.5 Detection of Bioluminescence Signal Produced by ddNTP-Incorporation Reaction

1. We used a house-made dispenser for adding a small amount of ddNTP solution to the reaction chamber. Only 250 nl of PPase-treated ddNTP was dispensed at a time (*see* **Note 6**).

4 Method Validation

4.1 Detecting DNA Fragments from TPMT and UGT1A1 Genes

Pyrosequencing technology is based on step-by-step dNTP addition [33], and the signal intensity is proportional to the number of bases incorporated by DNA polymerase at a time. Genotype is determined from a pyrogram. However, a pyrogram becomes complex when the polymorphism is located in a homogeneous region. In contrast, as for the BATI method, the spectrum is simple because ddNTPs do not have a 3′ hydroxyl group for further

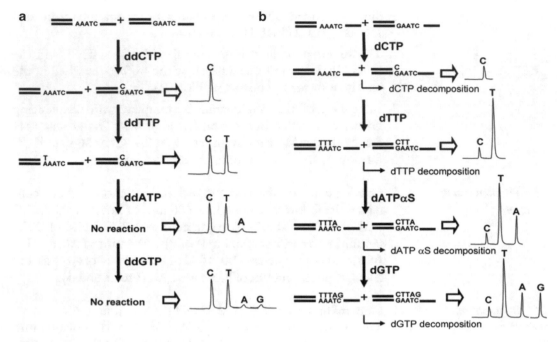

Fig. 2 Comparison of ddNTP-based BATI (**a**) with dNTP-based pyrosequencing (**b**)

extension. The differences in spectra are demonstrated in Fig. 2 for a sample having a sequence of -A/GAATC- (bold indicates the SNP type). As shown in Fig. 2a, the typed nucleotide pattern is 1C:1T:0A:0G, and the pattern of dNTP incorporation in Fig. 2b is 1C:5T:2A:2G. As the signal intensities obtained by the incorporation of >5 nt are probably not in linear proportion to the number of incorporated nucleotides in pyrosequencing, it is difficult to determine the base sequence from the observed pyrogram, even though the expected peak ratio is 1C:5T: 2A:2G. On the contrary, the difficulty will not occur with the BATI method based on ddNTP incorporation because SNPs are determined by a spectral pattern: a homozygote gives a single peak and a heterozygote gives two peaks in the spectrum. This means that a typing spectrum obtained by BATI gives straightforward information on SNPs.

Usually, the detection limit in the BATI method is determined by the signals from a luciferase reaction with substrates like dNTPs, ddNTPs, APS, or AMP. The amounts of these substrates are very large compared with the target DNA amount. The other component affecting the detection limit of ATP with a bioluminescent assay is the reaction of luciferase with the substrates such as APS and AMP. There are two possible ATP production reactions: APS–ATP sulfurylase reaction and AMP–PPDK reaction. Although the reaction activities of these substrates are small, a large background signal will appear if a large amount of such substances are added to the reaction mixture. A detection system using the AMP–PPDK reaction gives a smaller background; therefore, we used such a system instead of an APS–ATP sulfurylase system commonly used in pyrosequencing.

For stable and reliable SNP typing, the minimum amount of template DNA was 10 fmol (i.e., ten times higher than the detection limit). Usually the amount of ddNTPs or dNTPs required for completing extension reactions is 30 times larger than that of template DNA, so 300 fmol of ddNTPs or dNTPs is dispensed. This amount of ddATP gives a small background signal, which is negligible; however, the signal produced by the same amount of dATP is three times larger than that produced by nucleotide incorporation reactions of 10 fmol of DNA templates and is not negligible. It is therefore impossible to use dATP for pyrosequencing, but it is possible to use dATPαS.

The background signals were manufacturer-specific (as shown in Fig. 3). It was found that the signal produced with ddCTP from Toyobo was very large. However, ddCTP from Amersham Bioscience did not give a large signal. According to the manufacturer's instructions, the purities of ddTTP, ddGTP, and ddCTP were 98 %, 98 %, and 94 % from Toyobo and 99.7 %, 99.9 %, and 99.5 % from Amersham Bioscience, respectively. It is thought that the high background produced with ddCTP from Toyobo was originated in the impurities in the reagent. It is required to use highly purified ddNTPs for the present assay.

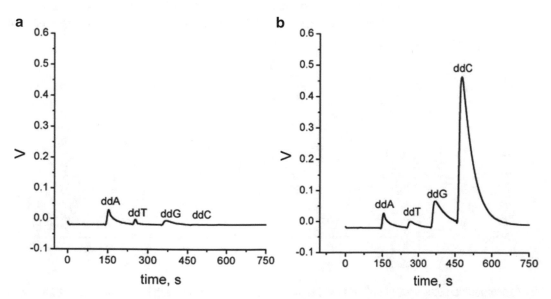

Fig. 3 Reaction profiles of ddTTP, ddGTP, and ddCTP from different manufacturers, (**a**) Amersham Bioscience and (**b**) Toyobo. ddATP was used as a reference and is from TaKaRa. The concentrations of all of four ddNTPs are 200 mM. The dispensing volume is 0.25 mL at a time, and the minisequencing mixture is 25 mL. The detection sensor is a photodiode array. The assignment of each ddNTP is marked at the *top of the peak*

As exonuclease-free DNA polymerase is required for the reaction, only two kinds of DNA polymerases are available, Exo⁻ Klenow (a fragment of *Escherichia coli* DNA polymerase I) and T7 DNA polymerase (Sequenase version 2.0). Exo⁻ Klenow is frequently used in DNA sequencing using chain terminators (ddNTPs), and it incorporates a ddNTP at a rate of 1000 times slower than that for dNTP. On the contrary, the ddNTP incorporation rate by T7 DNA polymerase is only a few times lower than that for dNTP.

As shown in Fig. 4a, the rate of ddATP incorporation by Klenow is very low. To confirm the completion of incorporation reactions, each ddNTP was dispensed twice. The peaks marked by arrows in Fig.4a indicated that the ddATP or ddGTP incorporation reaction with Klenow was not completed before the degradation. On the contrary, the incorporation reaction of ddATP or ddGTP by Sequenase was completed, and two equal sharp peaks with the same intensity were observed (as shown in Fig. 4b). We therefore used T7 DNA polymerase with Mg^{2+}.

4.2 Multiplex SNP Typing

The BATI method can be applied for typing multiplexed SNPs on a template. We have successfully analyzed various two-plex and three-plex SNPs. First, a total of six SNPs on two templates (T-2 and G-2) were determined by uni-plex typing, and then a combination of different SNPs for two-plex and three-plex typing were carried out. In the two-plex typing, the simultaneous addition of two primers followed by incorporation reactions with four ddNTPs was carried out for three different SNP combinations: SNP-1 + SNP-4, SNP-2 + SNP-3, and SNP-5 + SNP-6. The observed spectra are

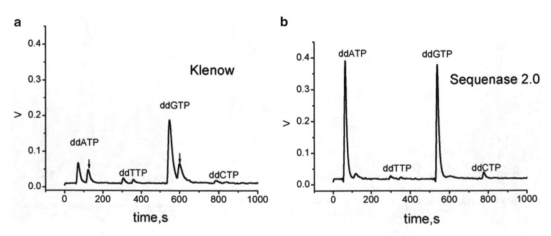

Fig. 4 Incorporation efficiency of ddNTPs by Klenow (**a**) and Sequenase (**b**) with Mg^{2+}. The concentration was 25 μM for ddATP, 50 mM for other three ddNTPs. The template was G-2 (a heterozygote of single-stranded PCR products of gene UGT1A1). The dispensing volume is 0.25 μL at a time, and the minisequencing mixture is 25 μL. The *left arrow* and the *right arrow* in (**a**) indicate the signals produced by the second addition of ddATP and ddGTP, respectively

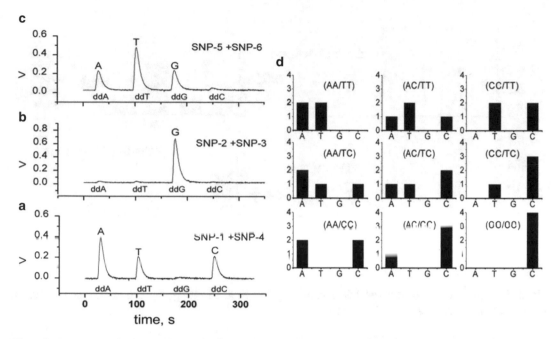

Fig. 5 SNP typing spectra for different combinations of SNPs by two-plex typing (**a–c**) and a set of possible patterns for two-plex typing by taking the SNPs from (**a**) as an example (**d**). The combination of each allele is indicated at the *top* of each pattern in (**d**). DNA template T-2 contains SNP-1, SNP-2, SNP-3, and SNP-4, and template G-2 contains SNP-5 and SNP-6. The marked code of SNP in each spectrum is explained in Sects. 2 and 3

shown in Fig. 5a, b, and c, respectively. To decode the allele for each SNP in the spectrum, the observed spectrum was compared with standard patterns.

The typing results of SNP-1 + SNP-4 in T-2 are indicated in Fig. 5a. By comparison, the genotypes of SNP-1 and SNP-4 on T-2 were determined to be AA and TC, respectively. Similarly, the genotypes at SNP-2 and SNP-3 on T-2 (Fig. 5b) were determined to be GG and GG, and those at SNP-5 and SNP-6 on G-2 (Fig. 5c) were determined to be AG and TT, respectively.

Figure 6 shows the three-plex typing profile for equal molar concentrations of template T-2 and G-2. By comparing the observed result with a set of 27 standard patterns (data not shown), the alleles of SNP-1, SNP-4, and SNP-5 in Fig. 6a were determined to be AA, TC, and AG, respectively, which coincided with the result by uni-plex typing. Similarly, the genotypes of SNP-2, SNP-4, and SNP-5 in Fig. 6b were accurately determined to be GG, TC, and AG, respectively.

Although multiplex typing is very efficient, the number of SNPs investigated simultaneously is limited to three. A combination of multiplex typing and successive typing by a step-by-step addition of sequencing primers improves the typing throughput and reduces the cost of SNP typing. Multiplex PCR products can be used as templates. The detection procedure is the same as that for uni-plex typing. The results of successive multiplex typing of

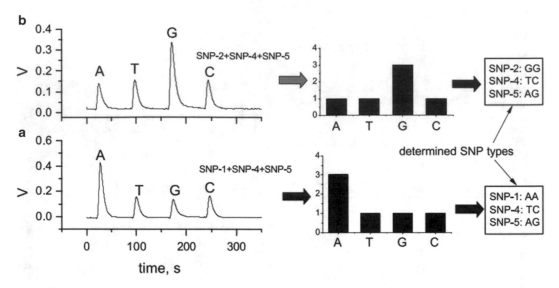

Fig. 6 SNP typing spectra for different combinations of SNPs by three-plex typing. The marked code of SNP in each spectrum is explained in Sects. 2 and 3

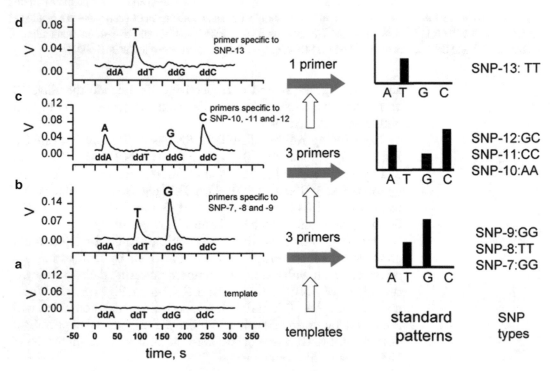

Fig. 7 Successive multiplex SNP typing by step-by-step addition of sequencing primers. (**a**) ddNTP addition by turns without primer addition; (**b**) adding a primer mixture for SNP-7, SNP-8 and SNP-9, followed by terminator incorporation reactions; (**c**) adding a primer mixture for SNP-10, SNP-11 and SNP-12, followed by terminator incorporation reactions; (**d**) adding a primer specific to SNP-13. The order of sequencing-primer addition is indicated by the *open arrows*. The standard patterns corresponding to the observed spectra were determined as those on the *right side of the solid arrows*

template mixtures, T-349 and T-454, are shown in Fig. 7. By comparing the observed spectra with the standard patterns for three-plex typing, SNP-7, SNP-8, and SNP-9 were determined as GG, TT, and GG, respectively, and SNP-10, SNP-11, and SNP-12 were determined as AA, CC, and GC, respectively. All of them were coincident with the results from uni-plex typing. SNP-13 was easily identified to be TT from the spectrum directly (Fig. 7d). Seven SNPs in a sample were typed easily by BATI.

5 Technical Notes

1. The template DNA was obtained by means of PCRs with primer pairs of TF and TR from human genome DNA to get 181 bp fragments of TPMT gene, with primers of GF and GR to get 151 bp fragments of UGT1A1 gene, with primers of PF1 and PR1 to get 349 bp fragments of TP53 gene (defined as T-349 fragment), and with primers of PF2 and PR2 to get 454 bp fragments of TP53 gene (defined as T-454 fragment).

2. Eight kinds of single-stranded DNA templates, named T-1,T-2, T-3, T-4, G-1, G-2, G-3, and G-4, were prepared from the PCR products of the TPMT gene and the UGT1A1 gene amplified by the combination of an unmodified primer and a biotin-primer. T-1 and G-1 are the liquid phase of sense strands of the TPMT gene and the UGT1A1 gene, respectively. T-2 and G-2 are the liquid phase of anti-sense strands of the TPMT gene and the UGT1A1 gene, respectively. T-3and G-3 are the beaded phase of sense strands of the TPMT gene and the UGT1A1 gene, respectively. T-4 and G-4 are the beaded phase of anti-sense strands of the TPMT gene and the UGT1A1 gene, respectively.

3. In conventional pyrosequencing, PPi released by the nucleotide incorporation reaction is converted into ATP by APS–ATP sulfurylase system, and luminescence is produced by ATP through a luciferase-catalyzed reaction with luciferin [30]. An alternative way for converting PPi into ATP is to use PPDK-catalyzed reaction, which was used for determining AMP by adding PPi and PEP [31]. Here, we added AMP to convert PPi into ATP in the presence of PPDK.

4. As APS is a substrate of a luciferin–luciferase reaction, a large background signal appears when a large amount of luciferase is added to increase the detection sensitivity. Unlike APS, AMP does not give any luminescence in the luciferin–luciferase reaction [32], therefore, a highly sensitive DNA detection can be carried out by adding a large amount of luciferase.

5. If PPase is used to remove the background from the detection solution instead of apyrase, PPase is added to the reaction mixture before the addition of AMP, and the solution of AMP is treated by PPase separately [34–36].

References

1. Miller RD, Phillips MS, Jo I, Donaldson MA, Studebaker JF, Addleman N, Alfisi SV, Ankener WM, Bhatti HA, Callahan CE et al (2005) High-density single-nucleotide polymorphism maps of the human genome. Genomics 86:117–126

2. Syvanen AC (2005) Toward genome-wide SNP genotyping. Nat Genet 37:S5–S10

3. Kwok PY (2000) High-throughput genotyping assay approaches. Pharmacogenomics 1:95–100

4. Ronaghi M, Uhlen M, Nyren P (1998) A sequencing method based on real-time pyrophosphate. Science 281:363–365

5. Pastinen T, Kurg A, Metspalu A, Peltonen L, Syvanen AC (1997) Minisequencing: a specific tool for DNA analysis and diagnostics on oligonucleotide arrays. Genome Res 7:606–614

6. Tyagi S, Bratu DP, Kramer FR (1998) Multicolor molecular beacons for allele discrimination. Nat Biotechnol 16:49–53

7. Shapero MH, Zhang J, Loraine A, Liu W, Di X, Liu G, Jones KW (2004) MARA: a novel approach for highly multiplexed locus-specific SNP genotyping using high-density DNA oligonucleotide arrays. Nucleic Acids Res 32:e181

8. Livak KJ (1999) Allelic discrimination using fluorogenic probes and the 5′ nuclease assay. Genet Anal 14:143–149

9. O'Meara D, Ahmadian A, Odeberg J, Lundeberg J (2002) SNP typing by apyrase-mediated allele-specific primer extension on DNA microarrays. Nucleic Acids Res 30:e75

10. Zhou G, Kamahori M, Okano K, Chuan G, Harada K, Kambara H (2001) Quantitative detection of single nucleotide polymorphisms for a pooled sample by a bioluminometric assay coupled with modified primer extension reactions (BAMPER). Nucleic Acids Res 29:E93

11. Iannone MA, Taylor JD, Chen J, Li MS, Rivers P, Slentz_Kesler KA, Weiner MP (2000) Multiplexed single nucleotide polymorphism genotyping by oligonucleotide ligation and flow cytometry. Cytometry 39:131–140

12. Hardenbol P, Baner J, Jain M, Nilsson M, Namsaraev EA, Karlin-Neumann GA, Fakhrai-Rad H, Ronaghi M, Willis TD, Landegren U et al (2003) Multiplexed genotyping with sequence-tagged molecular inversion probes. Nat Biotechnol 21:673–678

13. Olivier M (2005) The Invader assay for SNP genotyping. Mutat Res 573:103–110

14. Chen X, Sullivan PF (2003) Single nucleotide polymorphism genotyping: biochemistry, protocol, cost and throughput. Pharmacogenomics J 3:77–96

15. Ye F, Li MS, Taylor JD, Nguyen Q, Colton HM, Casey WM, Wagner M, Weiner MP, Chen J (2001) Fluorescent microsphere-based readout technology for multiplexed human single nucleotide polymorphism analysis and bacterial identification. Hum Mutat 17:305–316

16. Xiao M, Kwok PY (2003) DNA analysis by fluorescence quenching detection. Genome Res 13:932–939

17. Rockenbauer E, Petersen K, Vogel U, Bolund L, Kolvraa S, Nielsen KV, Nexo BA (2005) SNP genotyping using microsphere-linked PNA and flow cytometric detection. Cytometry A 64:80–86

18. Shen R, Fan JB, Campbell D, Chang W, Chen J, Doucet D, Yeakley J, Bibikova M, Wickham Garcia E, McBride C et al (2005) High-throughput SNP genotyping on universal bead arrays. Mutat Res 573:70–82

19. Griffin TJ, Smith LM (2000) Single-nucleotide polymorphism analysis by MALDI-TOF mass spectrometry. Trends Biotechnol 18:77–84

20. Gut IG (2004) DNA analysis by MALDI-TOF mass spectrometry. Hum Mutat 23:437–441

21. Zhou GH, Shirakura H, Kamahori M, Okano K, Nagai K, Kambara H (2004) A gel-free SNP genotyping method: bioluminometric assay coupled with modified primer extension reactions (BAMPER) directly from double-stranded PCR products. Hum Mutat 24:155–163

22. Kakihara F, Kurebayashi Y, Tojo Y, Tajima H, Hasegawa S, Yohda M (2005) MagSNiPer: a new single nucleotide polymorphism typing method based on single base extension, magnetic separation, and chemiluminescence. Anal Biochem 341:77–82

23. Jansson V, Jansson K (2004) An enzymatic bioluminescent assay of DNA ligation. Anal Biochem 324:307–308

24. Boon EM, Ceres DM, Drummond TG, Hill MG, Barton JK (2000) Mutation detection by electrocatalysis at DNA-modified electrodes. Nat Biotechnol 18:1096–1100

25. Li ZP, Tsunoda H, Okano K, Nagai K, Kambara H (2003) Microchip electrophoresis of tagged probes incorporated with one-colored ddNTP for analyzing single-nucleotide polymorphisms. Anal Chem 75:3345–3351

26. Ahmadian A, Gharizadeh B, Gustafsson AC, Sterky F, Nyren P, Uhlen M, Lundeberg J (2000) Single-nucleotide polymorphism analysis by pyrosequencing. Anal Biochem 280:103–110

27. Ronaghi M (2003) Pyrosequencing for SNP genotyping. Methods Mol Biol 212:189–195

28. Ronaghi M (2001) Pyrosequencing sheds light on DNA sequencing. Genome Res 11:3–11

29. Pourmand N, Elahi E, Davis RW, Ronaghi M (2002) Multiplex pyrosequencing. Nucleic Acids Res 30, e31

30. Zhou G, Kamahori M, Okano K, Harada K, Kambara H (2001) Miniaturized pyrosequencer for DNA analysis with capillaries to deliver deoxynucleotides. Electrophoresis 22:3497–3504

31. Sakakibara T, Murakami S, Eisaki N, Nakajima M, Imai K (1999) An enzymatic cycling method using pyruvate orthophosphate dikinase and firefly luciferase for the simultaneous determination of ATP and AMP (RNA). Anal Biochem 268:94–101

32. Kamahori M, Harada K, Kambara H (2002) A new single nucleotide polymorphisms typing method and device by bioluminometric assay coupled with a photodiode array. Meas Sci Technol 13:1779–1785

33. Elahi E, Ronaghi M (2004) Pyrosequencing: a tool for DNA sequencing analysis. Methods Mol Biol 255:211–219

34. Kristensen T, Vass H, Ansorge W, Prydz H (1990) DNA dideoxy sequencing with T7 DNA polymerase: improved sequencing data by the addition of manganese chloride. Trends Genet 6:2–3

35. Tabor S, Richardson CC (1990) DNA sequence analysis with a modified bacteriophage T7 DNA polymerase. Effect of pyrophosphorolysis and metal ions. J Biol Chem 265:8322–8328

36. Tabor S, Richardson CC (1989) Effect of manganese ions on the incorporation of dideoxynucleotides by bacteriophage T7 DNA polymerase and Escherichia coli DNA polymerase I. Proc Natl Acad Sci U S A 86:4076–4080

Chapter 12

Improvement of Pyrosequencing Sensitivity by Capturing Free Adenosine 5′-Phosphosulfate with Adenosine Triphosphate Sulfurylase

Haiping Wu, Wenjuan Wu, Zhiyao Chen, Weipeng Wang, Bingjie Zou, Qinxin Song, Guohua Zhou, and Hideki Kambara

Abstract

In pyrosequencing chemistry, four cascade enzymatic reactions with the catalysis of polymerase, ATP sulfurylase, luciferase, and apyrase are employed. The sensitivity of pyrosequencing mainly depends on the concentration of luciferase which catalyzes photoemission reaction. However, the side reaction of adenosine 5′-phosphosulfate (APS, an analogue of ATP) with luciferase resulted in an unavoidable background signal; hence, the sensitivity cannot be much higher due to the simultaneous increase of the background signal when using a larger amount of luciferase. In this, study, we demonstrated a sensitive pyrosequencing by using a large amount of ATP sulfurylase to lower the concentration of free APS in the pyrosequencing mixture. As the complex of ATP sulfurylase and APS does not react with luciferase, a large amount of luciferase can be used to achieve a sensitive pyrosequencing reaction. This sensitivity-improving pyrosequencing chemistry allows the use of an inexpensive light sensor photodiode array for constructing a portable pyrosequencer, a potential tool in point-of-care test (POCT).

Key words Highly sensitive pyrosequencing, ATP sulfurylase, Photodiode array, Portable pyrosequencer

1 Introduction

Pyrosequencing, which is based on the real-time bioluminometric quantification of pyrophosphate (PPi) released from dNTP incorporation [1], has been widely applied to SNP typing [2], microbe genotyping [3], gene expression analysis [4], and gene methylation analysis [5]. The next-generation sequencing platform was firstly constructed using pyrosequencing chemistry as 454 GS FLX [6]. So pyrosequencing technology has offered us a powerful tool in the field of post-genomic research. In the conventional pyrosequencing chemistry, four enzymatic reactions are employed, polymerization with Klenow, conversion of PPi

Guohua Zhou and Qinxin Song (eds.), *Advances and Clinical Practice in Pyrosequencing*, Springer Protocols Handbooks, DOI 10.1007/978-1-4939-3308-2_12, © Springer Science+Business Media New York 2016

to ATP with ATP sulfurylase in the presence of adenosine 5′-phosphosulfate (APS), photoemission through luciferase reaction, and degradation of ATP and excess dNTPs with apyrase. This chemistry arises from the enzymatic luminometric PPi detection assay (ELIDA) [7–9] but has a lower background than ELIDA because ATP generated from PPi contamination in the reagents is degraded by the coexisting apyrase. So the background signal of pyrosequencing is only from the side reaction of APS (an analogue of ATP) with luciferase [10]. The sensitivity of pyrosequencing mainly depends on the background level and the luciferase concentration. Although the signal intensity in pyrosequencing increases in proportion to luciferase concentration, the background due to free APS in the sequencing mixture increases with luciferase as well [10]. Therefore, the sensitivity of conventional pyrosequencing chemistry is greatly limited. To use an inexpensive and compact photodiode (PD) array-based instrument for pyrosequencing [11], the sensitivity of pyrosequencing chemistry should be improved to compensate the sensitivity insufficiency of PD sensor. We have previously reported a method enabling pyrosequencing with a high sensitivity by using pyruvate orthophosphate dikinase (PPDK) instead of ATP sulfurylase to convert PPi into ATP in the presence of AMP which does not react with luciferase [12]. Although several fmols of DNA template have been successfully sequenced in the PD-sensor pyrosequencer, it is difficult to obtain the commercialized PPDK on market for the moment. In addition, the optimum temperature for PPDK-catalyzed reaction is 55–60 °C, and the activity of PPDK drops to 25 % of the maximum value at room temperature [13]; so PPDK-AMP-based chemistry is not in good accordance with the other three enzymatic reactions in pyrosequencing. Furthermore, we found that the yield of PPDK expressed from *Microbispora rosea* subsp. *aerata* in *E. coli* is much lower than that of ATP sulfurylase [14], suggesting that PPDK-AMP-based pyrosequencing may require expensive reagents. Accordingly, the widespread application of the PD array pyrosequencer in molecular diagnosis is greatly limited by the reagents. It is preferable to take the advantage of the low cost of conventional pyrosequencing chemistry while keeping a higher sensitivity. Because the sensitive pyrosequencing using ATP sulfurylase and APS needs a low background, a straightforward way is to use a small amount of APS; however, this is not practical due to the decrease in the rate of PPi conversion reaction. Here, we improved the conventional pyrosequencing chemistry by using a large amount of ATP sulfurylase to capture the free APS, allowing the use of a high concentration of luciferase in the sequencing mixture for increasing pyrosequencing sensitivity (Fig. 1).

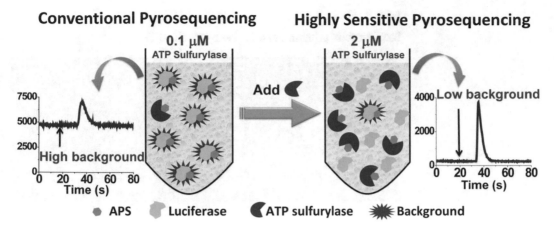

Fig. 1 Use a large amount of ATP sulfurylase to capture the free APS, allowing the use of a high concentration of luciferase in the sequencing mixture for increasing pyrosequencing sensitivity

---

2   Materials

1. ATP sulfurylase and Klenow fragment were obtained by gene engineering in our lab.

2. DNA polymerase was purchased from Takara (Dalian, China).

3. Polyvinylpyrrolidone (PVP) and QuantiLum recombinant luciferase were purchased from Promega (Madison, WI).

4. Bovine serum albumin (BSA), APS, and apyrase VII were obtained from Sigma (St. Louis, MO).

5. Dynabeads M-280 streptavidin was from Dynal Biotech ASA (Oslo, Norway).

6. Sodium 2′-deoxyadenosine-5′-O-(1-triphosphate) (dATPαS), 2′-deoxyguanosine-5′-triphosphate(dGTP),2′-deoxythymidine-5′-triphosphate (dTTP), and 2′-deoxycytidine-5′-triphosphate (dCTP) were purchased from MyChem (San Diego, CA).

7. Other chemicals were of a commercially extra-pure grade. All solutions were prepared with deionized and sterilized water.

---

3   Methods

3.1 Primers and Target Sequences

1. Three pairs of gene-specific primers were designed for the amplification of a 106-bp DNA fragment in the membrane protein gene (the M gene), a 195-bp DNA fragment in the nucleocapsid protein gene (the NP gene), and a 116-bp DNA fragment in the hemagglutinin gene (the HA gene), respectively. The primer sequences are listed in Table 1.

Table 1

Sequences of primers used for gene-specific PCR

Gene	Primer	Sequence (5′ to 3′)
M	InfA forward	gaccratcctgtcacctctgac
	InfA reverse	biotin-agggcattytggacaaakcgtcta
NP	SW InfA forward	gcacggtcagcacttatyctrag
	SW InfA reverse	biotin-gtgrgctgggttttcatttggtc
HA	SW H1 forward	gtgctataaacaccagcctycca
	SW H1 reverse	biotin-cgggatattccttaatcctgtrgc

3.2 RNA Reverse Transcription

1. Total RNA in RNase-free water was heated to 65 °C for 5 min and snap chilled on ice for at least 1 min.

2. A reaction mixture containing 0.5 mM of each dNTP, 1× RT buffer, 1 μM random primer, 0.5 U/μL RNase inhibitor, and 0.2 U/μL Omniscript reverse transcriptase was added to each tube containing RNA and mixed gently.

3. Collected by a brief centrifugation and incubated at 37 °C for 60 min, followed by 93 °C for 5 min to terminate the reaction.

3.3 PCR

1. Fifty microliters of each PCR reaction mixture contained 1.5 mM $MgCl_2$, 0.2 mM of each dNTP, 1.25 U of Taq polymerase, 20 pmol of the biotinylated PCR primer, and 20 pmol of the other PCR primer.

2. Amplification was performed on an EDC-810 thermocycler PCR system according to the following protocol: denaturing at 94 °C for 2 min, followed by 35 thermal reaction cycling (94 °C for 30 s, 56 °C for 60 s, 72 °C for 60 s). After the thermal cycle reaction, the product was incubated at 72 °C for 7 min to ensure the complete extension of the amplified DNA.

3.4 ssDNA Preparation

1. Streptavidin-coated magnetic Dynabeads M-280 were used to prepare ssDNA template for pyrosequencing (*see* **Note 1**).

2. Biotinylated PCR products were captured onto the magnetic beads (*see* **Note 2**).

3.5 Pyrosequencing

1. Pyrosequencing was performed in 100 μL of pyrosequencing mixture containing 0.1 M Tris–acetate (pH 7.7), 2 mM EDTA, 10 mM magnesium acetate, 0.1 % BSA, 1 mM dithiothreitol, 2 μM APS, 0.4 mg/mL PVP, 0.4 mM D-luciferin, 0.1–5 μM ATP sulfurylase, 5.7×10^8 RLU QuantiLum™ recombinant

luciferase, 18 U/mL *Exo–* Klenow fragment, and 1.6 U/mL apyrase (*see* **Note 3**).

2. Sequencing reaction starts by a stepwise elongation of primer strands through sequential additions of four kinds of deoxynucleotide triphosphates (*see* **Note 4**).

---

4 Method Validation

4.1 Genotyping the 2009 Influenza A Virus (2009 H1N1)

The effect of ATP-sulfurylase concentration on the background due to APS and the signals from DNA extension reaction was investigated. As shown in Fig. 2a, the background signal intensities due to APS decreased dramatically when the concentration of ATP sulfurylase increased from 0.1 μM to 2 μM, and no obvious decrease of the background is observed when the concentration of ATP sulfurylase is more than 2 μM, which is equal to that of the added APS. On the other hand, the signal intensity due to dNTP incorporation also increased a little with the concentration of ATP sulfurylase (around 80 % from 0.1 μM to 1 μM) and stayed constant after 1 μM (see Fig. 2a for details). These results indicate that a highly sensitive pyrosequencing is possible by optimizing the ATP-sulfurylase concentration to allow a low background and the largest signal; therefore, the best concentration of ATP sulfurylase was selected as 2 μM in the case of 2 μM APS.

To further investigate the optimum ratio in concentration between APS and ATP sulfurylase, pyrosequencing with different amounts of ATP sulfurylase was individually performed at the APS concentration of 0.5 μM, 1 μM, 2 μM, 5 μM, and 7.5 μM,

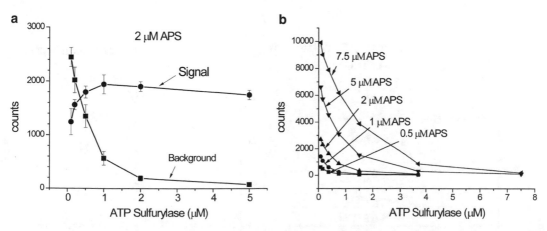

Fig. 2 Effect of the concentration of ATP sulfurylase on both signals and background of pyrosequencing at 2 μM APS (**a**) and on background of pyrosequencing at various concentrations of APS (0.5, 1, 2, 5, 7.5 μM), respectively (**b**). The sequences of the template (50 fmol) and the sequencing primer are 5′-CAG ATG AGA GAA CAA GAA GTG GGG-3′ and 5′-CCC CAC TTC TTG TTC TCT CAT-3′, respectively

respectively. As shown in Fig. 2b, the background signals at each APS concentration decreased with the increase of ATP-sulfurylase concentration. By using the background signal of 300 as a criteria, the optimum concentrations of ATP sulfurylase are around 0.5 µM, 1 µM, 2 µM, 5 µM, and 7.5 µM at 0.5 µM, 1 µM, 2 µM, 5 µM, and 7.5 µM APS, respectively; we thus concluded that a sensitive pyrosequencing reaction could be achieved by keeping ATP-sulfurylase concentration as high as that of APS in a sequencing mixture. From the viewpoint of reagent cost, a small amount of ATP sulfurylase is preferable; hence, APS concentration in pyrosequencing should be optimized. Pyrosequencing on various amounts of APS showed that sequencing signals become constant when more than 1 µM APS was employed (data not showed), indicating that 2 µM APS is enough for a pyrosequencing reaction.

As the concentration of free APS was significantly reduced by adding a large amount of ATP sulfurylase, the sensitivity of conventional pyrosequencing can be increased by using a high concentration of luciferase. For comparison, pyrosequencing on 50 fmol of synthesized ssDNA at various amounts of luciferase (0.57×10^8 RLU, 1.1×10^8 RLU, 2.8×10^8 RLU, 5.7×10^8 RLU, and 11.3×10^8 RLU) was carried out at 0.1 µM and 5.3 µM ATP sulfurylase, respectively. The results in Fig. 3a showed that the backgrounds increased significantly with the increase of luciferase concentration when 0.1 µM ATP sulfurylase was employed, resulting in a low signal-to-noise ratio and a low detection sensitivity. On the other hand, pyrosequencing with 5.3 µM ATP sulfurylase (Fig. 3b) gave a very low background and a higher signal-to-noise ratio, while the signal increased in proportion to the luciferase concentration. Therefore, it is feasible to employ a higher ATP-sulfurylase concentration to achieve a sensitive pyrosequencing.

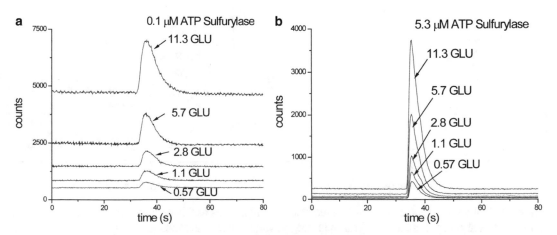

Fig. 3 Pyrosequencing sensitivity at various amounts of luciferase with the ATP-sulfurylase concentration of 0.1 µM (**a**) and 5.3 µM (**b**), respectively. GLU means 10^8 relative light units

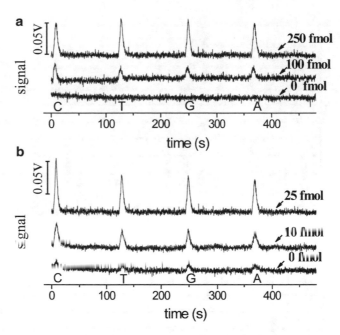

Fig. 4 Pyrograms of different amounts of synthesized ssDNA with conventional pyrosequencing system (**a**) and improved pyrosequencing system (**b**). The amount of template was indicated in each pyrogram. Pyrosequencing was performed in 100 µL of mixture by using a PD array-based portable bioluminescence analyzer

We have constructed a prototype of 8-channel pyrosequencer by using a PD array sensor with the dimension of $140W \times 158H \times 250D$ (mm) [11, 15]. Different amounts of ssDNA template were detected by conventional and improved pyrosequencing system, respectively. As shown in Fig. 4, about 250 fmol of DNA template were required for an accurate sequencing with conventional pyrosequencing chemistry, while 25 fmol of DNA template gave the similar sequencing intensity with the improved pyrosequencing chemistry. Therefore, the pyrosequencing sensitivity increased ten times in the improved pyrosequencing chemistry, resulting in a tenfold reduction in the amount of DNA template for pyrosequencing.

We have applied this chemistry in the 8-channel pyrosequencer for genotyping the 2009 influenza A virus (2009 H1N1) by sequencing the segments of the M gene, the NP gene, and the HA gene which are species specific. The results were showed in Fig. 5, and it is observed that the pyrograms contain some unexpected signals (short peaks). The pyrogram of a negative control (data not showed) suggests that these short peaks are from the contributions of both dNTP's impurities and the background due to incompletely extended templates. Comparison between the theoretical histograms and the obtained pyrograms indicates that these short peaks have less impact on the base-calling accuracy. Therefore, the sensitive pyrosequencing system coupled with PD array-based portable DNA analyzer is feasible.

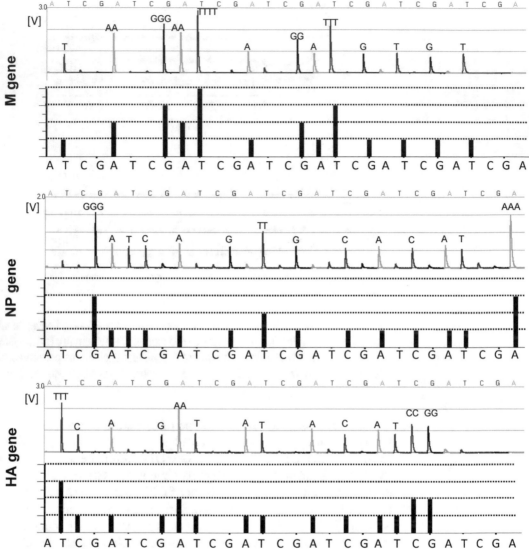

Fig. 5 Typical pyrograms and the corresponding theoretical sequence histograms of the M gene, the NP gene, and the HA gene of influenza A 2009 virus (H1N1). The detected sequence is on the *top* of each peak. Each dNTP was dispensed with the order of A-T-C-G

---

5 Technical Notes

1. After sedimentation, the remaining components of the PCR reaction can be removed by washing to obtain pure double-stranded DNA followed by alkali denaturation to yield ssDNA [16–18].

2. The immobilized biotinylated strand was used as the sequencing template.

3. At the condition of 2 µM APS and 2 µM ATP sulfurylase, the concentration of free APS in the pyrosequencing mixture was theoretically calculated to be 0.38 µM by taking the Kd of 0.09 µM into consideration. The background signal from this amount of APS corresponds to the signal from 0.09 nM ATP, much lower than the template amount (2 nM) used in conventional pyrosequencing.

4. We used portable bioluminescence analyzer (HITACHI, Ltd., Central Research Laboratory, Japan) for pyrosequencing [15]. This apparatus has a portable size of 140 mm (W) × 158 mm (H) × 250 mm (D), which used an array of eight photodiodes (S1133; Hamamatsu Photonics K.K) to detect photo signals, and employed four separate capillaries for dispensing small amounts of dNTPs into the reaction chamber [19–21]. To vibrate the reaction chamber, a cell phone motor fixed on the base support was employed, and a plate holding the reaction chambers was vibrated with the motor. In addition, a commercialized pyrosequencing platform of PyroMark ID System (Biotage Co., Sweden) together with the pyrosequencing kit (Qiagen, Germany) was used for the method evaluation.

References

1. Ronaghi M, Uhlen M, Nyren P (1998) A sequencing method based on real-time pyrophosphate. Science 281(363):365

2. Ahmadian A, Gharizadeh B, Gustafsson AC, Sterky F, Nyren P, Uhlen M, Lundeberg J (2000) Single-nucleotide polymorphism analysis by pyrosequencing. Anal Biochem 280:103–110

3. Gharizadeh B, Oggionni M, Zheng B, Akom E, Pourmand N, Ahmadian A, Wallin KL, Nyren P (2005) Type-specific multiple sequencing primers: a novel strategy for reliable and rapid genotyping of human papillomaviruses by pyrosequencing technology. J Mol Diagn 7:198–205

4. Zhang X, Wu H, Chen Z, Zhou G, Kajiyama T, Kambara H (2009) Dye-free gene expression detection by sequence-tagged reverse-transcription polymerase chain reaction coupled with pyrosequencing. Anal Chem 81:273–281

5. Tost J, Gut IG (2007) DNA methylation analysis by pyrosequencing. Nat Protoc 2:2265–2275

6. Chi KR (2008) The year of sequencing. Nat Methods 5:11–14

7. Nyren P, Lundin A (1985) Enzymatic method for continuous monitoring of inorganic pyrophosphate synthesis. Anal Biochem 151:504–509

8. Nyren P (1987) Enzymatic method for continuous monitoring of DNA polymerase activity. Anal Biochem 167:235–238

9. Ronaghi M, Karamohamed S, Pettersson B, Uhlen M, Nyren P (1996) Real-time DNA sequencing using detection of pyrophosphate release. Anal Biochem 242:84–89

10. Hyman ED (1988) A new method of sequencing DNA. Anal Biochem 174:423–436

11. Kambara H, Zhou G (2009) DNA analysis with a photo-diode array sensor. Methods Mol Biol 503:337–360

12. Zhou GH, Kajiyama T, Gotou M, Kishimoto A, Suzuki S, Kambara H (2006) Enzyme system for improving the detection limit in pyrosequencing. Anal Chem 78:4482–4489

13. Eisaki N, Tatsumi H, Murakami S, Horiuchi T (1999) Pyruvate phosphate dikinase from a thermophilic actinomyces *Microbispora rosea* subsp. *aerata*: purification, characterization and molecular cloning of the gene. Biochim Biophys Acta 1431:363–373

14. Zou B, Chen Z, Zhou G (2008) Expression of PPDK from *Microbispora rosea* subsp. *aerata* in *Escherichia coli* and its application in pyrosequencing. Chin J Biotech 24:679–683

15. Song Q, Jing H, Wu H, Zhou G, Kajiyama T, Kambara H (2010) Gene expression analysis on a photodiode array-based bioluminescence analyzer by using sensitivity-improved SRPP. Analyst 135:1315–1319

16. Mashayekhi F, Ronaghi M (2007) Analysis of read length limiting factors in pyrosequencing chemistry. Anal Biochem 363:275–287

17. Lalor DJ, Schnyder T, Saridakis V, Pilloff DE, Dong A, Tang H, Leyh TS, Pai EF (2003) Structural and functional analysis of a truncated form of *Saccharomyces cerevisiae* ATP sulfurylase: C-terminal domain essential for oligomer formation but not for activity. Protein Eng 16:1071–1079

18. Foster BA, Thomas SM, Mahr JA, Renosto F, Patel HC, Segel IH (1994) Cloning and sequencing of ATP sulfurylase from Penicillium chrysogenum. Identification of a likely allosteric domain. J Biol Chem 269:19777–19786

19. Karamohamed S, Nilsson J, Nourizad K, Ronaghi M, Pettersson B, Nyren P (1999) Production, purification, and luminometric analysis of recombinant *Saccharomyces cerevisiae* MET3 adenosine triphosphate sulfurylase expressed in *Escherichia coli*. Protein Expr Purif 15:381–388

20. Luo J, Wu WJ, Zou BJ, Zhou GH (2007) Expression and purification of ATP sulfurylase from Saccharomyces cerevisias in Escherichia coli and its application in pyrosequencing. Chinese J Biotech 23:623–627

21. Lee HJ, Ho MR, Bhuwan M, Hsu CY, Huang MS, Peng HL, Chang HY (2010) Enhancing ATP-based bacteria and biofilm detection by enzymatic pyrophosphate regeneration. Anal Biochem 399:168–173

Chapter 13

Using Polymerase Preference Index to Design imLATE-PCR Primers for an Efficient Pyrosequencing

Qinxin Song, Xiemin Qi, Yiyun Shen, Yiru Jin, Bingjie Zou, and Guohua Zhou

Abstract

To simplify pyrosequencing protocol, we improved linear-after-the-exponential-PCR (imLATE-PCR) for yielding single-stranded DNA templates directly for pyrosequencing reaction. However, it is very critical for designing qualified primers for imLATE-PCR. To achieve a high amplification efficiency in imLATE-PCR, the polymerase preference index (PPI) value together with conventional melting temperature-dependent method were employed to design the primers. Issues frequently occurring in pyrosequencing based on conventional LATE-PCR, such as a low signal intensity or a high non-specific peak, were well solved by the PPI technology. The new strategy is validated by using pyrosequencing for various application, including resequencing, quantitative SNP genotyping, and relative gene expression analysis. Successful detection of gene sequence of genetically modified organisms, copy number variations of samples from Down's syndrome (trisomy-21) patients, and gene expression levels in tissues from patients of breast cancer demonstrates the feasibility of this method for real application. Compared with pyrosequencing based on conventional LATE-PCR, the merits lie on a flexible primer design, increased yield of ssDNA, and good quality of pyrograms.

Key words Pyrosequencing, imLATE-PCR (Improved linear-after-the-exponential-PCR), Polymerase preference index (PPI), Quantitative genotyping, Gene expression analysis

1 Introduction

Pyrosequencing is widely used in clinical DNA sequencing as the gold standard for molecular diagnosis [1], however it requires the preparation of single-stranded DNA (ssDNA) as sequencing templates. In conventional pyrosequencing protocols, a biotin-modified PCR primer and streptavidin-coated beads are needed to prepare ssDNA. Potential issues caused from ssDNA preparation include high cost, tedious process, and a high risk of DNA cross-contamination due to aerosol. To overcome this issue, we proposed a new method based on nicking endonuclease (NEases) which nicks a specific strand of PCR products and pyrosequencing

Guohua Zhou and Qinxin Song (eds.), *Advances and Clinical Practice in Pyrosequencing*, Springer Protocols Handbooks, DOI 10.1007/978-1-4939-3308-2_13, © Springer Science+Business Media New York 2016

could therefore directly start along with the nick position by strand-displacement reaction [2]. Although this method was successfully used for quantitative genotyping and differential gene expression analysis, there are following restrictions: a very limited set of NEases commercially available now, about an extra hour for nicking reaction, a very limited readable length (around 10 bp) due to the inefficient activity of strand displacement by polymerase Klenow used in pyrosequencing.

Recently, linear-after-the-exponential-PCR, a modified type of asymmetric PCR, has been developed to generate ssDNA directly by PCR [3, 4], but there is a very strict criteria for primer design, and length of amplicons is short. To improve this method, we proposed imLATE-PCR (improved linear-after-the-exponential-PCR) to optimize primer design for general use (Fig. 1) [5]. However, the

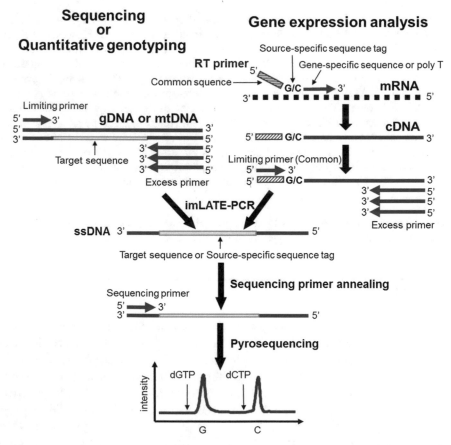

Fig. 1 Schematic overview of the method of pyrosequencing on ssDNA generated by improved linear-after-the-exponential-PCR (imLATE-PCR). Pyrosequencing directly on ssDNA products produced by imLATE-PCR on genomic DNA (gDNA) or mitochondrial DNA (mtDNA) in case of sequencing or quantitative genotyping, and pyrosequencing on ssDNA products produced by sequence-tagged reverse-transcription polymerase chain reaction coupled with imLATE-PCR in case of relative gene expression levels analysis on messenger RNA (mRNA)

efficiency of imLATE-PCR still depends on the melting temperature (T_m) values of asymmetric PCR primers. In some cases, although T_m of the primer well fits the requirement of amplification and GC content is not so high, we cannot obtain ssDNA products from PCR with a desirable yield. To improve amplification efficiency and signal intensity, here the polymerase preference index (PPI) value was introduced into the design of PCR primers for pyrosequencing in addition to T_m and GC measurements.

2 Materials

1. GMO Materials: Certified Reference Materials (CRMs) produced by the European Union (EU) Joint Research Center, Institute for Reference Materials and Measurements (IRMM), were purchased from Fluka, Buchs, Switzerland. 1 % genetically modified Bt11 maize, 2 % genetically modified Bt176 maize, and 2 % genetically modified Roundup ready soya were used.

2. Biospin Plant Genomic DNA Extraction Kit (Bioer Technology Co., Ltd., Hangzhou, China) (*see* **Note 1**).

3. TransStart Taq DNA Polymerase was purchased from TransGen Biotech (Beijing, China).

4. Exo⁻ Klenow Fragment, polyvinylpyrrolidone (PPV), and QuantiLum recombinant luciferase were purchased from Promega (Madison, WI).

5. ATP sulfurylase, apyrase, D-luciferin, bovine serum albumin (BSA), and adenosine 5′-phosphosulfate (APS) were obtained from Sigma (St. Louis, MO).

6. 2′-Deoxyadenosine-5′-O-(1-thiotriphosphate) sodium salt (dATP-α-S) was purchased from Amersham Pharmacia Biotech (Amersham, UK).

7. dGTP, dTTP, and dCTP were purchased from Amersham Pharmacia Biotech (Piscataway, NJ).

8. Homemade PD array eight-channel pyrosequencer.

9. All of the oligomers were synthesized and purified by Invitrogen (Shanghai, China) (*see* **Note 2**).

3 Methods

3.1 imLATE-PCR

1. Each 25 μL of PCR mixture contained 3.0 mM $MgCl_2$, 0.1 mM of each dNTP, 1.0 μM of the excess primer, 0.1 μM of the limiting primer, 1 μL of DNA template, and 0.1 U of Hotstar*Taq* DNA polymerase (Qiagen). Sometimes 0.5 % BSA (w/v) and 12.5 % glycerol (v/v) were added as PCR Enhancer.

2. Amplification was performed on a PTC-225 thermocycler PCR system (MJ research) according to the following imLATE-PCR program: initial heating step at 95 °C for 15 min, followed by 30 cycles (denaturation at 90 °C for 10 s, annealing at 55 °C for 10 s, elongation at 72 °C for 40 s), then followed by another 30 cycles (denaturation at 90 °C for 10 s, annealing at 65 °C for 10 s, elongation at 72 °C for 40 s), followed by a final 10 min elongation step at 72 °C.

3. imLATE-PCR: 95 °C, 15 min; followed by 30 cycles (94 °C for 10 s; 60 °C for 10 s; 72 °C for 20 s); followed by 30 cycles (94 °C for 10 s; 66 °C for 10 s; 72 °C for 20 s), 72 °C for 10 min; 16 °C hold.

4. Breast cancer imLATE-PCR: 95 °C, 5 min, 25 cycles (87 °C, 15 s; 52 °C, 10 s; 72 °C, 20 s), 35 cycles (87 °C, 15 s; 63 °C, 10 s; 72 °C, 20 s) 72 °C, 10 min.

3.2 Pyrosequencing

1. The reaction volume of pyrosequencing was 40 µL, containing 0.1 M Tris–acetate (pH 7.7), 2 mM EDTA, 10 mM magnesium acetate, 0.1 % BSA, 1 mM dithiothreitol (DTT), 2 µM adenosine 5′-phosphosulfate (APS), 0.4 mg/mL PVP, 0.4 mM D-luciferin, 200 mU/mL ATP sulfurylase, 3 µg/mL luciferase, 18 U/mL Klenow fragment, and 1.6 U/mL apyrase.

2. Five microliters of imLATE-PCR products were added into 40 µL pyrosequencing buffer first to remove the residual SNPs in a imLATE-PCR mixture by apyrase coupled with ATP sulfurylase for 5 min before pyrosequencing. And then 10 pmol sequencing primer was added into the buffer anneal to the ssDNA template for 5 min at room temperature.

3. Pyrosequencing was carried out on an eight-channel Prototype of Portable Bioluminescence Analyzer (Hitachi, Japan) according to the manufacturer's protocols. The sequencing procedure was carried out by a stepwise elongation of the primer strand through sequential additions of four kinds of dNTPs, degradation of nucleotides by apyrase, and simultaneous detection of resulting light emission by using a PD array sensor.

4   Method Validation

4.1 Primer Design Based on PPI and T_m

Recent studies have shown that DNA polymerase priming bias has an effect on priming efficiencies in addition to T_m and GC content, which is evaluated by an index value termed polymerase preference index or ‚PPI for a sliding eight base pair window [6]. By the example of 1555A>G mutation of inherited deafness on mitochondrial DNA (400 bp), the PPI value was calculated with the aid of the online iC-Architect software (http://icubate.com/index.php/2011/03/ppi-helps-you-design-better-pcr-primers/).

Figure 2a presents sense and anti-sense strand PPI profiles displayed from 5′ to 3′ and 3′ to 5′, respectively, in which maximum positions are the optimal placement for the 3′ end of the primer while minimum positions should be avoided. These results together with T_m were utilized to design two sets of imLATE-PCR primer. Higher PPI values of the good primer pair results in the remarkable difference between two PAGE electropherograms that the obtained ssDNA with the good primer pair is more prominent than that with the poor one (Fig. 2b). Therefore, a PCR primer with higher PPI value can provide better amplification efficiency. Furthermore, the signal intensity of the pyrogram obtained by good primer pair (Fig. 2d) is significantly stronger in comparison with the one obtained by poor primer pair (Fig. 2c), thus increasing the quantification accuracy of pyrosequencing. As a result, we can employ this software to guide primer design by positioning the 3′ end of the primer in places where the PPI value of the template is high and avoiding secondary structural elements like hairpins so as to generate sufficient ssDNA products with high amplification efficiency for pyrosequencing.

4.2 Sequencing Analysis of GMO

With the development of GMOs technology, many methods have been established for DNA sequencing analysis [7]. In order to evaluate the performance of our method in this field, five genes (zSSIIb, Bt11, and Bt176 gene of the genetically modified maize; Lectin and 35S-CTP4 gene of the genetically modified roundup ready soya) extracted from plant tissue were used. We designed the primers of five different genes and then carried out imLATE-PCR amplification. Pyrosequencing was directly executed on the target sequence of ssDNA products generated by imLATE-PCR. Figure 3 shows typical programs for zSSIIb, Bt11, Bt176, Lectin, and 35S-CTP4 gene where the detected sequence is on the top of each peak. Since the GM sequences were successfully detected, the method is feasible for DNA sequencing.

4.3 Quantitative Genotyping of Down's Syndrome

Conventional SNP typing can qualitatively identify homotype and heterotype. However, for the diagnosis of aneuploidy diseases, the allele-specific peak intensity is required to be accurately proportional to the amount of allele-specific template. To demonstrate the capability of this method for quantitative genotyping on the genome DNA, we selected two SNPs (rs2839110 and rs1042917 located in chromosome 21) with a high heterozygote rate from NCBI and analyzed them for the diagnosis of Down's syndrome (trisomy-21). A series of single cells from normal persons and Down's syndrome patients was used for detection. As a result, we obtained representative programs of SNP-rs2839110 and SNP-rs1042917 from normal persons and patients.

In theory, the allelic ratio of the SNP in chromosome 21 is 2:1 or 1:2 because a trisomy-21 patient has an additional third

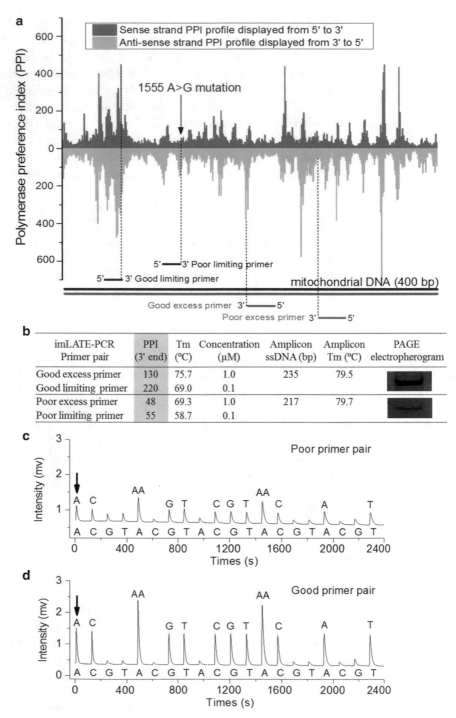

Fig. 2 Primer design based on polymerase preference index (PPI) and T_m. (**a**) A graphical display of the output of the ic-Architect online software for mitochondrial DNA template (400 bp) with assigned PPI. Maximum positions indicate the optimal placement for the 3′ end of the primer, while minimum positions should be avoided. (**b**) Two imLATE-PCR primer pairs with different PPI values. PAGE electropherograms show that the ssDNA obtained from imLATE-PCR using the good primer pair with higher PPI value is more prominent than that using the poor one. The signal intensity of the pyrogram obtained by good primer pair (**d**) is significantly stronger in comparison with the one obtained by poor primer pair (**c**)

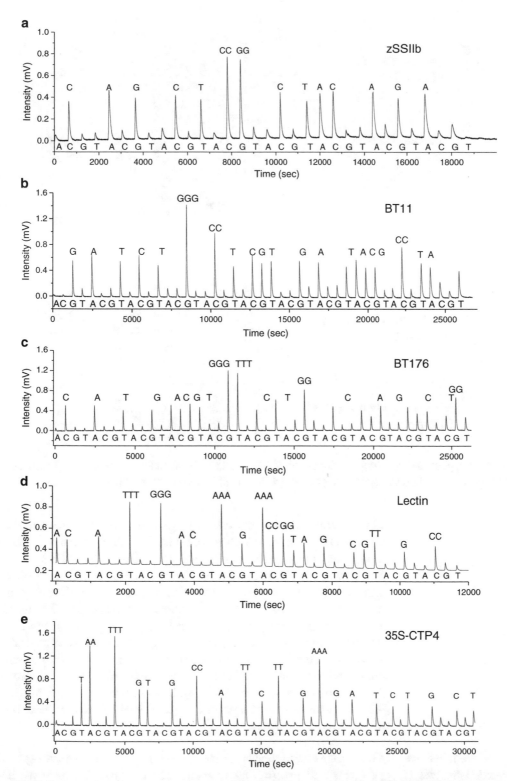

Fig. 3 Typical pyrograms of pyrosequencing on ssDNA directly generated by imLATE-PCR. zSSIIb (**a**), Bt-11 (**b**), and Bt-176 gene (**c**) of the genetically modified maize; Lectin (**d**) and 35S-CTP4 gene (**e**) of the genetically modified roundup ready soya. The detected sequence is on the *top* of each peak. Each dNTP was dispensed with the order of A-C-G-T

162   Qinxin Song et al.

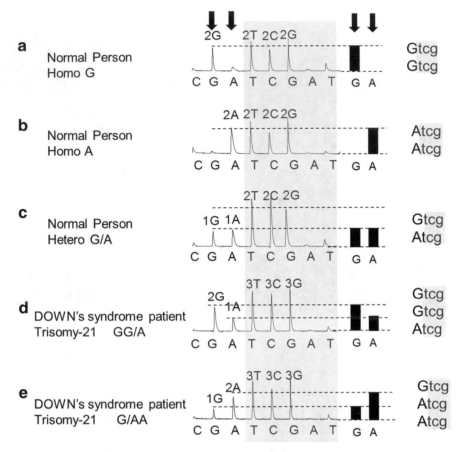

Fig. 4 Homozygous and heterozygote pyrograms of SNP-rs2839110 located in chromosome 21 from normal persons (**a**, **b**, **c**) and Down's syndrome patients (**d**, **e**). The SNP types were indicated by *arrows*

chromosome 21 compared with a normal people. As shown in Figs. 4 and 5, the genotypes are GG, AA, GA for normal homozygous and heterozygotes (Figs. 4a–c and 5a–c), but GGA or GAA for Down's syndrome patients (Figs. 4d, e and 5d, e). In addition, Fig. 6 indicates the allelic ratio of SNP can be quantitatively measured through this method. The allelic ratios are 1:0, 0:1 and 1:1 for normal homozygous and heterozygotes (Fig. 6a–c), but 2:1 or 1:2 for Down's syndrome patients (Fig. 6d, e). More importantly, it was successfully demonstrated that sequencing a homopolymetric stretch or a single cell containing an extremely small amount of DNA templates worked well while maintaining good accuracy. Thus it promises to be a practical and efficient tool for the diagnosis of aneuploid diseases.

4.4 Differential Gene Expression Analysis

Gene expression levels prove to be relevant to carcinogenesis, progress and prognosis of various cancers [8]. Recently we have developed a sensitive and inexpensive method, SRPP (Sequence-tagged Reverse-transcription PCR coupled with Pyrosequencing)

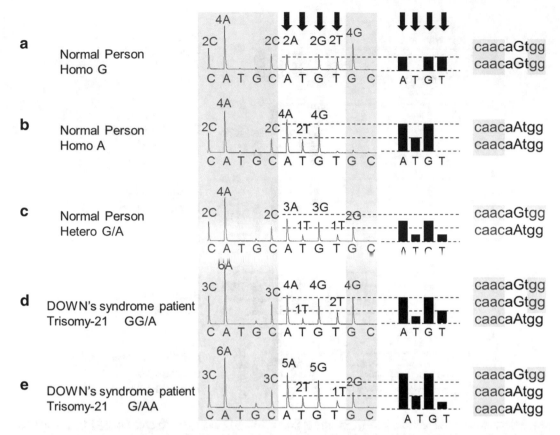

Fig. 5 Homozygous and heterozygote pyrograms of SNP-rs1042917 located in chromosome 21 from normal persons (**a**, **b**, **c**) and Down's syndrome patients (**d**, **e**). The SNP types were indicated by *arrow*

to quantitatively detect gene expression levels [9, 10]. In this study, we verified that a sufficient amount of ssDNA generated by imLATE-PCR coupled with pyrosequencing could be applied in SRPP.

First, two kinds of reverse-transcription (RT) primers (RT-G and RT-C) were designed to prepare cDNAs of normal and tumor breast tissues. The sequences are 5′-CCA TCT GTT GG GGATC TGTC *g*atc ttt ttt ttt ttt ttt VN-3′ for RT-G, and 5′-CCA TCT GTT GG GGATC TGTC *c*atg ttt ttt ttt ttt ttt VN-3′ for RT-C (underlined italics: gene source-specific bases). After reverse transcription from different amount of total RNA with RT primers, imLATE-PCR was carried out followed by quantitative decoding of the source-specific sequence tags in amplicons by pyrosequencing. The ratios of two source-specific cDNAs in the artificial templates were 1:1, 1:2, 1:5, and 1:10 (G:C), respectively (Fig. 7a). Based on the comparison of the peak intensities in the pyrograms, the correlation between the theoretical ratios of the two sources and the observed ratios by the imLATE-PCR method is satisfying ($r^2 = 0.9923$) (Fig. 7b). Moreover, Fig. 7c presents the comparison

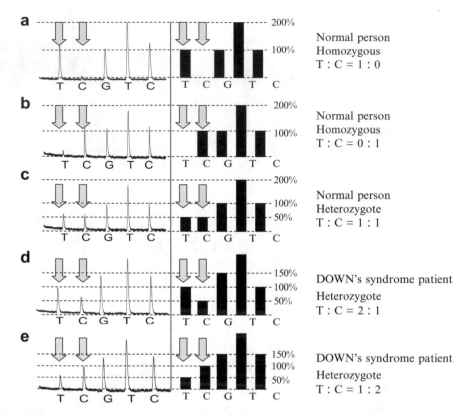

Fig. 6 Homozygous and heterozygote pyrograms of SNP-rs1042917 located in chromosome 21 from single cell of normal persons (**a**, **b**, **c**) and Down's syndrome patients (**d**, **e**). The SNP types were indicated by *arrows*

between real-time PCR, the gold standard for quantitative gene expression analysis, and the imLATE-PCR for quantification of the expression levels of three prognostic marker genes (MMP9, AF052162, and ESM1) in a patient suffering from breast cancer ($n = 3$). Differential expression levels between tumor tissue and normal tissue adjacent to tumor tissue indicates a relatively high risk of metastasis for this patient. Since no significance difference between two methods was observed, the results indicate our method is reliable for gene expression analysis by SRPP.

5   Technical Notes

1. 1–30 μg genomic DNA can be acquired from up to 100 mg plant tissue by using this Kit. The quantity and quality of DNA in the samples were measured and evaluated according to the absorbance measurements at 260 nm wavelength and 1 % agarose gel electrophoresis.

2. For the evaluation, five genes of GMO (zSSIIb, Bt11, and Bt176 gene of the genetically modified maize; Lectin and 35S-

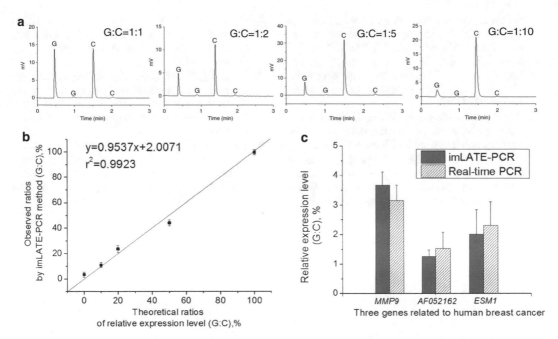

Fig. 7 (**a**) Typical pyrosequencing pyrograms of imLATE-PCR from artificial samples prepared by pooling cDNAs transcribed from different amounts of total RNA. The ratios of two source-specific cDNAs in the artificial templates were 1:1, 1:2, 1:5, and 1:10 (G:C), respectively. (**b**) Correlation between the theoretical ratios of the two sources and the observed ratios by the imLATE-PCR method based on the comparison of the peak intensities in the pyrograms. The ratios were calculated with the formula of "G/C × 100", where "G" and "C" denote the peak intensity. (**c**) Comparison between nicked dsDNA-based SRPP (*gray*) and real-time PCR (*white*) for the quantification of the expression levels of MMP9, AF052162, and ESM1 gene in a patient suffering from breast cancer (*n* = 3). Differential expression levels between tumor tissue and normal tissue adjacent to tumor tissue were denoted by fold changes (tumor tissue/normal tissue)

CTP4 gene of the genetically modified Roundup ready soya), three SNPs (rs1053315, rs2839110, and rs1042917) in chromosome 21 and three genes of breast cancer (MMP9, AF052162, and ESM1 gene) were selected as examples for the method. Two kinds of reverse-transcription primers (RT-G and RT-C) were designed to individually reverse-transcribe normal and tumor breast tissues. The sequences are 5′-CCA TCT GTT GG GGATC TGTC *g*atc ttt ttt ttt ttt ttt VN-3′ for RT-G, and 5′-CCA TCT GTT GG GGATC TGTC *c*atg ttt ttt ttt ttt ttt VN-3′ for RT-C (underlined italics: gene source-specific bases).

References

1. Zhou G, Kajiyama T, Gotou M et al (2006) Enzyme system for improving the detection limit in pyrosequencing. Anal Chem 78:4482–4489

2. Song Q, Wu H, Feng F et al (2010) Pyrosequencing on nicked Dsdna generated by nicking endonucleases. Anal Chem 82:2074–2081

3. Sanchez JA, Pierce KE, Rice JE et al (2004) Linear-after-the-exponential (late)-Pcr: an advanced method of asymmetric Pcr and its uses in quantitative real-time analysis. Proc Natl Acad Sci U S A 101:1933–1938

4. Pierce KE, Sanchez JA, Rice JE et al (2005) Linear-after-the-exponential (late)-Pcr: primer

design criteria for high yields of specific single-stranded DNA and improved real-time detection. Proc Natl Acad Sci U S A 102:8609–8614

5. Song Q, Yang H, Zou B et al (2013) Improvement of late-Pcr to allow single-cell analysis by pyrosequencing. Analyst 138:4991–4997

6. Pan W, Byrne-Steele M, Wang C et al (2014) DNA polymerase preference determines Pcr priming efficiency. BMC Biotechnol 14:10

7. Song Q, Wei G, Zhou G (2014) Analysis of genetically modified organisms by pyrosequencing on a portable photodiode-based bioluminescence sequencer. Food Chem 154:78–83

8. Chen Z, Fu X, Zhang X et al (2012) Pyrosequencing-based barcodes for a dye-free multiplex bioassay. Chem Commun (Camb) 48:2445–2447

9. Zhang X, Wu H, Chen Z et al (2009) Dye-free gene expression detection by sequence-tagged reverse-transcription polymerase chain reaction coupled with pyrosequencing. Anal Chem 81:273–281

10. Song Q, Jing H, Wu H et al (2010) Gene expression analysis on a photodiode array-based bioluminescence analyzer by using sensitivity-improved Srpp. Analyst 135:1315–1319

Part III

Reagents Preparation

Chapter 14

Preparation of Thermal-Stable Biotinylated Firefly Luciferase and Its Application in Pyrosequencing

Shuhui Zhu, Bingjie Zou, Haiping Wu, Yinjiao Ma, Ying Chen, Qinxin Song, and Guohua Zhou

Abstract

The next-generation pyrosequencing system requires stable and immobilized luciferase. In order to get stable and immobilized luciferase for the large-scale pyrosequencing platform, the genes coding the *Photinus pyralis* firefly luciferase and 87 C-terminal residues of biotin carboxyl carrier protein (BCCP87) were inserted into plasmid to express biotinylated fusion protein in *E. coli* BL21 (DE3), and the gene of luciferase was mutated to get thermo-stable biotinylated luciferase. The fusion protein was immobilized on streptavidin-coated beads and applied to pyrosequencing. The results of activity detection showed that mutant luciferase had a good tolerance to heat, and still showed activities at 50 °C. The activities of mutant LUC remains 80 % at 43 °C for 10 min. Western blot analysis indicated that the fusion protein was successfully biotinylated in *E. coli*. The biotinylated luciferase immobilized by magnetic beads coated with streptavidin showed catalytic activity of 2.1×10^5 RLU/μL beads and the activity was nearly constant even if bead-LUC suffered from multiple washing processes. The DNA was accurately and quantitatively sequenced by using luciferase and ATP sulfurylase co-immobilized on magnetic beads. This study provides an efficient and thermal-stable enzyme for the large-scale chip-based pyrosequencing system.

Key words Biotinylated luciferase, Large-scale pyrosequencing, Biotin carboxyl carrier protein

1 Introduction

Firefly luciferase (EC 1.13.12.7) catalyzes the bioluminescence reaction in the presence of luciferin, ATP, O_2, and magnesium ions [1]. Many kinds of biological assays, such as pyrosequencing [2], have been established based on the bioluminescence reaction.

Pyrosequencing is a real-time sequencing method that employed four enzymes, DNA polymerase, ATP sulfurylase, luciferase, and apyrase, to detect PPi from DNA extension for the analysis of template DNA [3]. At present, pyrosequencing has been applied to discrimination of single-nucleotide polymorphism (SNP) [4], detection of virus and microorganism [5, 6], and measurement of differential gene expression [7]. Currently, the

Guohua Zhou and Qinxin Song (eds.), *Advances and Clinical Practice in Pyrosequencing*, Springer Protocols Handbooks,
DOI 10.1007/978-1-4939-3308-2_14, © Springer Science+Business Media New York 2016

development of high-throughput picoliter-upgrade pyrosequencing technology with the capability of good sensitivity, short time-consuming, and analysis of one billion base pairs simultaneously is a new revolution in the history of sequencing technology. The whole human genome sequences can be sequenced in couple of months using this technology. This will greatly facilitate the process of post-genome studies [8]. One of the key points of this technology is to gain immobilized luciferase with good thermal stability.

Traditionally, chemical method is used to get biotin-modified enzyme to make enzyme immobilize on the streptavidin-coated beads surface with the specific binding characteristics between biotin and streptavidin. However, the method of chemical modification has shortcomings, such as no specification, affection of the active site of enzyme, tedious operations, and uneven products. Biotin ligase can catalyze biotin to attach covalently to the ε-NH$_2$ of the Lys122 of biotin carboxyl carrier protein (BCCP), which is the unique receptor of biotin in *E. coli* [9, 10]. Exogenous protein fused with the C-terminal 87 amino acids of BCCP (BCCP87) will be biotinylated in *E. coli* [11, 12] with high activity due to the BCCP87 as a linker to make the unique biotinylated site far away from active site. Biotinylated firefly luciferase had been expressed in *E. coli* through the fusion with BCCP [13]. However, this biotinylated luciferase similar to wild-type luciferase has a poor thermal stability especially when the external environment temperature exceeds 40 °C [14]. The thermal stability of North American firefly luciferase (*Photinus pyralis*) can be enhanced by site-directed mutagenesis [15]. However, to the best of our knowledge, the expression of thermal-stable biotinylated North American firefly luciferase has not been reported.

In order to prepare immobilized luciferase with high stability and good reusability for application to solid-phase or large-scale pyrosequencing, the fusion protein consisted of BCCP87 and thermal-stable mutant North American firefly luciferase was biotinylated and expressed in *E. coli*. The biotinylated thermal-stable luciferase had properties of good stability, easily immobilized, and successfully applied to solid-phase pyrosequencing.

2   Materials

1. Ultra-Weak Chemiluminescence Analyzer System (Institute of Biophysics Chinese Academy of Science).

2. EDC-810-type gene amplification instrument (Dongsheng Innovation Biotech Co., Ltd., China).

3. PowerPac 1000 high-voltage power supply (BIO-RAD company, USA).

4. GenGenius gel imager (Syngene Corporation, USA).

5. Gene Spe III 7A0-0038 UV–visible spectrophotometer (NaKa Instruments Corporation, Japan).

6. Beckman 21R-type refrigerated centrifuge (Beckman Coulter Co., Ltd., USA).

7. Restriction endonucleases of *Bam*H I, *Hind* III, and *Nde* I were purchased from Dalian TakaRa Company.

8. APS (adenosyl sulfuric acid), Apyrase, Luciferin, and luciferase were purchased from Sigma (St. Louis, MO) Company.

9. Dynabeads TM-280 Streptavidin (streptavidin–biotin-coated magnetic beads) were purchased from Shanghai Invitrogen Corporation.

10. Plasmid pGEM-Luc was purchased from Promega (Madison, WI) Company.

11. Deoxy-α-sulfide adenosine triphosphate (dATPαS), dGTP, dTTP, and dCTP were purchased from Amersham Pharmacia, Biotech Company.

12. Klenow DNA polymerase (ex-) and ATP sulfurylase were prepared in laboratory.

13. *E. coli* BL21 (DE3) was conserved in our laboratory.

14. Primers were synthesized by Shanghai Invitrogen Corporation; other chemical reagents were of analytical pure grade, all reagents were configured to use sterile deionized water.

3 Methods

3.1 Construction of pET28a-BCCP87-LUC Plasmid and Site-Directed Mutagenesis of Luciferase Gene

1. The luciferase gene (*luc*) was amplified using primers, 5′-GTGCGGATCCATGGAAGACG-CCAAA-3′ (*Bam*H I) and 5′-GCGTGCAAGCTTTT ACAATTTGGACTTTCC GCCCT-3′ (*Hind* III), with pGEM-LUC plasmid as a template.

2. The BCCP87 gene from *E. coli* was amplified using primers, 5′-CA-TCATATGGAAGCGCCAGCAGC-3′ (*Nde* I), and 5′-GTGTGTGGATCCCTCGATGAC-GACCAG-3′ (*Bam*H I).

3. The BCCP87 gene was inserted into the plasmid pET28a (+), and then *luc* gene was inserted into the downstream of BCCP87 gene.

4. Site-directed mutagenesis was performed by the method of Overlap Extension PCR (OE-PCR) [16]. The primers, 5′-biotin-CCTTCCGCATAGAACTCTCTGCGTCAGATTCTCG-3′ and 5′-biotin-CGAGAATCTGACGCAGAGAGTTCTATG CGGAAGG-3′, were used to introduce the mutation at 215 site (A215L) of luciferase.

5. The primers, 5′-biotin-CTATTCTGATTACACCCAAGGGG GATGATAAACC-3′ and 5′-biotin-CGGTTTATCATCCCCC TTGGGTGTAATCAGAATAG-3′, were used to introduce the mutation at 354 site (E354K) of luciferase (*see* **Note 1**).

6. The recombinant plasmid was transformed into *E. coli* BL21 (DE3). The positive clones were screened by PCR and sequenced by Shanghai Invitrogen Corporation.

3.2 Western Blot Analysis and Activity Assay of Fusion Protein (BCCP87-LUC)

1. The positive clone was inoculated into LB medium (kan⁺, 30 mg/L) and induced overnight (16 °C, 200 r/min) with IPTG.

2. The bacteria were harvested and broken by ultrasonic, and then centrifuged for 30 min at $12,000 \times g$ to get supernatant for SDS-PAGE (12 %) analysis.

3. Western blot was performed using horseradish peroxidase-labeled avidin to analyze whether the fusion protein was biotinylated in vivo.

4. The fusion protein was purified by nickel ion affinity chromatography.

5. 1 μL of different concentrations of commercial luciferase was added to 10 μL of reaction buffer (0.1 mol/L Tris-Ac pH 7.9, 0.5 mmol/L EDTA, 5 mmol/L Mg(Ac)₂, 0.4 mg/mL PVP, 0.02 % BSA, 1 mmol/L DTT, 0.4 mmol/L D-luciferin, 5 μmol/L ATP) to measure signal intensity, respectively, to get the standard curve of "signal intensity-activity units."

6. The signal of fusion protein with an optimal concentration was detected under the same conditions to calculate the specific activity. The concentration of the fusion protein was measured by ultraviolet spectrophotometry.

3.3 The Thermal Stability of BCCP87-LUC

1. Thermal stability of mutant luciferase (BCCP-LUC) was detected by placing the enzyme at 40 °C, 42 °C, 45 °C, 47 °C, 49 °C, and 50 °C for 10 min, respectively, and at 43 °C for 10 min, 15 min, 20 min, 25 min, 30 min, 35 min and 40 min, respectively, to detect remaining, activity (*see* **Notes 2–3**).

3.4 Activity Assay and Washing Tolerance of the BCCP-LUC

1. 10 μL of streptavidin-coated magnetic beads were washed with 50 μL of washing buffer (0.1 mol/L Tris-Ac pH 7.9, 0.5 mmol/L EDTA, 5 mmol/L Mg(Ac)₂, 0.4 mg/mL PVP, 0.02 % BSA, 1 mmol/L DTT) twice.

2. Resuspended in 40 μL of washing buffer, and then 10 μL of BCCP-LUC were added.

3. After incubation at 4 °C for 1 h, the mixture was placed on the magnet for 1 min to discard the supernatant, and the beads were washed twice.

4. Resuspended in 10 μL of washing buffer to get bead-immobilized luciferase (bead-LUC).

5. Detected the activity of bead-LUC.

6. To examine the washing tolerance of the bead-LUC, the bead-LUC was washed nine times, and the remaining activity was detected after every three times of washing (*see* **Note 5**).

7. The relative activity of washed bead-LUC was calculated with the initial activity of bead-LUC as 100 %.

3.5 Application of Bead-LUC to Pyrosequencing

1. A synthesized DNA template (*see* **Note 5**) was sequenced using sequencing mixture containing 2 μL of bead-LUC, 1 μL of solid-phase single-strand DNA template, and 10 μL of sequencing buffer (0.1 mol/L Tris-Ac pH 7.9, 0.5 mmol/L EDTA, 5 mmol/L Mg(Ac)$_2$, 0.4 mg/mL PVP, 0.02 % BSA, 1 mmol/L DTT, 4 μmol/L APS, 0.4 mmol/L D-luciferin, 90 U/mL Klenow (exo⁻) DNA polymerase, 0.2 U/mL ATP sulfurylase).

2. Signal was detected by BPLC when the corresponding dNTP was added one by one (*see* **Notes 6–7**).

3.6 Application of Biotinylated ATP Sulfurylase Combined with Bead-LUC to Pyrosequencing

1. The biotinylated ATPS prepared by our laboratory [17] (ATP sulfurylase, ATPS, EC 2.7.7.4) and biotinylated luciferase were co-immobilized on beads to get the bead-ATPS-LUC. The bead-ATPS-LUC was also applied to pyrosequencing, and the protocol was as proposed in Sect. 2.2.5. The only difference was that ATP sulfurylase was absent in sequencing buffer.

4 Method Validation

The sequencing result of positive recombinant plasmid demonstrated that the BCCP87-LUC was successfully mutated at the site of 215 (A215L) and 354 (E354K). The result of SDS-PAGE analysis showed that the soluble fusion protein with the molecular weight of 77 kDa could be obtained in the supernatant. Western blot analysis (Fig. 1, lane 2) indicated that a specific reaction was occurred between the fusion protein and the horseradish peroxidase (HRP)-conjugated streptavidin, which indicated that the fusion protein was biotinylated in *E. coli*. The specific activity of the purified BCCP87-LUC was detected and calculated as 2.03×10^9 RLU/mg.

In order to verify whether the thermal stability of the mutant luciferase (BCCP87-LUC) was enhanced, the activities of the luciferase placed in various temperatures for 10 min were measured. The results (Fig. 2a) showed that the activity of wild-type luciferase decreased rapidly while the temperature was higher than 38 °C and no activity was detected when the temperature was at 45 °C. However, the activity of mutant luciferase was decreased slowly from 37 °C to 46 °C, and the remaining activity was more than 50 % while the temperature was at 45 °C. In addition, the activity of luciferase at 43 °C for different time period was measured.

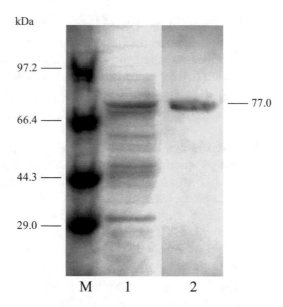

Fig. 1 SDS-PAGE and Western blot analysis of the fusion protein expressed in *E. coli* BL21 (DE3) M: protein marker; *Lane 1*: Supernatant of the lysate of clones after being induced with IPTG for 12 h; *Lane 2*: Western blot analysis of biotinylated fusion protein with horseradish peroxidase-conjugated streptavidin (HRP)

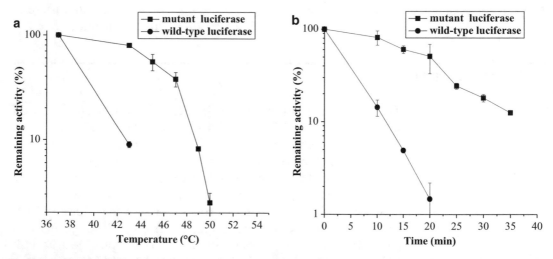

Fig. 2 Comparison of thermostability of mutant luciferase (BCCP87-LUC) and wild-type luciferase. (**a**) Remaining activities of mutant luciferase and wild-type luciferase were detected after being incubated at various temperatures for 10 min. (**b**) Remaining activities of mutant luciferase and wild-type luciferase were detected after being incubated at 43 °C for different time periods. Every experiment was carried out three times

The results (Fig. 2b) showed that the activity of the wild-type luciferase was only retained 10 % after placing in 43 °C for 10 min, and was inactivated after 20 min. But the activity of mutant-type luciferase was retained 80 % after placed at 43 °C for 10 min and more than 50 % after 20 min. These results suggested that the thermal stability of the mutant-type luciferase was improved significantly.

The fusion protein (BCCP87-LUC) was immobilized on the streptavidin-coated magnetic beads through the affinity between streptavidin and biotin. The immobilized BCCP87-LUC (bead-LUC) could be separated from the solution by magnets. The activity of bead-LUC detected by the method proposed in Sect. 2.2.3 was 2.1×10^5 RLU/μL beads.

The beads in chip-based pyrosequencing would be washed many times to remove the influence of prior dNTPs. Therefore, washing tolerance is acquired for the bead-LUC. In this experiment, the bead-LUC was washed for nine times, and the remaining activity was detected after every three times of washing. The remaining activity of bead-LUC after washed three times, six times, and nine times was 95.2 %, 90.1 %, and 83.4 %, respectively. The loss activity of every three times of washing was from 5 % to 7 %. The loss of beads during manual washing process was considered as the main course of activity decreasing, therefore, mild operation was needed in washing steps to reduce the loss of beads during pyrosequencing.

Large-scale chip-based pyrosequencing requires not only immobilized luciferase but also immobilized ATP sulfurylase. We had successfully expressed biotinylated ATP sulfurylase (BCCP-ATPS) previously, which could also be immobilized on streptavidin-coated magnetic beads [17]. The BCCP-ATPS and BCCP87-LUC were co-immobilized on streptavidin-coated magnetic beads to carry out pyrosequencing with the same protocol as that of pyrosequencing using bead-LUC. The results of pyrosequencing were shown in Fig. 3. Another experiment showed that the signal

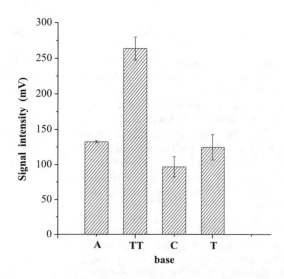

Fig. 3 The results of pyrosequencing with LUC and ATPS co-immobilized on beads

intensity was increased by using more bead-ATPS-LUC. The correct sequencing results indicated that BCCP-ATPS and BCCP87-LUC were able to be co-immobilized on beads and applied to pyrosequencing with a good quantitative capacity. These characters met the needs of large-scale chip-based pyrosequencing.

5 Technical Notes

1. The bold represented the mutant bases.
2. The wild-type luciferase served as a control. Each experiment was carried out three times in parallel.
3. The activity of bead-LUC was detected as described in Sect. 2.2.2.
4. The loss of beads during manual washing process was considered as the main course of activity decreasing, therefore, mild operation was needed in washing steps to reduce the loss of beads during pyrosequencing.
5. The sequence of the DNA template was A-T-T-C-T.
6. Before each addition of the dNTP, the beads were washed three times with sequencing buffer to eliminate the effect of prior dNTPs. Parallel experiment was carried out three times.
7. The result of sequencing was consistent with the sequence of template and showed a good quantitative capacity. Multiple washing of bead-LUC has no influence on the operations of pyrosequencing.

References

1. Deluca M (1976) Firefly luciferase. Adv Enzymol Relat Areas Mol Biol 44:37–68
2. Elahi E, Ronaghi M (2004) Pyrosequencing: a tool for DNA sequencing analysis. Methods Mol Biol 255:211–219
3. Hyman ED (1988) A new method of sequencing DNA. Anal Biochem 174:423–436
4. Zhang XD, Wu HP, Zhou GH (2006) Pyrosequencing and its application in genetical analysis. Chinese J Anal Chem 34:582–586
5. Wang WP, Wu HP, Zhou GH (2008) Detection of avian influenza A virus using pyrosequencing. Chinese J Anal Chem 36:775–780
6. Yang HY, Xi T, Liang C, Chen ZY, Xu DB, Zhou GH (2009) Preparation of single-stranded DNA for pyrosequencing by linear-after-the-exponential-polymerase chain reaction. Chinese J Anal Chem 37:489–494
7. Zhang XD, Wu HP, Chen ZY, Zhou GH (2009) Differential gene expression analysis by combin-

ing sequence-tagged reverse-transcription polymerase chain reaction with pyrosequencing. Chinese J Anal Chem 37:1107–1112
8. Chi KR (2008) The year of sequencing. Nat Methods 5:11–14
9. Li SJ, Cronan JE Jr (1992) The gene encoding the biotin carboxylase subunit of Escherichia coli acetyl-CoA carboxylase. J Biol Chem 267:855–863
10. Reed KE, Cronan JE Jr (1991) *Escherichia coli* exports previously folded and biotinated protein domains. J Biol Chem 266:11425–11428
11. Weiss E, Chatellier J, Orfanoudakis G (1994) In vivo biotinylated recombinant antibodies: construction, characterization, and application of a bifunctional Fab-BCCP fusion protein produced in *Escherichia coli*. Protein Expr Purif 5:509–517
12. Smith PA, Tripp BC, DiBlasio-Smith EA, Lu Z, LaVallie ER, McCoy JM (1998) A plasmid

expression system for quantitative in vivo biotinylation of thioredoxin fusion proteins in *Escherichia coli*. Nucleic Acids Res 26: 1414–1420

13. Wang CY, Hitz S, Andrade JD, Stewart RJ (1997) Specific immobilization of firefly luciferase through a biotin carboxyl carrier protein domain. J Biol Chem 246:133–139

14. Tafreshi NKH, Hosseinkhani S, Sadeghizadeh M, Sadeghi M, Ranjbar B, Naderi-Manesh H (2007) The influence of insertion of a critical residue (Arg356) in structure and bioluminescence spectra of firefly luciferase. J Biol Chem 282:8641–8647

15. White PJ, Squirrell DJ, Arnaud P, Lowe CR, Murray JA (1996) Improved thermostability of the North American firefly luciferase: saturation mutagenesis at position 354. Biochem J 319:34–350

16. Urban A, Neukirchen S, Jaeger KE (1997) A rapid and efficient method for site-directed mutagenesis using one-step overlap extension PCR. Nucleic Acids Res 25:2227–2228

17. Zou BJ, Luo J, Wu HP (2009) Expression, immobilization and application of biotinylated ATP sulfurylase. Prog Biochem Biophys 36:923–928

Chapter 15

Expression of Thermostable Recombinant *Luciola lateralis* Luciferase and Its Function on Setting Up of Heat-Stable Pyrosequencing System

Shu Xu, Bingjie Zou, Qinxin Song, and Guohua Zhou

Abstract

Pyrosequencing is a technology to determine DNA sequence based on extending. The poor stability of luciferase in pyrosequencing reaction mixture leads to disappointed results, which limits the application and promotion of pyrosequencing. In order to set up a heat-stable pyrosequencing system, we used genetic engineering technology to express recombinant thermostable *Luciola lateralis* luciferase (rt-LlL) with His-tag on N-end. The crude protein was purified with Ni-affinity chromatography. The rt-LlL was obtained, whose molecular mass was about 60 kDa. With commercial *Photinus pyralis* luciferase (PpL) to be standard, the activity detection demonstrated that the specific activity of rt-LlL was 4.29×10^{10} RLU/mg, which was higher than that of PpL. Another result indicated that rt-LlL kept high activity at 50 °C and more than 90 % of original activity at 40 °C for 25 min. We got correct results and better signals when substituting the commercial PpL with rt-LlL in pyrosequencing system, which laid the foundation of building stable and reliable pyrosequencing system.

Key words *Luciola lateralis* luciferase, Mutation, Good thermostability, High specific activity, Pyrosequencing

1 Introduction

Pyrosequencing is a technology to determine DNA sequence based on extending [1, 2], which is under the action of DNA polymerase, ATP sulfurylase [3, 4] or pyruvate phosphate dikinase (PPDK) [5], luciferase [6, 7], and apyrase. Due to its convenience, high throughput, and automation, pyrosequencing is largely applied on analysis of single nucleotide polymorphism (SNP) [8, 9], rapid detection of viruses and bacteria [10, 11], and analysis of difference on gene expression [12–14]. However, commercial *Photinus pyralis* luciferase (PpL) is used in conventional pyrosequencing reagent, whose poor heat stability makes the reaction mixture lose its activity in room temperature so that the signal of pyrosequencing result is undermined seriously. What's more, the measures taken to keep the

Guohua Zhou and Qinxin Song (eds.), *Advances and Clinical Practice in Pyrosequencing*, Springer Protocols Handbooks, DOI 10.1007/978-1-4939-3308-2_15, © Springer Science+Business Media New York 2016

activity of reagent greatly increase the difficulty and cost of transportation and operation. Therefore, replacing the commercial PpL in traditional reagent with kinds of thermostable luciferase will make great contribution to the establishment of a stable and reliable pyrosequencing system. This system will be extremely beneficial to the promotion of pyrosequencing technology.

Actually, site mutations on commercial PpL have been done in order to improve its heat stability [6, 7]. However, the poor special activity and low soluble expression amount of mutant PpL limit the application in large quantity. According to literatures, *Luciola lateralis* luciferase (LlL) has greater special activity than PpL. The thermostability of LlL is greatly increased when 217 Ala was mutated into Leu [15]. However, the mutant LlL can only be purchased in Japan, so we can only express it by ourselves.

On the basis of code preference [16], the gene of recombinant thermostable *Luciola lateralis* luciferase (rt-LlL) was synthesized and inserted into expression vector. The rt-LlL was expressed and purified. Special activity and heat stability was also determined. The results of pyrosequencing with rt-LlL demonstrated better stability than conventional ones.

2 Materials

1. ArcticExpress strain was used for the expression luciferase.

2. pET28a(+) plasmid was restored in our lab.

3. *Hin*dIII and *Nde*I restriction endonucleases were purchased from Takara.

4. ATP sulfurylase, apyrase, and D-luciferin were obtained from Sigma.

5. Commercial *Photinus pyralis* luciferase was obtained from Promega.

6. dATPαS, dGTP, dTTP, and dCTP were obtained from Amersham Pharmacia Biotech.

3 Methods

3.1 Construction of Recombinant Bacteria and Expression of rt-LlL

1. The whole gene of rt-LlL was synthesized with mutation of Ala217Leu, which was then inserted into pET28a (+) plasmid after digested by *Hin*dIII and *Nde*I.

2. The recombinant plasmid was transformed into ArcticExpress.

3. The nucleotide sequence of transformants was determined. Transformants were cultured in the presence of 0.1 mM IPTG (*see* **Note 1**).

3.2 Purification of rt-LlL and Activity Assay

1. ArcticExpress cells expressing the rt-LlL were grown and harvested by centrifugation.

2. The supernatant of the crude extract was loaded onto a column of Ni-NTA. The column was eluted with buffer containing 30 mM and 50 mM imidazole, respectively.

3. Fractions with rt-LlL were obtained by buffer containing 300 mM imidazole and were ultrafiltrated.

4. The commercial PpL was diluted into different concentrations. One microliter of the diluted commercial luciferase was added to 10 μL assay-measured solution (Tris-EDTA, Mg(Ac)$_2$, PVP, DTT, BSA, APS, D-luciferin, ATP, respectively).

5. The mixed solution was tested in BPCL to test counts and make counts-units standard chart. The rt-LlL was tested in the same activity and condition.

3.3 Comparison of the Thermostability of the rt-LlL and Wild Commercial Photinus pyralis Luciferase

1. The rt-LlL was incubated at 25, 30, 35, 40, 45, and 50 °C for 10 min, respectively. The residual luciferase activity was measured at various times.

2. On the other way, the rt-LlL was incubated at 40 °C for 0, 5, 10, 15, 20, and 25 min, respectively. The residual luciferase activity was measured at various times.

3.4 Thermostability of Pyrosequencing with rt-LlL

1. In order to verify the thermostability of pyrosequencing with rt-LlL, rt-LlL was added into reaction mixture (Tris-EDTA, Mg(Ac)$_2$, PVP, DTT, BSA, APS, D-luciferin, ATP sulfurase, Klenow (exo$^-$), luciferase, apyrase) and incubated at 37 °C for 0, 30, and 60 min, respectively.

2. After that, the artificial single-strand DNA template (AGTTAA GCTATATAAGAAGCTGAAAAGAGAA) was sequenced with traditional pyrosequencing reaction mixture as comparison.

4 Method Validation

4.1 Expression of rt-LlL

The recombinant bacteria were cultured and expressed. The protein of ArcticExpress transformed with recombinant plasmid was analyzed by SDS-PAGE with the protein of ArcticExpress transformed with pET28a(+) as comparison (Fig. 1). The protein with mass of 60 kDa can be observed in lanes 1 and 2. This protein had same mass as rt-LlL and could be treated as rt-LlL.

4.2 Purification of rt-LlL and Assay of Activity

After purification, fractions containing high rt-LlL activity were obtained by buffer containing 300 mM imidazole. The protein was ultrafiltrated to concentrate. The SDS-PAGE result showed the product is the rt-LlL (Fig. 2). With standard commercial PpL, the activity test demonstrated the specific activity of the rt-LlL was

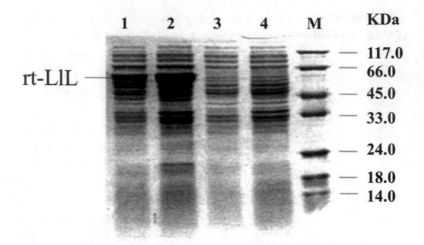

Fig. 1 SDS-PAGE analysis of rt-LIL. *Lane 1*, supernatant of the lysate of ArcticExpress transformed with pET28a(+)-LIL after induced; *Lane 2*, total protein of the ArcticExpress transformed with pET28a(+)-LIL after induced; *Lane 3*, supernatant of the lysate of ArcticExpress transformed with pET28a(+) after induced; *Lane 4*, total protein of the ArcticExpress transformed with pET28a(+) after induced; *M*, protein marker

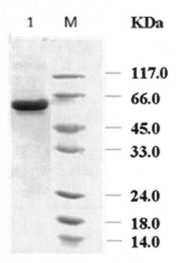

Fig. 2 SDS-PAGE analysis of purified rt-LIL. *M*, protein marker; *Lane 1*, purified rt-LIL

4.29×10^{10} RLU/mg (Fig. 3), which was higher than that of commercial PpL (3.9×10^{10} RLU/mg). The rt-LIL guaranteed the quantity of signal of pyrosequencing.

4.3 Thermostability of rt-LIL

In order to compare the thermostability of rt-LIL and commercial PpL, we incubated them at different temperature for 10 min and assayed the activity, respectively. On the other way, we incubated them at 40 °C for different time and assayed the activity, respectively (Fig. 4). The activity of commercial PpL decreased

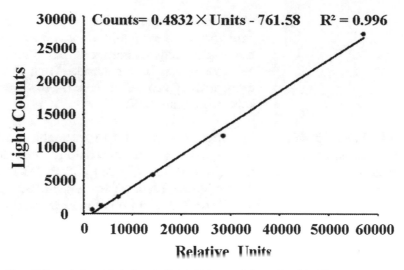

Fig. 3 The relationship between light counts and the units of luciferase

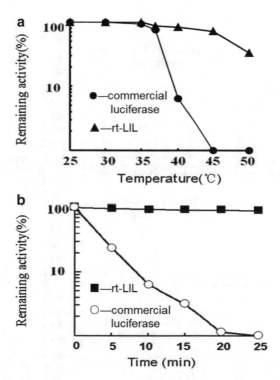

Fig. 4 Thermostability of rt-LIL and commercial *Photinus pyralis* luciferase. (**a**) Remaining activity of rt-LIL and commercial *Photinus pyralis* luciferase after incubated at various temperatures for 10 min, respectively. (**b**) Remaining activity of rt-LIL and commercial *Photinus pyralis* luciferase after incubated at 40 °C for different time, respectively

when incubated at temperature more than 37 °C. When incubated at 40 °C for 5 min, the commercial PpL remained 30 % of the original activity. For more than 5 min, only 10 % of the original activity can be measured. When incubated for 20 min, no more activity can be observed. However, the activity of rt-LlL kept more than 90 %.

4.4 Thermostability of Pyrosequencing with rt-LlL

In order to verify the thermostability of pyrosequencing with rt-LlL, rt-LlL and commercial PpL were added into reaction mixture (Tris-EDTA, Mg(Ac)$_2$, PVP, DTT, BSA, APS, D-luciferin, ATP sulfurase, Klenow (exo$^-$), luciferase, apyrase) and incubated at 37 °C for 0, 30, and 60 min, respectively. After that, the artificial single-strand DNA template (AGTTAAGCTATATAAGAAGCTG AAAAGAGAA) was sequenced (Fig. 5). The signal of traditional pyrosequencing decreased more than 80 % after incubated at 37 °C for 30 min and cannot be observed after incubated for 60 min. However, the signal of pyrosequencing with rt-LlL was still reliable and clear when incubated at 37 °C for 60 min.

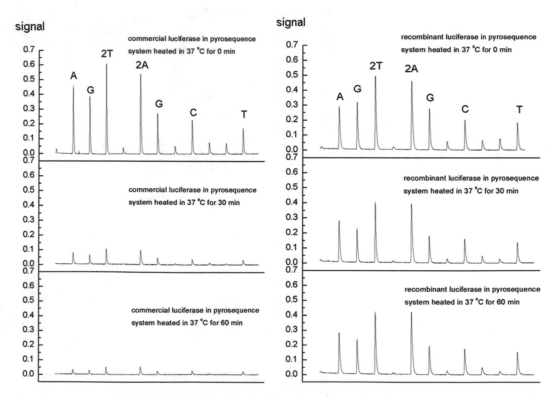

Fig. 5 Pyrograms of artificial single-strand DNA template by using conventional pyrosequencing reagent and the rt-LlL contained pyrosequencing reagent incubating at 37 °C for different time. The order of dNTP dispensing is C-A-G-T

5 Technical Notes

1. To obtain more products, the temperature was 25 °C when cultured in the presence of 0.1 mM IPTG. The expression level was too low when cultured in 37 °C.

References

1. Zhou GH, Kajiyama T, Gotou M et al (2006) Enzyme system for improving the detection limit in pyrosequencing. Anal Chem 78(13):4482–4489
2. Wu HP, Wu WJ, Zhou GH et al (2011) Highly sensitive pyrosequencing based on the capture of free adenosine 5′ phosphosulfate with adenosine triphosphate sulfurylase. Anal Chem 89(9):3600–3605
3. Luo J, Wu WJ, Zou BJ et al (2007) Expression and purification of ATP sulfurylase from *Saccharomyces cerevisiae* in *Escherichia coli* and its application in pyrosequencing. Chin J Biotechnol 23(4):623–627
4. Zou BJ, Luo J, Wu HP et al (2009) Expression, immobilization and application of biotinylated ATP sulfurylase. Prog Biochem Biophy 36(7): 923–928
5. Zou BJ, Chen ZY, Zhou GH (2008) Expression of PPDK from *Microbispora rosea* subsp. *aerata* in *Escherichia coli* and its application in pyrosequencing. Chin J Biotechnol 24(4):679–683
6. Rong JJ, Cheng ZY, Zhou GH (2007) Immobilization of luciferase by cloning and expression of biotinylated luciferase. China Biotechnology 27(9):41–46
7. Zhu SH, Zou BJ, Wu HP et al (2010) Preparation of thermostable biotinylated firefly luciferase and its application to pyrosequencing. Chinese J Anal Chem 38(4):458–463
8. Huang H, Wu HP, Zhou GH et al (2009) Single nucleotide polymorphism typing based on pyrosequencing chemistry and acryl-modified glass chip. Electrophoresis 30(6): 991–998
9. Zhou ZY, Limor J, Goldman I et al (2006) Pyrosequencing—a high-throughput method for detecting single nucleotide polymorphisms (SNPs) in the dihydrofolate reductase and dihydropteroate synthetase genes of *Plasmodium falciparum*. J Clin Microbiol 44:3900–3910
10. Wang WP, Wu HP, Zhou GH (2008) Detection of avian influenza A virus using pyrosequencing. Anal Biochem 36(6): 775–780
11. Yang HY, Xi T, Liang C et al (2009) Preparation of single-stranded DNA template for pyrosequencing by linear-after-the exponential-polymerase chain reaction. Anal Biochem 37(4):489–494
12. Zhang XD, Wu HP, Chen ZY et al (2009) Dye-free gene expression detection by sequence-tagged reverse-transcription polymerase chain reaction coupled with pyrosequencing. Anal Chem 81(1):273–281
13. Song QX, Jing H, Zhou GH et al (2010) Gene expression analysis on a photodiode array-based bioluminescence analyzer by using sensitivity-improved SRPP. Analyst 135: 1315–1319
14. Song QX, Wu HP, Zhou GH et al (2010) Pyrosequencing on nicked dsDNA generated by nicking endonucleases. Anal Chem 82(5):2074–2081
15. Kajiyama N, Nakano E (1994) Enhancement of thermostability of firefly luciferase from *Luciola lateralis* by a single amino acid substitution. Biosci Biotechnol Biochem 58(6):1170–1171
16. Tatsumi H, Kajiyama N, Nakano E (1992) Molecular cloning and expression in *Escherichia coli* of a cDNA clone encoding luciferase of a firefly, *Luciola lateralis*. Biochim Biophys Acta 1131(2):161–165

Expression and Purification of ATP Sulfurylase from *Saccharomyces cerevisias* in *Escherichia coli* and Its Application in Pyrosequencing

Juan Luo, Wenjuan Wu, Bingjie Zou, Qinxin Song, and Guohua Zhou

Abstract

ATP sulfurylase (ATPS, C 2.7.7.4) reversibly catalyzes the reaction between ATP and sulfate to produce APS and pyrophosphate (PPi), and has been used in pyrosequencing. The gene coding ATP sulfurylase was amplified from the genomic DNA of *Saccharomyces cerevisias* (CICC 1202), and cloned into prokaryotic expression plasmid pET28a(+) to provide a recombinant expression plasmid pET28a(+)-ATPS. Upon IPTG induction, ATP sulfurylase was produced by *E. coli* BL21(DE3) harboring the recombinant expression plasmid pET28a(+)-ATPS. The relative molecular weight of recombinant ATP sulfurylase with His tag was about 60 kD. Including the extra desalting step, only two purification steps are required to obtain the recombinant ATPS with electrophoretic pure grade. The specific activity of the purified recombinant ATP sulfurylase was as high as 5.1×10^4 U/mg. The successful application of the enzyme in pyrosequencing was also demonstrated.

Key words ATP sulfurylase, *Saccharomyces cerevisias*, Expression, Purification, Pyrosequencing

1 Introduction

ATP sulfurylase (ATPS, EC 2.7.7.4) is a ubiquitous enzyme found in plants, animals, and microorganisms, and plays different roles in different organisms. In plants and some microorganisms, ATPS catalyzes the reaction between ATP and sulfate to produce adenosine phosphosulfate (APS) and pyrophosphate (PPi). This is the first step in the biological assimilation of inorganic sulfate. In some chemoautotrophic bacteria [1] and chemolithotroph bacteria [2], ATPS catalyzes the final step in the overall oxidation of sulfide to sulfate (the backward direction of the following reaction).

$$ATP + SO_4{}^{2-} \leftrightarrow APS + PPi$$

ATPS has been extracted and purified from *Penicillium chrysogenum* [3], rat liver [4], and cabbage [5]. ATPS genes have been cloned from prokaryotes [6], lower eukaryotes [7], animals [8], as

Guohua Zhou and Qinxin Song (eds.), *Advances and Clinical Practice in Pyrosequencing*, Springer Protocols Handbooks, DOI 10.1007/978-1-4939-3308-2_16, © Springer Science+Business Media New York 2016

well as plants [9], and expressed in different hosts. The *E. coli* ATPS is a heterodimer that is activated by GTP [6], whereas ATPS from yeast, fungi, and plant are monomers or homooligomers [5, 7]. Moreover, the structure–function studies, using amino acid modification, provide us more information about its function at molecular level [7].

ATPS coupled with luciferase has various applications, e.g., quantitative analysis of PPi [10], real-time studies of RNA synthesis [11], DNA sequencing [12], and the activity detection of DNA polymerase [13]. In the previous studies, pCR II [7] and pSVL [8] were used as expression vectors, but it is very difficult to purify the expressed protein. In our studies, pET28a(+) (Novagen Corporation) was used as an expression vector, which can express the recombinant protein with a His-Tag. Including the extra desalting step, only two purification steps are required to obtain the recombinant ATPS with electrophoretic pure grade. The successful application of the enzyme in pyrosequencing was also demonstrated.

2   Materials

1. *Saccharomyces cerevisias* (CICC 1202) was purchased from CICC in China. *E. coli* BL2(DE3) and plasmid pET28a(+) were gifts from Dr. Diao Zheng-Yu (Huadong Research Institute for Medicine and Biotechnics, Nanjing 210002, China).

2. Restriction enzyme, *Taq* DNA polymerase, T4DNA ligase, λ-Eco T14 I digest DNA Marker, Protein Marker, and DNA Fragment Purification Kit Ver.2.0 were purchased from TaKaRa Corporation.

3. Klenow (exo-) DNA polymerase, D-luciferin, and luciferase were purchased from Promega Corporation.

4. Apyrase was purchased from Sigma Corporation.

5. Yeast Extract and Tryptone were purchased from Oxoid Corporation.

6. IPTG and Lysozyme were purchased from Amresco Corporation.

7. His·Bind Resin and His·Bind Columns were purchased from Novagen Corporation.

8. The 10 kD ultrafiltration tube was purchased from Millipore.

3   Methods

3.1   Plasmid Construction

1. Genomic DNA of *Saccharomyces cerevisias* was prepared using the method of Phenol-Chloroform. The forward oligonucleotide primer ATPS-P1 (5′-GTGTGT **GGATCC** ATGCC TGCTCCTCACGGTGGTA-3′) and the bold letters underlined represent the Bam H I site, and the reverse primer

ATPS-P2(5′-GTGTGT**AAGCTT**CTACTTTTGAGATGGGA GCATT-3′) and the bold letters underlined represent the Hind III site; these were designed according to the MET3 gene [14] and were synthesized by Invitrogen Co.

2. Using these primers and the Genomic DNA of *Saccharomyces cerevisias*, a 1597 bp DNA fragment was amplified by the polymerase chain reaction (PCR). The reaction volumes were 25 μL, and contained 1× Taq PCR reaction buffer, 1.5 mmol/L $MgCl_2$, 0.2 mmol/L each dNTP, 0.4 μmol/L each primer, 0.5 U of Taq polymerase (TaKaRa), and 10–20 ng of genomic DNA.

3. Thermal cycling was carried out at an initial denaturation of 3 min at 94 °C, followed by 30 cycles of 10 s at 94 °C, 20 s at 58 °C, 90 s at 72 °C, and a terminal extension of 7 min at 72 °C.

4. The fragment was purified using the DNA Fragment Purification Kit and digested with Bam H I and Hind III, and then inserted into the Bam H I site and the Hind III site of the pET28a(+), yielding the recombinant plasmid pET28a(+)-ATPS. The *E. coli* BL21(DE3) was transformed with pET28a(+)-ATPS. The clone was screened by digesting plasmids extracted from the clones with Bam H I and Hind III, and then the positive clone was sequenced by Invitrogen Co.

3.2 Expression of ATPS

1. The *E. coli* BL21 (DE3) [pET28a(+)-ATPS] was spread and grown on an LB plate (containing 30 μg/mL Kan) at 37 °C overnight. Single colony was inoculated in 5 mL of LB (containing 30 μg/mL Kan) and incubated at 37 °C with 200 rpm/min (2233 × *g*) shaking overnight, and then 0.5 mL of the overnight cultures was inoculated in 50 mL of LB (containing 30 μg/mL Kan) and incubated at 37 °C with 200 rpm/min (2233 × *g*) shaking, until the cultures reached an OD600 of 0.6–0.7.

2. At this time, 1 mL of the cultures was collected for SDS-PAGE analysis, and then 0.1 mmol/L IPTG was added and incubated at 30 °C with 200 rpm/min (2233 × *g*) shaking for 5 h. During this period, 1 mL of the cultures was collected for SDS-PAGE analysis at the incubation time of 1, 3, and 5 h, respectively.

3.3 Expression Form and Purification of ATPS

1. One hundred milliliters of the cultures incubated for 5 h with the induction of IPTG were centrifuged for 1 min at 12,000 rpm/min (13,400 × *g*) and washed with PBS, and then resuspended in 10 mL of 1× Binding Buffer containing 100 μg/mL lysozyme and 0.1 % Triton X-100.

2. Cells were broken by freezing and thawing the cells for three times, and were then sonicated in an ice bath. The broken

crude was 4 °C-centrifuged at 12,000 rpm/min (13,400 × g) for 20 min, and then the supernatant (*see* **Note 1**) and precipitate were collected, respectively, for SDS-PAGE analysis. The crude ATPS was purified by His·Bind Resin affinity chromatography. The detailed protocol can be found in Novegen His·Bind Resin Manual.

3.4 The Determination of the Protein Concentration

The protein concentration was determined by ultraviolet spectrophotometry at OD280. The standard curve was drawn with BSA.

3.5 Activity Detection

The activity was detected by coupling ATPS with luciferase [15]. The activity assay mixture contained 0.1 mol/L Tris-Ac (pH 7.75), 0.5 mmol/L EDTA, 5 mmol/L Mg (Ac)2, 0.4 mg/mL PVP, 0.02 % BSA, 1 mmol/L DTT, 4 μmol/L APS, 4 μmol/L PPi, 0.4 mmol/L D-luciferin, and 1.46 μg/mL luciferase. The ATPS from Sigma was used as a positive control (*see* **Note 2**).

3.6 The Application of the Recombinant ATPS in Pyrosequencing

Pyrosequencing [12] is a DNA sequencing method that employs multiple enzymatic reactions to monitor DNA synthesis. The standard pyrosequencing solution contains 90 U/mL Klenow (exo-) DNA polymerase, 2 U/mL Apyrase, 0.1 mol/L Tris-Ac (pH 7.75), 0.5 mmol/L EDTA, 5 mmol/L Mg(Ac)2, 0.4 mg/mL PVP, 0.02 % BSA, 1 mmol/L DTT, 4 μmol/L APS, 0.4 mmol/L D-luciferin, 1.46 μg/mL luciferase, and 0.2 U/mL ATPS. The target sequence of the single-strand DNA template is 5'-**GGTTCCAAGTCA** CCCCGCCCGC-3', and the bold letters underlined represent the sequence to be determined.

4 Method Validation

4.1 Plasmid Construction

Using these primers and genomic DNA of *Saccharomyces cerevisias*, a DNA fragment of 1597 bp was amplified by PCR (Fig. 1). The positive clone was screened by extracted plasmid and then digested it with *Bam*H I and *Hind* III, and both the 1597-bp fragment and the 5300-bp fragment representing the vector were obtained (Fig. 2). The sequencing results indicated that the fragment inserted in pET28a(+)-ATPS was MET3 gene [14] which encodes ATPS enzyme.

4.2 Expression of ATPS

The *E. coli* BL21(DE3) was transformed with pET28a(+)-ATPS. After IPTG induction, SDS-PAGE analysis was performed on the expressed products at different incubation times. As seen in Fig. 3, a recombinant protein band with 60 kD was successfully expressed after IPTG induction.

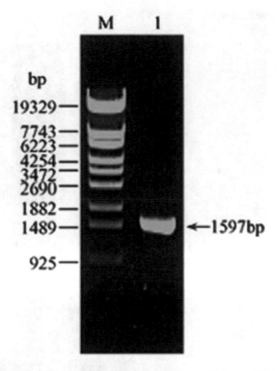

Fig. 1 The result of PCR amplification of ATPS gene *M*: λ-Eco T14 digest DNA marker; *lane 1*: PCR products of ATPS gene

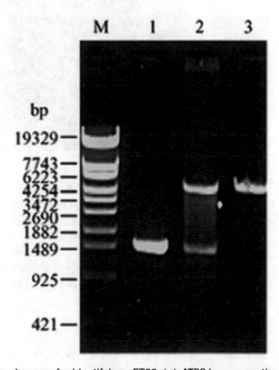

Fig. 2 Electrophogram for identifying pET28a(+)-ATPS by enzymatic digestion *M*: λ-Eco T14 digest DNA Marker; *lane 1*: PCR products of ATPS gene; *lane 2*: pET28a(+)-ATPS digested with Bam H I and Hind III; *lane 3*: pET28a(+) digested with Bam H I and Hind III

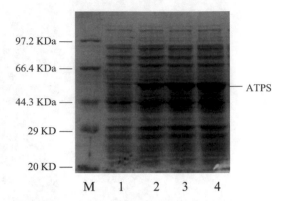

Fig. 3 SDS-PAGE analysis of recombinant ATPS expressed in *E. coli* BL (DE3) *M*: Protein Marker; *Lane 1*: Total protein of *E. coli* BL (DE3) transformed with pET28a(+)-ATPS without IPTG induction; *Lane 2–4*: Total protein of *E. coli* BL (DE3) transformed with pET28a(+)-ATPS after being induced with IPTG of 1 h, 3 h, and 5 h; respectively

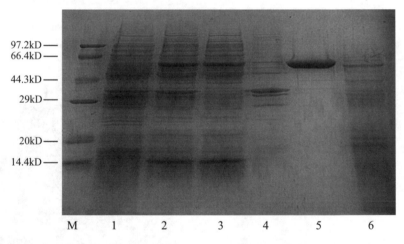

Fig. 4 SDS-PAGE analysis of expression pattern and purification of recombinant ATPS *M*: Protein Marker; *Lane 1*: Total protein of *E. coli* BL (DE3) transformed with pET28a(+)-ATPS without IPTG induction; *Lane 2*: Total protein of *E. coli* BL (DE3) transformed with pET28a(+)-ATPS after being induced with IPTG for 5 h; *Lane 3*: Supernatant of the lysate of *E. coli* BL21 (DE3) transformed with pET28a(+)-ATPS; *Lane 4*: Precipitate of the lysate of *E. coli* BL21 (DE3) transformed with pET28a(+)-ATPS; *Lane 5*: Purified recombinant ATPS; *Lane 6*: Commercial ATP sulfurylase

4.3 Expression Form and Purification of ATPS

Cells were broken by freeze–thaw for three times and sonication in an ice bath. This was centrifuged at 4 °C, 12,000 rpm/min ($13,400 \times g$) for 20 min and collected cellular and supernatant, respectively, for SDS-PAGE analysis. The result of SDS-PAGE analysis indicated that most of the recombinant ATPS was expressed as a soluble form (Fig. 4). The ATPS was purified by His·Bind Resin affinity chromatography. The supernatant was applied to the His·Bind column and washed with a buffer containing 60 mmol/L imidazole to remove hybrid protein, and then eluted with a buffer containing 200 mmol/L imidazole. The recombinant ATP sulfurylase with electrophoretic pure grade was obtained after ultrafiltration with the 10-kDa molecular weight cut-off membrane (Fig. 4). The recombinant ATPS had the same molecular weight, but is purer than the commercial one (see lane 6 in Fig. 4).

4.4   The Application of the Enzyme in Pyrosequencing

The successful application of the enzyme in pyrosequencing was demonstrated. Pyrosequencing is actually based on the detection of the PPi from a DNA strand extension reaction. Four kinds of dNTPs are added into the reaction solution one by one. When the added dNTP is complementary to the base in a template strand hybridized with a sequencing primer, a strand extension reaction occurs. It is followed by ATP production and luciferase reaction. A light signal is detected as a peak in a pyrogram. The relative intensity of each peak is proportional to the number of incorporated nucleotides. The principle of pyrosequencing can be described as follows:

$$\left(DNA\right)_n + dNTP \xrightarrow{\text{Polymerase}} PPi + \left(DNA\right)_{n+1} \tag{1}$$

$$PPi + APS \xrightarrow{\text{Sulfurylase}} ATP + SO_4^{2-} \tag{2}$$

$$ATP + Luciferin + O_2 \xrightarrow{\text{Luciferase}} AMP + CO_2 + Oxyluciferin + PPi + h\nu \tag{3}$$

$$ATP + dNTP \xrightarrow{\text{Apyrase}} ADP + dNDP + 2Pi \tag{4}$$

$$ADP + dNDP \xrightarrow{\text{Apyrase}} AMP + dNMP + 2Pi \tag{5}$$

The DNA template is an artificial single-strand oligonucleotide. The sequence of the template is ACTGAACCTTGG (the complementary sequence was TGACTTGGAACC). The dNTP dispensing order is G-A-C-T-G. The result can be seen in Fig. 5. Because the first base of the template is A, no extension signal but background signal was detected when the other three nucleotides were added. The first extension signal was obtained when dTTP was added, and the other signals can be obtained in a same way. Twelve extension peaks were obtained using the recombinant ATPS, and DNA sequence was determined as "ACTGAACCTTGG."

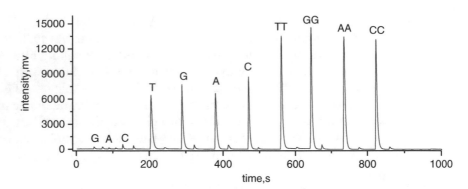

Fig. 5 Pyrogram of DNA sequencing with homemade ATPS Template: artificially synthesized oligonucleotide; order of dNTP dispensing: G-A-C-T-G with the double dispensing of each dNTP species

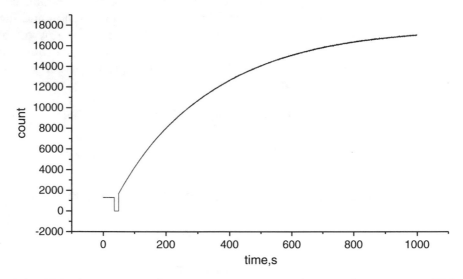

Fig. 6 Real-time bioluminescent traces for determining the activity of homemade recombinant ATPS

5   Technical Notes

1. Most of the recombinant ATPS was expressed as a soluble form.

2. ATPS from Sigma Chemical Co. was used as a standard for the detection, and the specific activity of ATPS was measured as 5.1×10^4 U/mg (Fig. 6).

References

1. Renosto F, Martin RL, Borrell JL et al (1991) ATP sulfurylase from trophosome tissue of Riftia pachyptila (hydrothermal vent tube worm). Arch Biochem Biophys 290:66–78

2. Hanna E, MacRae IJ, Medina DC et al (2002) ATP sulfurylase from the hyperthermophilic chemolithotroph Aquifex aeolicus. Arch Biochem Biophys 406:275–288

3. Renosto F, Martin RL, Wailes LM et al (1990) Regulation of inorganic sulfate activation in filamentous fungi. Allosteric inhibition of ATP sulfurylase by 3'-phosphoadenosine-5'-phosphosulfate. J Biol Chem 265:10300–10308

4. Yu M, Martin RL, Jain S et al (1989) Rat liver ATP-sulfurylase: purification, kinetic characterization, and interaction with arsenate, selenate, phosphate, and other inorganic oxyanions. Arch Biochem Biophys 269:165–174

5. Osslund T, Chandler C, Segel IH (1982) ATP sulfurylase from higher plants: purification and preliminary kinetics studies on the cabbage leaf enzyme. Plant Physiol 70:39–45

6. Leyh TS, Suo Y (1992) GTPase-mediated activation of ATP sulfurylase. J Biol Chem 267:542–545

7. Foster BA, Thomas SM, Mahr JA et al (1994) Cloning and sequencing of ATP sulfurylase from Penicillium chrysogenum. Identification of a likely allosteric domain. J Biol Chem 269:19777–19786

8. Li H, Deyrup A, Mensch JR et al (1995) The isolation and characterization of cDNA encoding the mouse bifunctional ATP sulfurylase-adenosine 5'-phosphosulfate kinase. J Biol Chem 270:29453–29459

9. Klonus D, Riesmeier JW, Willmitzer L (1995) A cDNA clone for an ATP-sulfurylase from Arabidopsis thaliana. Plant Physiol 107:653–654

10. Nyren P, Nore BF, Baltscheffsky M (1986) Studies on photosynthetic inorganic pyrophosphate formation in Rhodospirillum rubrum chromatophores. Biochim Biophys Acta 851:276–282

11. Nyren P, Karamouhamed S, Ronagshi M (1996) Real-time sequence-based DNA analyses using bioluminescence. In: Hastings et al (ed) Bioluminescence and chemiluminescence molecular reporting with photons, p 466–469

12. Ahmadian A, Ehn M, Hober S (2006) Pyrosequencing: history, biochemistry and future. Clin Chim Acta 363:83–94

13. Nyren P (1987) Enzymatic method for continuous monitoring of DNA polymerase activity. Anal Biochem 167:235–238

14. Cherest H, Kerjan P, Surdin-Kerjan Y (1987) The Saccharomyces cerevisiae MET 3 gene: nucleotide sequence and relationship of the 5' non-coding region to that of MET25. Mol Gen Genet 210:307–313

15. Karamohamed S, Nyren P (1999) Real-time detection and quantification of adenosine triphosphate sulfurylase activity by a bioluminometric approach. Anal Biochem 271:81–85

Chapter 17

Characterization of Recombinant *Escherichia coli* Single-Strand Binding Protein and Its Application in Pyrosequencing

Jianping Wang, Bingjie Zou, Qinxin Song, and Guohua Zhou

Abstract

We expressed recombinant single-strand binding protein (r-SSBP) from *Escherichia coli* with the molecular weight of 24-kDa by using genetic engineering strategy and demonstrated the single-stranded DNA (ssDNA)-binding activity of the r-SSBP by electrophoretic mobility shift assay (EMSA). To further characterize the r-SSBP, we studied the effects of the r-SSBP on melting temperature (T_m) of DNA. The results showed that the r-SSBP can bind to ssDNA and can lower the T_m of DNA, especially for single-base mismatched DNA. Therefore, the r-SSBP can significantly increase the T_m difference between single-base mismatched DNA and perfect matched DNA. These results are very beneficial for single-nucleotide polymorphism detection. Moreover, we applied the r-SSBP in high sensitive pyrosequencing system developed by our group. The results suggested that the r-SSBP can decrease unspecific signals, correct the proportion of signal peak height, and improve the performance of pyrosequencing. This research laid the foundation for the development of high sensitive pyrosequencing regents.

Key words *Escherichia coli*, Single-strand binding protein, Electrophoretic mobility shift assay, Pyrosequencing

1 Introduction

The single-strand binding protein (SSBP) of *Escherichia coli* plays a central role by participating in replication, repair, and recombination by stabilizing single-stranded DNA intermediates that are generated during DNA processing and are essential for the survival of the cell [1].

Since SSBP can prevent the formation of secondary structures and degradation by nuclease after interacting with ssDNA [2], the SSBP can be exploited in many biotechnical applications, such as capillary electrophoresis [3], Polymerase Chain Reaction [4], and Pyrosequencing [5]. Pyrosequencing is a new DNA sequencing method [6–8] that employs enzymatic reactions to detect inorganic

Guohua Zhou and Qinxin Song (eds.), *Advances and Clinical Practice in Pyrosequencing*, Springer Protocols Handbooks, DOI 10.1007/978-1-4939-3308-2_17, © Springer Science+Business Media New York 2016

pyrophosphate (PPi) released to ATP in the presence of adenosine 5′ phosphosulfate (APS) by ATP sulfurylase and subsequently visible light is generated in a luciferase reaction during which luciferin is oxidized by consuming ATP. In the previous study we have successfully expressed ATP sulfurylase [9, 10], luciferase [11], Pyruvate phosphate dikinase [12], and initially established the high sensitive pyrosequencing system, which has been applied in SNP analysis [13], gene expression analysis [14], etc. But for some ssDNA template having complex structure, we can't get accurate results, since SSBP can stabilize formation of ssDNA secondary structures, the SSBP can decrease unspecific signals, correct the proportion of signal peak height, and improve the performance of pyrosequencing [5, 6].

In this chapter, we have expressed recombinant SSBP (r-SSBP) from *E. coli* by using genetic engineering strategy and demonstrated ssDNA-binding activity of the r-SSBP by electrophoretic mobility shift assay (EMSA). To further characterize the r-SSBP, we studied the effects of the r-SSBP on melting temperature (T_m) of DNA. Moreover, we applied the r-SSBP in high sensitive pyrosequencing system developed by our group for improving the performance of pyrosequencing.

2 Materials

1. Expression vector pET28a (+), host cell ArcticExpress (DE3) were from our laboratory.

2. All of oligonucleotides and primer sequences were synthesized by Invitrogen (Shanghai).

3. Taq DNA polymerase, *Hin*d III and *Bam*H I restriction enzymes, T4 DNA ligase, and PCR product purification kits were purchased from TaKaRa Company (Dalian).

4. Peptone purchased from Oxoid.

5. Isopropyl-β-D-thiogalactoside (IPTG) was purchased from Amresco Inc.

6. Beads (Dynabeads M-280 streptavidin) were purchased from Invitrogen.

7. α-sulfide deoxy adenosine triphosphate (dATPαS), dGTP, dTTP, and dCTP were purchased from Amersham Pharmacia, Biotech.

3   Methods

3.1 Construction of Recombinant Vector pET28a (+)-ssb and Expression of r-SSBP

1. According to the SSBP coding sequence from GeneBank, the primers were designed with incorporation of the restriction sites for cloning ssb-1 and ssb-2 (Table 1) and were synthesized to amplify ssb gene with *E. coli* BL21 (DE3) genomic DNA as a template (*see* **Note 1**).

2. The PCR product was purified by PCR product purification kit and then cloned into pET28a (+) vector. The recombinant plasmid was sequenced by the Beijing Genomics Institute (shanghai) for screening the positive expressed cell ArcticExpress™.

3. Overnight cultures were transferred into the fresh LB medium (kan⁺, 30 mg/L) at the ratio 1:100, and then were allowed to grow at 37 °C for 3 h with rotary shaking (160 r/min) before 0.01 mmol/L IPTG; cultures were further grown at 30 °C for 4.5 h.

4. The cells were harvested by centrifugation ($8000 \times g$ for 3 min at 4 °C), then were resuspended in 40 mL 1× Binding buffer (0.5 mol/L NaCl, 20 mmol/L Tris–HCl, 5 mmol/L Imidazole, pH 7.9), added 1 µL lysozyme (100 g/L) into the buffer for 0.5 h at room temperature.

5. The cells were disrupted by gentle sonication on ice and centrifuged ($10,000 \times g$ for 30 min at 4 °C); the supernatants were purified by His•Bind Resin affinity chromatography. The purity of the protein preparations was assessed by SDS-PAGE.

3.2 Electrophoretic Mobility Shift Assay

The different concentrations of r-SSBP (0, 2.5, 7.5, 12.5, 25 µmol/L) were respectively added into the 10 µL of r-SSBP buffer (6 mmol/L Tris–HCl, 150 mmol/L NaCl, 0.3 mmol/L EDTA, 0.3 mmol/L DTT, 1 µmol/L ssDNA S-1 [Table 1]), incubated for 10 min at room temperature, added an equal volume of 2× loading buffer (0.08 % bromophenol blue, 13 % sucrose), the product was analyzed by 10 % of polyacrylamide gel electrophoresis (110 V, 40 min), silver staining [15], compared with the interaction product without ssDNA S-1 (Table 1).

3.3 Melting Temperature Analysis

1. 1.2 µmol/L of T-2, T-3, T-4, T-5 (Table 1) was added into the 10 µL of r-SSBP buffer (6 mmol/L Tris–HCl, 150 mmol/L NaCl, 0.3 mmol/L EDTA, 0.3 mmol/L DTT, 1 µmol/L T-1 (Table 1), 1× SYBR Green I 2 µL), respectively.

2. The different concentrations of r-SSBP (0, 7.5, 22.5, 30, 37.5 µmol/L) were added to the buffer, incubated for 10 min at room temperature. T_m was measured by real-time PCR instrument.

Table 1
Oligonucleotides sequences used in this study

No.	Sequences (5′–3′)	Description
ssb-1	GCGCGGATCCATGGCCAGCAGAGGCGTAAACAA	Upstream primer for amplifying the *ssb* gene
ssb-2	GCGCAAGCTTTCAGAAACGGAATGTCATCAAA	Downstream primer for amplifying the *ssb* gene
S-1	AGGCAAATACGCTCGCGGTATTCTGGCGAACTACGGCATTGAACGATC	The oligonucleotide used for electrophoretic mobility shift assay
T-1	CTATTGCACCAGGCCAGATGAGAGAACCAAGGGGAAGTGACAT	The template used for the detection of T_m
T-2	ATGTCACTTCCCCTTGGTTCTCTC	The matched probe used for the detection of T_m
T-3	ATGTCACTTCCCgTTGGTTCTCTC	The G/G mismatched probe used for the detection of T_m
T-4	ATGTCACTTCCCtTTGGTTCTCTC	The T/G mismatched probe used for the detection of T_m
T-5	ATGTCACTTCCCaTTGGTTCTCTC	The A/G mismatched probe used for the detection of T_m
35s-1	bio-TGATGTGATATCTCCACTGACG	Upstream primer for amplifying fragment of *35s* gene
35s-2	ACAACATGGCACAAGGGATACA	Downstream primer for amplifying fragment of *35s* gene
35s-3	TGATGTGATATCTCCACTGACG	Sequencing primer of the *35s* gene fragment
H-1	bio-TATGCATACAAAATTGTCAAG	Upstream primer for amplifying fragment of HA gene
H-2	ACCTGCTATAGCTCCAAATAG	Downstream primer for amplifying fragment of HA gene
H-3	CTATTTGGAGCTATAGCAGGT	Sequencing primer of the HA gene fragment

The sequences of *GGATCC* and *AAGCTT* in italic are the restriction sites of *Bam*H I and *Hind* III, respectively; T-2 is a probe complementary to the 3′ end of T-1; T-3, T-4, T-5 have one different base (marked with lowercase letter) from T-2 at the same position

3.4 Pyrosequencing

1. *35s* gene and the fragment of *HA* gene were amplified as the primers with genomic DNA from transgenic soybean and the synthetic fragment of HA gene of the H5N1 bird flu virus as the template.

2. Thermal cycling for the PCR primer pairs *35s*-1/*35s*-2 (Table 1) and H-1/H-2 (Table 1) was performed with an initial activation for 5 min at 94 °C, succeeded by 35 cycles of denaturation for 30 s at 94 °C, primer annealing for 30 s at 55 °C, and synthesis for 45 s at 72 °C. A final primer extension was conducted for 5 min at 72 °C.

3. The products were purified by PCR product purification kit.

4. The ssDNA was prepared with Streptavidin-coated superparamagnetic beads, added 2 μL sequencing primer (*35s*-3 and H-3, Table 1), denaturation for 30 s at 95 °C, primer annealing for 3 min at 55 °C.

5. 1 μL of sample was added into pyrosequencing reaction buffer (0.7 mol/L Tris-HAc, 0.35 mmol/L EDTA, 0.35 mmol/L $Mg(Ac)_2$, 0.28 mg/mL PVP, 1 mmol/L DTT, 0.02 % BSA, 0.4 mmol/L Luciferin, 0.16 U/mL Apyrase, 0.1 μL Klenow DNA polymerase (exo-), 2 μmol/L APS, 22.4 μg/mL Luciferase, 1.5 μL ATP Sulfurylase). 6 μmol/L r-SSBP (*see* **Note 2**) was added into the reaction buffer, compared with the reaction results without r-SSBP.

4   Method Validation

4.1 Expression and Purification of r-SSBP

Recombinant expressed cell ArcticExpress™ containing pET28a (+)-*ssb* was built with genetic engineering, then was cultured and induced with IPTG. The cells were collected by centrifugation and disrupted by gentle sonication. The supernatant was purified with His-Bind Resin affinity chromatography. The supernatant of the lysate and purified recombinant r-SSBP were assessed by SDS-PAGE, compared with the lysate of ArcticExpress™ and ArcticExpress™ transformed with pET28a(+)-*ssb* without IPTG induction (Fig. 1). The r-SSBP with the molecular weight of about 24 kDa was found near the 25 kDa of protein marker (Fig. 1, lane 3–5), and the r-SSBP was mostly expressed in soluble form (Fig. 1, lane 2–3); after purification with Ni^+ affinity chromatography column, the r-SSBP with electrophoretic pure grade was obtained (Fig. 1, lane 1).

4.2 Characterization of ssDNA-Binding Activity of r-SSBP

The ssDNA-binding activity of r-SSBP was demonstrated by analyzing the changes of electrophoretic bands after the various of concentration of r-SSBP binding to ssDNA; the results were shown in Fig. 2. With increasing r-SSBP concentration, the bands of the r-SSBP-ssDNA complex gradually deepened, and the bands of ssDNA became weaker. The results indicated r-SSBP has the activity binding to ssDNA.

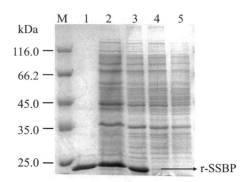

Fig. 1 SDS-PAGE electrophoretograms of r-SSBP expressed in recombinant ArcticExpress™. *M*: protein marker; *1*: purified recombinant SSBP; *2*: supernatant of the lysate of ArcticExpress™ transformed with pET28a(+)-*ssb*; *3*: total protein of the lysate of ArcticExpress™ transformed with pET28a(+)-*ssb*; *4*: total protein of the lysate of ArcticExpress™ transformed with pET28a(+)-*ssb* without IPTG induction; *5*: total protein of the lysate of ArcticExpress™

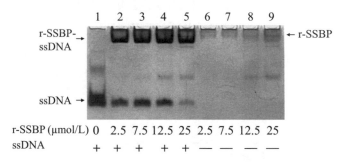

Fig. 2 Native gel electrophoretograms of the reaction mixtures of r-SSBP and ssDNA. *1*: ssDNA for reference; *2–5*: ssDNA with different concentrations of r-SSBP; *6–9*: different concentrations of r-SSBP

4.3 Effect of r-SSBP on the Melting Temperature DNA

The different single-base mismatched and the perfect matched DNA probes (T-2, T-3, T-4, T-5, Table 1) with ssDNA (T-1, Table 1) and the different concentration of r-SSBP were added into the buffer containing T-1, the T_m of DNA was measured by real-time PCR instrument, and the results were shown in Fig. 3. With r-SSBP, T_m of DNA decreased, and the difference of T_m was increasing between perfect matched DNA (C/G) and single-base mismatched DNA (G/G, T/G, A/G) with increasing r-SSBP concentration; this is related to the activity of r-SSBP binding to ssDNA. *E. coli* SSBP can bind to the ssDNA, and then decrease the nonspecific DNA hybridization and can stabilize formation of ssDNA secondary structures. It has cooperative effect promoting other SSBP molecules binding to ssDNA, so can reduce the T_m of DNA [16, 17]. Since the mismatched DNA can melt at low temperature, SSBP can be easier to bind to DNA, and has more effect on T_m. The effect of SSBP was the same for the different mis-

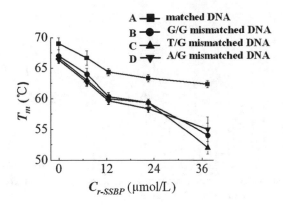

Fig. 3 The effects of r-SSBP with different concentrations on T_m of DNA. -■- (**A**): perfect matched DNA (C/G); (**B**) -●-, (**C**) -▲-, (**D**) -▼-: single-base mismatched DNA (G/G, T/G, A/G)

matched DNA, and this is related to the nonspecific activity of r-SSBP binding to ssDNA. The r-SSBP can increase the T_m difference between perfect matched DNA and single-base mismatched DNA [18–21]. The results are very beneficial for single-nucleotide polymorphism detection.

4.4 The Application of r-SSBP for Improving the Performances of Pyrosequencing

To investigate the effect of r-SSBP in pyrosequencing, we sequenced the single-stranded PCR product of the fragments of *35s* gene from transgenic plant and *HA* gene from the H5N1 bird flu virus. The r-SSBP was used for improving the performances of pyrosequencing, and the results were shown in Figs. 4 and 5. According to Fig. 4, the nonspecific signals were decreased, and the proportion of signal peak height was corrected. This is due to the unspecific 3′-end hybridization of the fragments of *35s* gene; the r-SSBP can prevent the 3′-end loops from forming and reduce the unspecific hybridization when the r-SSBP binds to the template, and then allow a more effective annealing of sequencing primer to the template. So r-SSBP can decrease the unspecific signals [6, 7].

The pyrograms of the fragment of *HA* gene from the H5N1 bird flu virus show (in Fig. 5) that the proportion of signal peak height of T: T: 5T: 2T is 0.49: 0.75: 2.76: 2.00, and 2C: C: C: C is 1.37: 1.25: 1.13: 1.00 without r-SSBP, that of the signal peak is 1.09: 1.32: 4.74: 2.00 and 2.32: 1.38: 1.21: 1.00 with r-SSBP. Apparently, in the presence of r-SSBP, the proportion of signal peak height is closer to the theoretical value, the homogeneity region extends more fully, and the sequencing results are more accurate. According to the analysis of secondary structure, we found 3′-end and 5′-end of the fragment of the HA gene can form the complex stem loop, which hind klenow (exo⁻) polymerase with binding to template. In the absence of r-SSBP, the template can form the secondary structure, the first T cannot be extended fully, the signal peak height is lower than the theoretical value, and when

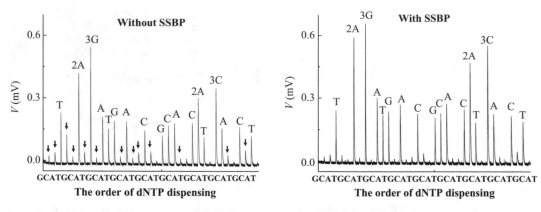

Fig. 4 Pyrograms of the fragment of *35s* gene from transgenic plant using high sensitive pyrosequencing system with and without r-SSBP. The order of dNTP dispensing was GCATG; the sequence of the template was 5′-TAAGGGATGACGCACAATCCCACT-3′. The *arrows* indicate the nonspecific signals

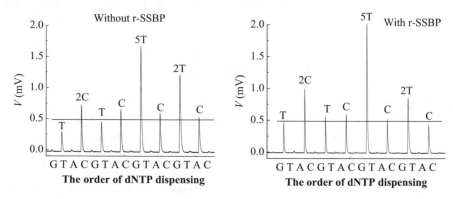

Fig. 5 Pyrograms of the fragment of *HA* gene from the H5N1 bird flu virus using high sensitive pyrosequencing system with r-SSBP and without r-SSBP. The dNTP dispending order was GTACG; the sequence of the template was 5′-TCCTCTTTTTCTTC-3′

the next T was extended, the extended signal was accumulated and was higher than the theoretical value. But in the presence of r-SSBP, r-SSBP can bind to the template, prevent the template from forming the unspecific hybridization, stabilize the single-stranded template, and every base can be fully extended, so r-SSBP can correct the proportion of signal peak height and improve the performance of pyrosequencing.

5   Technical Notes

1. Restriction sites *Bam*H I and *Hin*d II were introduced to the 5′- and 3′-terminal primer, respectively.
2. The r-SSBP can increase the T_m difference between perfect matched DNA and single-base mismatched DNA.

References

1. Witte G, Urbanke C, Curth U (2005) Single-stranded DNA-binding protein of Deinococcus radiodurans: a biophysical characterization. Nucleic Acids Res 33:1662–1670

2. Greipel J, Urbanke C, Maass G (1989) Physicochemical properties and biological functions. In: Saenger W, Heinemann U (eds) Protein–nucleic acid interaction. Macmillan, London, pp 61–86

3. Drabovich A, Krylo SN (2000) Single-stranded DNA-binding protein facilitates gel-free analysis of polymerase chain reaction products in capillary electrophoresis. J Chromatogr A 1051: 171–175

4. Awomir S, Browski D, Kur Józef (1999) Cloning, overexpression and purification of the recombinant His-tagged SSB protein of Escherichia coli and use in polymerase chain reaction amplification. Protein Expr Purif 16:96–102.

5. Ronaghi M (2002) Improved performance of pyrosequencing using single-stranded DNA-binding protein. Anal Biochem 286:282–288

6. Nordstrom T, Alderborn A, Nyren P (2002) Method for one-step preparation of double-stranded DNA template applicable for use with Pyrosequencing™ technology. J Biochem Biophy Meth 52:71–82

7. Ronaghi M (2001) Pyrosequencing sheds light on DNA sequencing. Gen Res 11:3–11

8. Zhou GH, Kajiyama T, Gotou M et al (2006) Enzyme system for improving the detection limit in pyrosequencing. Anal Chem 78:4482–4489

9. Luo J, Wu WJ, Zou BJ et al (2007) Expression and purification of ATP sulfurylase from Saccharomyces cerevisias in Escherichia coli and its application pyrosequencing. Chin J Biotech 423:623–627

10. Zou BJ, Luo J, Zhou GH et al (2009) Expression, immobilization and application of biotinylated ATP sulfurylase. Prog Biochem Biophys 36:923–928

11. Zhu SH, Zou BJ, Wu HP et al (2010) Preparation of thermostable biotinylated firefly luciferase and its application to pyrosequencing. Chinese J Anal Chem 38:458–463

12. Zou BJ, Chen ZY, Zhou GH (2008) Expression of PPDK from Microbispora rosea subsp. aerata in Escherichia coli and its application in pyrosequencing. Chin J Biotech 24: 679–683

13. Zhou GH, Kamahori M, Okano K et al (2001) Miniaturized pyrosequencer for DNA analysis with capillaries to deliver deoxynucleotides. Electrophoresis 22:3497–3504

14. Song QX, Jing H, Wu HP et al (2010) Gene expression analysis on a photodiode array-based bioluminescence analyzer by using sensitivity-improved SRPP. Analyst 135:1315–1319

15. Sambrook J, Fritsch EF, Maniatis T (2001) Molecular cloning: a laboratory manual, 3rd edn. Cold Spring Harbor Laboratory Press, New York

16. Sigal N, Delius H, Kornberg T et al (1972) A DNA unwinding protein isolated from Escherichia coli: its interaction with DNA and DNA polymerase. Proc Natl Acad Sci U S A 69:3537–3541

17. Witte G, Urbanke C, Curth U (2005) Single-stranded DNA-binding protein of Deinococcus radiodurans: a biophysical characterization. Nucl Acids Res 33:1662–1670

18. Gundry CN, Dobrowolski SF, Martin YR et al (2008) Base-pair neutral homozygotes can be discriminated by calibrated high-resolution melting of small amplicons. Nucl Acids Res 36:3401–3408

19. Zuo Z, Chen SS, Chandra PK et al (2009) Application of COLD-PCR for improved detection of KRAS mutations in clinical samples. Mod Pathol 22:1023–1031

20. Muyzer G, Smalla K (1998) Application of denaturing gradient gel electrophoresis (DGGE) and temperature gradient gel electrophoresis (TGGE) in microbial ecology. Anton Leeuw 73:127–141

21. Satokari RM, Vaughan EE, Akkermans ADL, Saarela M, DeVos WM (2001) Bifidobacterial diversity in human feces detected by genus specific PCR and denaturing gradient gel electrophoresis. Appl Environ Microbiol 67: 504–513

Chapter 18

Expression of PPDK from *Microbispora rosea* subsp. *aerata* in *E. coli* and Its Application in Pyrosequencing

Bingjie Zou, Qinxin Song, and Guohua Zhou

Abstract

Using the genomic DNA of *Microbispora rosea* subsp. *aerata* as the template, a DNA fragment encoding the gene of PPDK was amplified by PCR and inserted into the expression vector pET28a(+), yielding pET28a(+)-PPDK. The *E. coli* BL21 (DE3) was transformed with the pET28a(+)-PPDK. After inducing with IPTG, the *E. coli* BL21 (DE3) [pET28a(+)-PPDK]-expressed recombinant PPDK fused to an N-terminal sequence of 6-His tag. The molecular weight of PPDK was estimated to be 101 kDa by SDS-PAGE. The electrophoretic grade PPDK was obtained by His•Bind resin affinity chromatography and ultrafiltration using 10-kDa molecular weight cutoff membrane. The successful application of PPDK in pyrosequencing was also demonstrated.

Key words PPDK, *Microbispora rosea* subsp. *aerata*, *E. coli*, Pyrosequencing

1 Introduction

Pyruvate phosphate dikinase (PPDK, EC 2.7.9.1) is found in certain microorganisms and plants and catalyzes the conversion of AMP, PPi, and phosphoenolpyruvate (PEP) to ATP, Pi, and pyruvate. In C4 plants, PPDK is responsible for PEP production [1]. On the other hand, in *Giardia* [2], *Trypanosoma cruzi* [3], and *Entamoeba histolytica* [4], PPDK functions in the process of ATP synthesis. PPDK is also found in some bacteria such as *Clostridium symbiosum* [5].

PPDKs from various species are generally labile, but the PPDK from *Microbispora rosea* subsp. *aerata* strain NBRC 14047 is stable and has been applied in many fields, e.g., determination of ATP, ADP, and AMP [6], enumeration of bacterial cell numbers [7], bioluminescent enzyme immunoassay [8], and pyrosequencing [9].

In our studies, we expressed the PPDK from *Microbispora rosea* subsp. *aerata* using pET28a(+) (Novagen Corporation) as an expression vector, which can express the recombinant protein with

Guohua Zhou and Qinxin Song (eds.), *Advances and Clinical Practice in Pyrosequencing*, Springer Protocols Handbooks,
DOI 10.1007/978-1-4939-3308-2_18, © Springer Science+Business Media New York 2016

a His tag. Including the extra-desalting step, only two purification steps are needed to get the recombinant PPDK with electrophoretic pure grade. The successful application of the enzyme in pyrosequencing was also demonstrated.

2   Materials

1. *Microbispora rosea* subsp. *aerata*, NBRC 14047 (Japan's Technical Evaluation Research Institute of Biological Resource Center, NBRC).

2. *E. coli* strain BL21 (DE3), pET28a(+) (Novagen).

3. Restriction endonuclease, LA Taq DNA polymerase, $2 \times$ LA GC buffer, T4 DNA ligase, λ-EcoT14 I digest DNA marker, protein marker, and PCR products purification kit (Takara, China).

4. D-luciferin, luciferase, and Klenow(exo⁻) DNA polymerase (Promega, USA).

5. Apyrase (Sigma, USA).

6. Yeast extract and tryptone (Oxoid).

7. IPTG and lysozyme (Amresco).

8. His-bind resin and His-bind columns (Novagen).

9. The other chemicals were of a commercially extra-pure grade.

3   Methods

3.1   Plasmid Construction and Expression of PPDK

1. Using the genomic DNA of *Microbispora rosea* subsp. *aerata* as the template, a DNA fragment encoding the gene of PPDK was amplified by PCR (*see* **Note 1**).

2. The amplified fragment was inserted into the *Eco*RI site and the *Hin*dIII site of the pET28a(+), yielding pET28a(+)-PPDK.

3. Cells from the *E. coli* strain BL21 (DE3) made competent with $CaCl_2$ were transformed with the pET28a(+)-PPDK, and transformants were selected by digesting plasmids extracted from the clones with *Eco*RI and *Hin*dIII. For the expression assay, a bacterial colony was inoculated in LB medium containing 30 μg/mL Kan and incubated at 37 °C with shaking.

4. The culture was grown until it had an o.d.$_{600\,nm}$ of 0.6; at this time, 0.1 mmol/L IPTG was added and the incubation continued for 5 h (*see* **Note 2**).

3.2   Purification of PPDK

1. One hundred milliliters of the cultures incubated for 5 h with the induction of IPTG were centrifuged for 3 min at $8000 \times g$ and washed with PBS and then resuspended in 10 mL of 1× binding buffer containing 100 μg/mL lysozyme and 0.1 % *Triton* X-100.

2. Cells were broken by freezing and thawing the cells three times and then sonicated in an ice bath.

3. The broken crude was 4 °C centrifuged at 12,000 r/min (13225 g) for 20 min, and then supernatant was collected for SDS-PAGE analysis. The supernatant was applied to the His•Bind column and washed with 10 column volumes of 1× binding buffer and followed by a wash with five column volumes of 1× binding buffer containing 60 mmol/L imidazole.

4. The protein was eluted with two column volumes of 1× binding buffer containing 300 mmol/L imidazole (*see* **Note 3**).

3.3 Enzyme Assay

1. The activity was determined in the direction of ATP and _ pyruvate synthesis and was measured as the quantity of ATP formed in the reaction mixture using bioluminescent assay. The assay mixture (pH 6.8) contained 20 mmol/L HEPES, 25 mmol/L $(NH4)_2SO_4$, 3 mmol/L $MgSO_4$, 2 mmol/L DTT, 2 mmol/L PPi, 2 mmol/L PEP, and 0.1 mmol/L AMP.

2. Firstly, the standard curve of ATP signal was drawn by adding different concentrations of ATP into a determine buffer (pH 7.75) containing 0.1 mol/L Tris-Ac, 0.5 mmol/L EDTA, 5 mmol/L $Mg(Ac)_2$, 0.4 mg/mL PVP, 0.02 % BSA, 1 mmol/L DTT, 0.4 mmol/L D-luciferin, and 1.46 μg/mL luciferase and measuring signal using BPCL luminometer.

3. Then, the assay was started by the addition of 1 μL of enzyme to the assay mixture at 37 °C.

4. After appropriate incubation periods, the reaction mixture was boiled for 3 min and immediately cooled on ice (*see* **Note 4**).

3.4 The Application of the Enzyme in Pyrosequencing

1. Pyrosequencing is a DNA-sequencing method that employs multiple enzymatic reactions to monitor DNA synthesis. The standard-pyrosequencing solution contains 90 U/mL Klenow (exo⁻) DNA polymerase, 2 U/mL apyrase, 0.1 mol/L Tris-Ac (pH 7.75), 0.5 mmol/L EDTA, 5 mmol/L $Mg(Ac)_2$, 0.4 mg/mL PVP, 0.02 % BSA, 1 mmol/L DTT, 0.4 mmol/L AMP, 0.08 mmol/L PEP, 0.4 mmol/L D-luciferin, 1.46 μg/mL luciferase, and 0.22 U/mL PPDK (*see* **Note 5**).

4   Method Validation

4.1 Plasmid Construction and Expression of PPDK

Using the genomic DNA of *Microbispora rosea* subsp. *aerata* as the template, a DNA fragment of 2.6 kb was amplified by PCR (Fig. 1, lane 1). The transformants were selected by digesting plasmids extracted from the clones with *Eco*RI and *Hin*dIII, and both the 2.6-kb fragment and the 5.3-kb fragment representing the vector were obtained (Fig. 1, lane 2). The positive colony was inoculated in LB medium containing 30 μg/mL Kan. After IPTG induction,

210 Bingjie Zou et al.

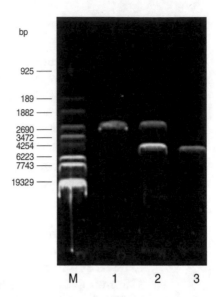

Fig. 1 Restriction enzyme digestion analysis of recombinant plasmid pET28a(+)-PPDK. *M*, λ-EcoT14 I digest DNA marker *1*—PCR products of PPDK gene; *2*—pET28a(+)-PPDK digested with *Eco*R I and *Hind* III; *3*—pET28a(+) digested with *Eco*RI and *Hind*IIII

SDS-PAGE analysis was performed on the expressed products at different incubation time. As shown in Fig. 2, a recombinant protein band with 101 kDa was successfully expressed after IPTG induction, and most of the recombinant ATPS was expressed as a soluble form (Fig. 2, lane 5).

4.2 Purification of PPDK

The recombinant PPDK with electrophoretic pure grade was obtained by His•Bind resin affinity chromatography and ultrafiltration using 10-kDa molecular weight cutoff membrane (Fig. 3).

4.3 Enzyme Assay

One unit of the enzyme is defined as the amount of enzyme, which produces 1 μmol of ATP per min at 37 °C and pH 6.8. The activity was determined in the direction of ATP and pyruvate synthesis and was measured as the quantity of ATP formed in the reaction mixture using bioluminescent assay. The specific activity of PPDK was measured as 0.1 U/mg.

4.4 The Application of the Enzyme in Pyrosequencing

The successful application of the enzyme in pyrosequencing was demonstrated. Pyrosequencing is actually based on the detection of the PPi from a DNA strand extension reaction. Four kinds of dNTPs are added into the reaction solution one by one. When the added dNTP is complementary to the base in a template strand hybridized with a sequencing primer, a strand extension reaction occurs. It is followed by ATP production and luciferase reaction. A light signal is detected as a peak in a pyrogram. The relative intensity of each peak is proportional to the number of incorporated nucleotides.

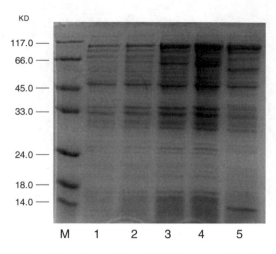

Fig. 2 SDS-PAGE analysis of recombinant PPDK expressed in *E. coli*. *M*, protein marker; *Lane 1*, total protein of *E. coli* BL21 (DE3) transformed with pET28a(+)-PPDK without IPTG induction; *Lane 2–4*, Total protein of *E. coli* BL21 (DE3) transformed with pET28a(+)-ATPS after being induced with IPTG for 1 h, 3 h, and 5 h, respectively; *Lane 5*, supernatant of the lysate of *E. coli* BL21(DE3) transformed with pET28a(+)-PPDK

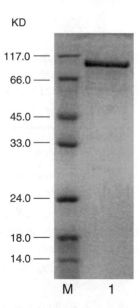

Fig. 3 SDS-PAGE analysis of purified recombinant PPDK. *M*, protein marker; *Lane 1*, purified recombinant PPDK

The DNA template is an artificial single-strand oligonucleotide. The sequence of the template is 5′-TCAGACTTTGACCGTA-3′, and the bold letters underlined represent the sequence to be determined. The dNTP dispensing order is A-T-G-C-T-G. The result can be seen in Fig. 4. Because the first base of the template is G, there was no extension signal but the background

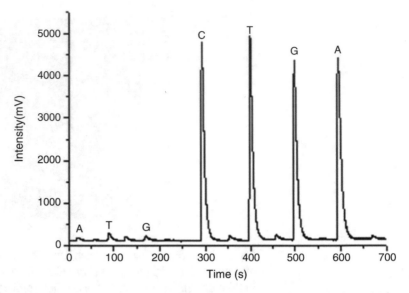

Fig. 4 Pyrosequencing on an artificial DNA template with recombinant PPDK. Template, artificially synthesized oligonucleotide (5′-TCAGACTTTGACCGTA-3′); order of dNTP dispensing, A-T-G-C-T-G with the double dispensing of each dNTP species

signal was detected when the other three nucleotides were added. The first extension signal was obtained when dCTP was added, and the other signals can be gotten in the same way.

5 Technical Notes

1. Expression was performed in the bacterial system pET (Novagen).

2. Expression of the protein was monitored by SDS-PAGE using bacterial lysates taken at different time intervals after induction.

3. A 10-kDa molecular weight cutoff membrane was used for desalting.

4. One microliter of reaction mixture was added into the determine buffer to measure the signal and calculated the concentration of ATP according to the standard curve of ATP signal.

5. The target sequence of single-strand DNA template is 5′-TCAGACTTTGACCGTA-3′.

References

1. Chastain CJ, Botschner M, Harrington GE et al (2000) Further analysis of maize C-4 pyruvate, orthophosphate dikinase phosphorylation by its bifunctional regulatory protein using selective substitutions of the regulatory Thr-456 and catalytic His-458 residues. Arch Biochem Biophys 37(1):165–170

2. Hiltpold A, Thomas RM, Kohler P (1999) Purification and characterization of recombinant pyruvate phosphate dikinase from *Giardia*. Mol Biochem Parasitol 104(2):157–169

3. Acosta H, Dubourdieu M, Quinones W et al (2004) Pyruvate phosphate dikinase and pyrophosphate metabolism in the glycosome of *Trypanosoma cruzi* epimastigotes. Comp Biochem Physiol B Biochem Mol Biol 138(4):347–356

4. Lua LS, Silva LR, Montfort RP (1998) Expression and characterization of recombinant pyruvate phosphate dikinase from *Entamoeba histolytica*. Biochimica et Biophysica Acta 1382:47–54

5. McGuire M, Carroll LJ, Yankie L et al (1996) Determination of the nucleotide binding site within *Clostridium symbiosum* pyruvate phosphate dikinase by photoaffinity labeling, site-directed mutagenesis, and structural analysis. Biochemistry 35:8544–8552

6. Ishii S, Sato Y, Terashima M et al (2004) A novel method for determination of ATP, ADP, and AMP contents of a single pancreatic islet before transplantation. Transplant Proc 36:1191–1193

7. Sakakibara T, Murakami S, Imai K (2003) Enumeration of bacterial cell numbers by amplified firefly bioluminescence without cultivation. Anal Biochem 312(1):48–56

8. Ito K, Nishimura K, Murakamib S et al (2000) Novel bioluminescent assay of pyruvate phosphate dikinase using firefly luciferase-luciferin reaction and its application to bioluminescent enzyme immunoassay. Anal Chim Acta 421:113–120

9. Zhou G, Kajiyama T, Gotou M et al (2006) Enzyme system for improving the detection limit in pyrosequencing. Anal Chem 78:4482–4489

Part IV

Pyrosequencing-Based Bio-Barcodes

Chapter 19

Construction of 3-Plex Barcodes for Differential Gene Expression Analysis with Pyrosequencing

Xiaodan Zhang, Haiping Wu, Zhiyao Chen, Guohua Zhou, and Hideki Kambara

Abstract

Presently most techniques for gene expression analysis are based on a dye label. Here, we describe a novel method for comparing gene expression levels among various tissues or cells by sequence-tagged reverse-transcription PCR coupled with pyrosequencing (termed "SRPP"). This method includes three steps: (1) reverse transcription of mRNA with source-specific RT primers consisting of a tail at the 5′-end for supplying a common PCR priming site, a source-specific sequence in the middle, and a poly-T stretch plus several degenerate bases at the 3′-end for annealing the mRNA strand, (2) PCR amplification of the templates produced by pooling sequence-labeled cDNAs equally from different sources, and (3) decoding and quantification of the source-specific sequences tagged in the amplicons by pyrosequencing. The signal ratio in the pyrogram is proportional to the amounts of mRNAs among different sources. As the signal is detected by observing bioluminescence, neither dye nor electrophoresis or laser source was used. The expression levels of six kinds of genes (Cdk2ap2, Vps4b, Fas, Fos, Cdk4, and Actb) among the kidney, the brain, and the heart tissues of a mouse were accurately detected, suggesting that the new method is promising in quantitatively comparing gene expression levels among different sources at a low cost.

Key words Gene expression analysis, DNA sequencing, Sequence-tagged PCR, Pyrosequencing, Dye-free labeling

1 Introduction

As the human genome sequencing has been completed, it is important to clarify gene functions and to utilize them for biomedical applications [1]. It is necessary to systematically understand the distribution and the amount of mRNA not only in a healthy tissue but also in a diseased tissue systematically. Changes in expression of target genes can be the markers of specific physiologic stages [2, 3]. A rapid and accurate comparison of gene expression levels in various tissues or cells is thus needed. For the moment, there are many methods based on various principles that have been developed for gene expression profiling; methods for global picturing include serial analysis of gene expression (SAGE) [4], cDNA microarray

Guohua Zhou and Qinxin Song (eds.), *Advances and Clinical Practice in Pyrosequencing*, Springer Protocols Handbooks, DOI 10.1007/978-1-4939-3308-2_19, © Springer Science+Business Media New York 2016

[5], sequencing of cDNA libraries [6], oligonucleotide microarray [7], and differential display polymerase chain reaction (PCR) (DD-PCR) [8]; methods for fine expression profiling of a select set of target genes include Northern blotting [9], real-time PCR [10, 11], matrix-assisted laser desorption/ionization time-of-flight (MALDI-TOF) mass spectrometry [12], and electronic microarray [13]. Each method has its advantages and disadvantages in terms of labor intensity, running cost, accuracy, sensitivity, and throughput. Almost all of the approaches for gene expression analysis are based on a dye-label method coupled with fluorescence detection except for mass spectrometry which needs an expensive mass spectrometer for the discrimination of molecular weights. As conventional dye-labeling techniques can be costly in reagents and instrumentation and are limited to the comparative analysis of two sample sources, typically one control and one sample, a dye-free method with an inexpensive readout is desirable for the comparative expression analysis of a few specific genes among more than two sources. Here, we propose a novel sequence-labeling method for quantitatively comparing gene expression levels from different sources by the use of sequence-tagged primers for reverse transcription (RT) prior to PCR. Each RT primer discriminates a gene source by a different tagged sequence, thus avoiding the use of a dye for the labeling. To decode and quantify the amplicons containing source-specific sequences labeled by the RT primers, a well-developed real-time sequencing technology, pyrosequencing [14, 15], is adapted. The signal intensities and the base order in a pyrogram correspond to the gene expression levels and the gene sources, respectively. Quantitative analysis of the relative expression levels of a target gene among three different sources was successfully achieved. The results demonstrate that gene expression analysis by sequence-tagged reverse-transcription PCR coupled with pyrosequencing (named "SRPP" for short) is well suited to the comparative expression analysis of selected target genes from multiple sample sources [16–18]. The major advantages of SRPP over existing dye-labeling methods include the low cost of instrumentation, the comparative gene expression analysis of multiple sample sources in a single assay [19–22], and a simple system setup without the use of a standard curve. The principle of SRPP is shown in Fig. 1. The key points of SRPP are how to label the gene source and how to decode the source-specific labels. Here we used a short source-specific sequence labeled in an RT primer for discriminating the gene sequence and pyrosequencing for quantitatively decoding the labeled sequences. The process consists of three steps: (1) reverse transcription of mRNA extracted from different sources by the source-specific RT primers. There are three parts in the source-specific RT primers: a common tail in the 5′-end for supplying a common priming site for the following PCR amplification, a source-specific sequence in the middle, and poly-T [15] plus several degenerate bases in the 3′-end for annealing the

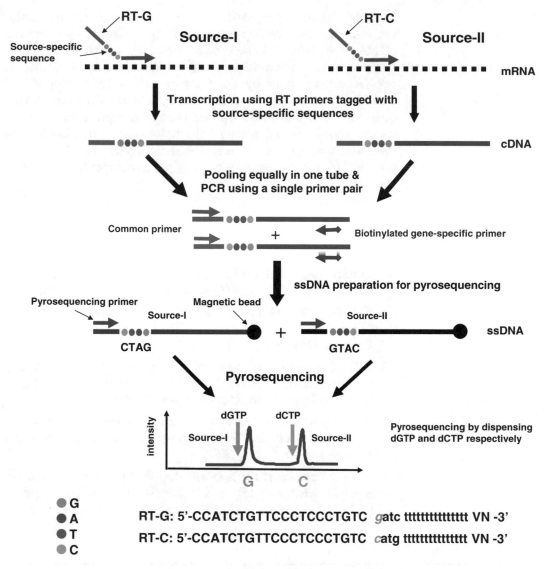

Fig. 1 A schematic of sequence-tagged reverse-transcription PCR coupled with pyrosequencing

mRNA strand. To fix the start position of the reverse transcription, two degenerate bases were added in the 3′-end of the RT primer. Each source-specific sequence has the same base content but a different base order; thus, Tm of cDNAs from different sources is completely identical. (2) PCR amplification of the templates and a pool of sequence-labeled cDNAs from different sources with a gene-specific primer and a common primer having the sequence identical to the common tail in the 5′-end of RT primers. Because of the specially designed RT primers, each source-specific amplicon has an identical Tm; unbiased PCR amplification on cDNA templates from different sources is thus achieved. Consequently the concentration ratio of amplicons from different sources can accurately reflect the expression level of a given gene among different sources. The cDNA produced by the labeled RT primers is a cDNA library which can be used for detecting any gene of interest. We can compare the abundance of any transcript among different mRNA sources only by changing a gene-specific primer. (3) Decoding and quantifying the source-specific amplicons by pyrosequencing. The base order in the pyrogram represents the gene source, and the peak intensity reflects the gene expression level in the corresponding gene source. The ratio of peak intensities is proportional to the relative abundance of the transcripts from different sources.

2   Materials

1. HotStarTaq DNA polymerase and Omniscript RT Kit were purchased from Qiagen (Qiagen GmbH, Hilden, Germany).

2. Exo-Klenow Fragment, polyvinylpyrrolidone (PVP), and QuantiLum Recombinant Luciferase were purchased from Promega (Madison, WI).

3. TRIzol reagent was from Invitrogen Inc. (Faraday Avenue, Carlsbad, CA), and Dynabeads M-280 Streptavidin (2.8 μm) was from Dynal Biotech ASA (Oslo, Norway).

4. ATP sulfurylase, apyrase, D-luciferin, bovine serum albumin (BSA), and adenosine 5′-phosphosulfate (APS) were obtained from Sigma (St. Louis, MO).

5. 2′-Deoxyguanosine-5′-triphosphate(dGTP),2′-deoxythymidine-5′-triphosphate (dTTP), and 2′-deoxycytidine-5′-triphosphate (dCTP) were purchased from Amersham Pharmacia Biotech (Piscataway, NJ).

3   Methods

3.1   Design of Source-Specific RT Primers

1. The source-specific RT primers are used for initiating cDNA synthesis, offering a common priming site for the following PCR, and discriminating the gene sources. The source-specific sequence is the key part in the RT primer. We used one base species to label one gene source. Since four kinds of dNTP are available, the expression level of a given gene among four different sources can be compared theoretically. Because of the high background signal from dATP in pyrosequencing, we employed bases T, G, and C for labeling the gene sources and put base A, which will not be dispensed in pyrosequencing, in a position next to these bases for blocking the extension. Unlike conventional pyrosequencing, the expensive reagent dATPαS was not used in SRPP [23–25]. To get an identical

melting temperature for every source-specific amplicon, it is preferable to balance the sequence composition in sequences of "gatc," "catg," and "tacg," respectively, but only dGTP, dCTP, and dTTP are dispensed. In the pyrogram, peaks "G," "C," and "T" represent the relative expression level of the target gene in each source.

2. Because mRNA has a long poly-A stretch, an RT primer with only a poly-T sequence will initiate the synthesis of cDNA at any site in the poly-A stretch of mRNA. To fix the start position of the reverse transcription, we have designed several RT primers with a different number of degenerate bases in the 3′-end. It was found that two degenerate bases in the 3′-end of the RT primer were enough to fix the start position of reverse transcription.

3. To facilitate the unbiased PCR amplification a priming sequence for PCR amplification is tagged in the 5′-end of the RT primer. As the PCR-primer sequence may affect the amplification efficiency [26–27], several kinds of candidate sequences were evaluated. The result indicates that a high GC content in 3′ termini of the common PCR primers is required. In the present research, P-2 with the GC content of 70 % is used.

3.2 RNA Extraction and Reverse Transcription

1. Total RNA from *Mus musculus* tissues was extracted by using a TRIzol reagent. The purity and concentration of the extracted RNA were determined by a UV–Vis spectrophotometer (Naka Instruments, Japan), and the concentration of these RNAs was adjusted to 1 µg/µL by RNase-free water.

2. An equal amount of the RNA (*see* **Note 1**) was used for the one-strand cDNA synthesis with different RT primers tagged with source-specific sequences (*see* **Note 2**).

3. First, total RNA in RNase-free water was heated to 65 °C for 5 min and snap chilled on ice for at least 1 min.

4. A reaction mixture containing 0.5 mM of each dNTP, 1× RT buffer, 1 µM RT primer, 0.5 U/µL RNase inhibitor, and 0.2 U/µL Omniscript reverse transcriptase (*see* **Note 3**) was added to each tube containing RNA, mixed gently, collected by brief centrifugation, and incubated at 37 °C for 60 min followed by 93 °C for 5 min to terminate the reaction.

3.3 Preparation of Template Pools

One-strand cDNAs from different sources which had been labeled by the sequences tagged in RT primers were diluted to 50 times. Aliquot of each source-specific cDNA was pooled and used as the template for PCR.

3.4 PCR

1. Each 50 µL PCR mixture contained 1.5 mM $MgCl_2$, 0.2 mM of each dNTP, 0.3 µM of each gene-specific primer, and the common primer MP, 1 µL of template pool, and 1.25 unit of HotStarTaq DNA polymerase (Qiagen) (*see* **Note 4**).

2. Amplification was performed on a PTC-225 thermocycler PCR system (MJ Research, Inc., MA) according to the following protocol: denatured at 94 °C for 15 min and followed by 35 thermal reaction cycles (*see* **Note 5**) (94 °C for 40 s; 60 °C for 40 s; 72 °C for 1 min). After the cycle, the product was incubated at 72 °C for 10 min and held at 4 °C before use.

3.5 Template Preparation for Pyrosequencing

1. Streptavidin-coated magnetic beads were used to prepare ssDNA template for pyrosequencing [14–17]. This technology enables biotinylated PCR products to be captured onto the magnetic beads. After sedimentation, the remaining components of the PCR reaction can be removed by washing to obtain a pure double-stranded DNA followed by alkali denaturation to yield ssDNA. Both the immobilized biotinylated strands and nonbiotinylated strands can be used as sequencing templates.

2. Then sequencing primers were added to hybridize the ssDNA. Here immobilized biotinylated strands were used as the sequencing templates.

3.6 Pyrosequencing

The reaction volume was 100 μL, containing 0.1 M tris-acetate (pH 7.7), 2 mM EDTA, 10 mM magnesium acetate, 0.1 % BSA, 1 mM dithiothreitol (DTT), 2 μM adenosine 5′-phosphosulfate (APS), 0.4 mg/mL PVP, 0.4 mM D-luciferin, 200 mU/mL ATP sulfurylase, 3 μg/mL luciferase, 18 U/mL Klenow fragment, and 1.6 U/mL apyrase. Pyrosequencing was carried out by the method reported by Ronaghi et al. [17] (*see* **Note 6**).

4   Method Validation

4.1 Quantitative Evaluation

As a method for quantitative analysis, accuracy should be the most important factor to be considered. To investigate the accuracy of SRPP, a series of templates pooled from two artificial sources were employed. The process was as follows: the total RNA from the *Mus musculus* liver was divided into two aliquots, and each aliquot was used as one source of the *Gapdh* gene. Two aliquots were transcribed with two source-specific primers, RT-G and RT-C, respectively, and then PCR-template pools were prepared by mixing two source-specific transcripts at the ratios of 10:0, 9:1, 8:2, 7:3, 6:4, 5:5, 4:6, 3:7, 2:8, 1:9, and 0:10, respectively. After PCR amplification using the common primer and the *Gapdh* gene-specific primer, pyrosequencing was performed. Usually, there is no peak appearing in a pyrogram when the added dNTP is not complementary to the template. However, dNTP is not so stable that a small amount of PPi due to dNTP degradation is produced. The noises by the unexpected PPi may interfere with the accuracy of SRPP even if the endogenous PPi in the original dNTP solution was degraded in advance with a small amount of beaded PPase. To eliminate the ambiguity due to the noises, each dNTP was dispensed twice to get two peaks corresponding to the strand extension and background signals, respectively. The typical pyrograms for the ratios of 10:0, 5:5, and 0:10 were seen in Fig. 2a, showing that almost no amplicon was yielded for RT-G (Fig. 2A-1) or for RT-C (Fig. 2A-3) when the template was only from one source, and nearly equal amounts of amplicons were observed when equally pooling two source-specific transcripts (Fig. 2A-2). Within the mixing range, the correlation between the measured and theoretical signal intensity ratios was as good as 0.9989 (R^2, $n=3$; see Fig. 2b). Since the RT primers could be labeled with three kinds of sequences ("gatc," "catg," and "tacg"), the ability of SRPP for quantifying the expression levels of the Cdk4 gene among three different sources was further investigated. The detection procedure was similar to that mentioned above, except for keeping two of the source-specific templates with a constant ratio while changing

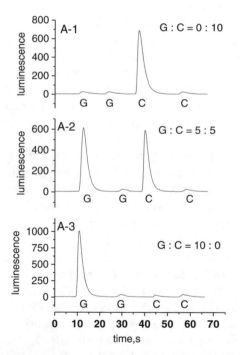

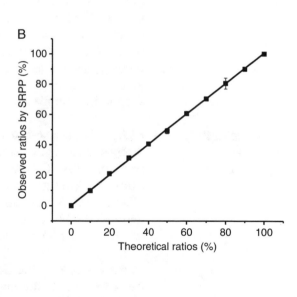

Fig. 2 (**a**) Pyrograms of artificial templates pooled with two source-specific cDNAs, each containing an equal amount of *Gapdh* transcripts at the ratios of 10:0, 5:5, and 0:10 (G:C), respectively. For convenience, two sources were termed as source-G and source-C, respectively, and the ratio of the amount of expressed gene between two sources was simply expressed as G:C. PCR was performed by using the common primer and the *Gapdh* gene-specific primer. Each dNTP was dispensed twice for detecting the background due to PPi impurity in dNTP solution. (**b**) Correlation between the theoretical ratios of the amounts of the *Gapdh* transcripts in two sources and the observed ratios by the SRPP method based on the comparison of the peak intensities in the pyrograms. The ratios were calculated with the formula of "G/(G + C) × 100" where G and C mean the peak intensity

the relative content of the third one. Three aliquots were first transcribed with three source-specific primers, RT-G, RT-T, and RT-C, respectively, and then the template pools were prepared by mixing the three source-specific transcripts at the ratios of 1:1:1, 1:2:1, 1:4:1, 1:6:1, 1:8:1, and 1:10:1. The typical pyrograms for the ratios of 1:2:1, 1:4:1, and 1:8:1 were shown in Fig. 3, and the statistical analysis for all the observed data was listed in Table 1, indicating that the ratio measured by comparing peak intensities in the pyrogram could accurately reflect the ratio between source-specific transcripts. Consequently, the source-specific sequence in the template did not cause a bias PCR amplification in SRPP, and the peaks decoded by pyrosequencing can quantitatively discriminate the source of a target gene. The dynamic range of SRPP is mainly dependent on that of pyrosequencing technology. By carefully reducing the noise due to dNTP, the transcripts as small as 5 % of the abundant transcripts can be accurately detected by measuring peak heights. SRPP is not competitive with the dye-based real-time PCR in a standpoint of dynamic range; however, the dynamic range can be readily extended by diluting the overexpressed transcripts with a high dilution ratio before the pooling process. We have successfully extended the dynamic range to three orders of magnitude by this strategy. Since differential gene expression analysis aims to compare the expression levels of the same target genes among different tissues but not different genes in a tissue, a dynamic range with one order of magnitude is enough to supply the data for explaining the biologic implication.

4.2 Effect of DNA Coexisting in the Transcripts on PCR

Although reverse-transcription process removes most DNAs, templates for PCR usually contain coexisting DNAs, which may result in a bias PCR amplification. To investigate the effect of coexisting DNA in the transcripts on PCR, two aliquots, each with 1 μg of a total RNA, were mixed with 0, 1, 2, and 3 μg of *Mus musculus* genomic DNA, respectively, and then transcribed by the RT primers, RT-G and RT-C, respectively. The amount of coexisting DNA is 0, 1, 2, and 3 times of that of the RNA sample, respectively. The expression level of the Cdk4 gene between the two artificial sources was detected for the investigation. If PCR was not biased by the coexisting DNA, the ratio measured by comparing peak intensities in a pyrogram should be close to 1:1. As shown in Fig. 4, the observed ratios are 1.1:1, 0.95:1, 0.92:1, and 1.1:1 for 0, 1, 2, and 3 μg of the spiked DNA, respectively, suggesting that the coexisting DNA did not result in a bias PCR in SRPP. This is because the coexisting DNA has no sequence complementary to the common PCR primer, and the exponential amplification should not occur even if the coexisting DNA contained the sequences complementary to the gene-specific primer. Most importantly, the undesired extension products due to the genomic DNA do not contain the source-specific sequences, so the source-specific amplification is not biased.

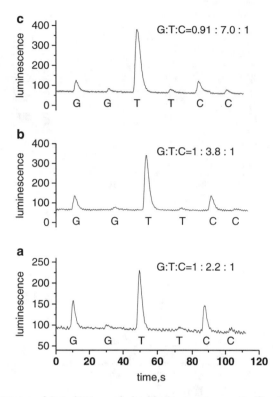

Fig. 3 Pyrograms of templates pooled with three source-specific cDNAs, each containing an equal amount of Cdk4 transcripts at the ratios (G:T:C) of 1:2:1 (A), 1:4:1 (B), and 1:8:1 (C), respectively. PCR was performed by using the common primer and the Cdk4 gene-specific primer. Each dNTP was dispensed twice for detecting the background due to PPi impurity in dNTP solution. The observed ratio of peak intensities was marked in each pyrogram as "G:T:C="

Table 1

Results for detecting the expression levels of the Cdk4 gene among the three sources, each containing different amount of Cdk4 transcripts

Template no.	Theoretic ratio (%) (G/T/C)[a]	Measured ratio (%) (G/T/C)[b]	RSD (%) (G/T/C)
1	25/50/25 (1:2:1)	25.2/49.6/25.2	0.6/0.6/0.6
2	16.7/66.7/16.7 (1:4:1)	17.6/65.2/17.1	3.7/1.6/1.7
3	12.5/75/12.5 (1:6:1)	13.3/73.6/13.1	4.4/1.3/3.3
4	10/80/10 (1:8:1)	10.3/78.5/11.3	2.1/1.3/8.6
5	8.3/83.3/8.3 (1:10:1)	8.2/82.0/9.8	0.9/1.1/11.7

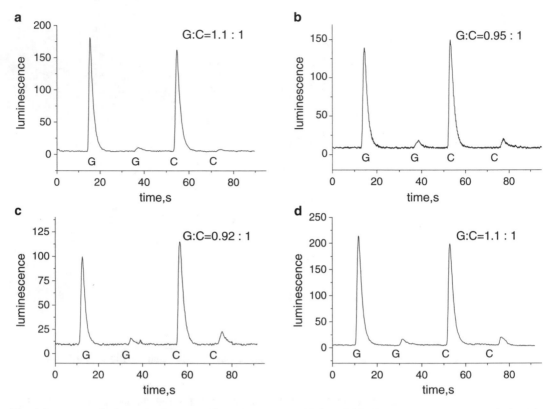

Fig. 4 Pyrograms for investigating the effect of coexisting DNA on PCR. The experiment was carried out by detecting the expression level of the Cdk4 gene between two identical sources which was prepared by spiking 0 (A), 1 (B), 2 (C), and 3 μg (D) of the *Mus musculus* genomic DNA into 1 μg of total RNA sample, respectively. The observed ratio of peak intensities was marked in each pyrogram as "G:C="

4.3 Determination of Gene Expression Levels

The SRPP method described here can compare the gene expression levels of two or three sources. To demonstrate the applicability of the established method, the relative expression levels of six kinds of genes (Cdk2ap2, Vps4b, Fas, Fos, Cdk4, and Actb) among the kidney, the brain, and the heart tissues of a mouse were detected. At first, equal amounts of total RNA from different tissues were transcribed with primers RT-G, RT-C, and RT-T, respectively. After PCR amplification on the pool of cDNAs, decoding and quantification of the source-specific sequence were carried out by pyrosequencing, and the pyrograms were shown in Fig. 5, indicating that all the six genes were expressed in the three organs of the mouse but with different expression levels. To confirm the accuracy of the SRPP in differential gene expression analysis, real-time PCR, which is a golden method for quantifying the gene expression levels, was used to detect the copy number of the six genes in each kind of the tissues. As shown in Table 1, the results from the two methods are quite similar. For example, the ratio of the expressed amounts of the Vps4b gene between the kidney, the brain, and the heart tissues of the mouse is 48.7:26.9:24.5

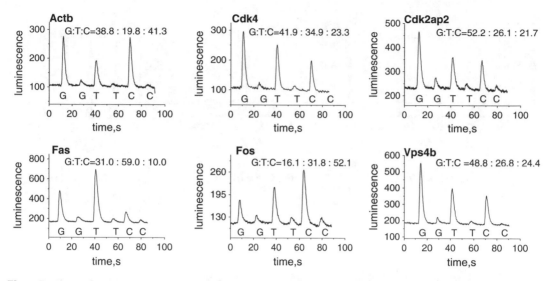

Fig. 5 Pyrograms for detecting the expression levels of the *Cdk2ap2*, *Vps4b*, *Fas*, *Fos*, *Cdk4*, and *Actb* genes among the kidney, the brain, and the heart tissues of a mouse. "G," "T," and "C" under the pyrogram mean the type of the dispensed dNTP and represent the tissue sources of kidney, heart, and brain, respectively. Each dNTP was dispensed twice for detecting the background due to PPi impurity in dNTP solution

by SRPP and 49.3:26:24.7 by real-time PCR, suggesting that our new method is accurate enough for quantitatively comparing gene expression levels among different sources.

4.4 Reproducibility and Sensitivity

For a quantitative analysis, a high reproducibility is necessary. The reproducibility of SRPP is evaluated by detecting the relative expression levels of three genes (Vps4b, Cdk4, and Actb) among the kidney, heart, and brain of a mouse independently at different days ($n=3$), showing RSD values ranging from 0.01 to 0.18 with the average of 0.06. Therefore, SRPP offers a superior reproducibility to conventional multiplex PCR. This is because SRPP is independent of a fluctuation of measuring conditions, such as PCR cycle numbers, PCR primer sequences, and PCR reaction conditions.

The main error in SRPP is believed from the step of quantification of RNA concentration by UV spectrophotometry because pyrosequencing is highly quantitative. This step could however be skipped if we employ housekeeping genes as the internal concentration control because the expression level of a housekeeping gene is almost constant among different tissues. The measured data for the target genes could be calibrated by several housekeeping genes, which is regularly used in the microarray-based method.

To evaluate the amount of total RNA samples required for an SRPP assay, the relative expression levels of two genes (Actb and Cdk4) between two identical sources artificially prepared with various amounts of total RNA (0.05, 0.2, and 1 μg, respectively) were analyzed. As indicated in Fig. 6, the measured ratios of the

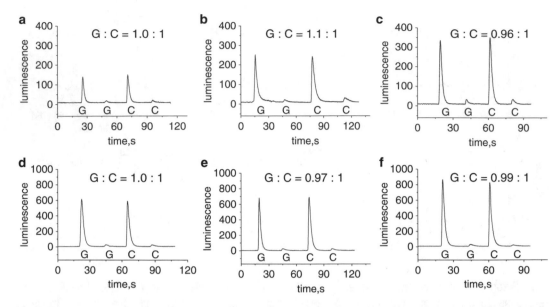

Fig. 6 Pyrograms for detecting the expression levels of the Cdk4 (**a–c**) and Actb (**d–f**) genes between two identical sources with 0.05 (**a, d**), 0.2 (**b, e**), and 1 μg (**c, f**) of total RNA, respectively. Each RNA sample was individually transcribed by RT primers RT-G and RT-C. The ten-times dilution of each cDNA sample was pooled as the PCR template. The ratios by measuring the peak intensities are marked in each pyrogram. The observed ratio of peak intensities was marked in each pyrogram as "G:C="

expression amounts of both genes between the two identical sources are close to 1:1 for all tested samples. Therefore, SRPP is highly sensitive, and 50 ng of total RNA is enough for an accurate SRPP assay.

As SRPP isdependent on PCR amplification, more PCR cycles are beneficial to the sensitivity. To demonstrate the effect of PCR cycles on the accuracy of SRPP, PCR of the *Gapdh* gene with various cycles was carried out on a template mix which was artificially prepared by pooling two source-specific transcripts at the ratio of 1:2. The detected ratios of the expression levels between two artificial sources are 1:1.8, 1:2.1, 1:2.1, 1:1.9, and 1:1.9 for PCR with the cycles of 20, 25, 30, 35, and 40, respectively. Therefore, the accuracy of SRPP is independent of PCR cycles, and more PCR cycles can be used for increasing the sensitivity. As more PCR cycles may cause nonspecific amplicons, 35 PCR cycles are recommended for a routine assay.

5   Technical Notes

1. SRPP is highly sensitive, and 50 ng of total RNA is enough for an accurate SRPP assay.

2. Because of the high background signal from dATP in pyrosequencing, we employed bases T, G, and C for labeling the gene sources and put base A, which will not be dispensed in

pyrosequencing, in a position next to these bases for blocking the extension.

3. A reverse transcriptase with a good quality should give a high efficiency of reverse transcription. We have tried AMV Reverse Transcriptase (TaKaRa), SuperScript III RNase H-Reverse Transcriptase (Invitrogen), and Omniscript RT Kit (Qiagen) for reverse transcription, respectively. The results indicated that AMV Reverse Transcriptase was not suitable for our method, and there was insignificant difference in RT efficiency between the other two kits.

4. It is difficult to escape the poly-T stretch in the target sequence used in SRPP as the RT primer having poly-T_{15} for reverse transcription. To enable efficient PCR for difficult templates, we tried several *Taq* polymerases, including TaKaRa *rTaq* polymerase, Promega *Taq* polymerase, and Qiagen HotStarTaq DNA polymerase. The results indicated that Qiagen HotStarTaq DNA polymerase is suitable for amplifying the template containing a poly-T tract in SRPP.

5. The accuracy of SRPP is independent of PCR cycles, and more PCR cycles can be used for increasing the sensitivity. As more PCR cycles may cause nonspecific amplicons, 35 PCR cycles are recommended for a routine assay.

6. To eliminate the ambiguity due to the noises, each dNTP was dispensed twice to get two peaks corresponding to the strand extension and background signals, respectively.

7. The ratio measured by comparing peak intensities in the pyrogram could accurately reflect the ratio between source-specific transcripts. Consequently, the source-specific sequence in the template did not cause a bias PCR amplification in SRPP, and the peaks decoded by pyrosequencing can quantitatively discriminate the source of a target gene.

8. The main error in SRPP is believed from the step of quantification of RNA concentration by UV spectrophotometry because pyrosequencing is highly quantitative. This step could however be skipped if we employ housekeeping genes as the internal concentration control, because the expression level of a housekeeping gene is almost constant among different tissues.

References

1. Chin D, Boyle GM, Theile DR, Parsons PG, Coman WB (2006) The human genome and gene expression profiling. J Plast Reconstr Aesthet Surg 59:902–911

2. van't Veer LJ, Dai H, van de Vijver MJ, He YD, Hart AA, Mao M, Peterse HL, van der Kooy K, Marton MJ, Witteveen AT, Schreiber GJ, Kerkhoven RM, Roberts C, Linsley PS, Bernards R, Friend SH (2002) Gene expression profiling predicts clinical outcome of breast cancer. Nature 415:530–536

3. Morris SR, Carey LA (2007) A gene expression profiling in breast cancer. Curr Opin Oncol 19(547):551

4. Velculescu VE, Zhang L, Vogelstein B, Kinzler KW (1995) Serial analysis of gene expression. Science 270:484–487

5. Schena M, Shalon D, Davis RW, Brown PO (1995) Quantitative monitoring of gene expression patterns with a complementary DNA microarray. Science 270:467–470

6. Fu GK, Stuve LL (2003) Quantitative monitoring of gene expression patterns with a complementary DNA microarray. Biotechniques 34:764–766

7. Lockhart DJ, Dong H, Byrne MC, Follettie MT, Gallo MV, Chee MS, Mittmann M, Wang C, Kobayashi M, Horton H, Brown EL (1996) Expression monitoring by hybridization to high-density oligonucleotide arrays. Nat Biotechnol 14:1675–1680

8. Liang P, Pardee AB (1992) Differential display of eukaryotic messenger RNA by means of the polymerase chain reaction. Science 257:967–971

9. White BA, Bancroft FC (1982) Cytoplasmic dot hybridization. Simple analysis of relative mRNA levels in multiple small cell or tissue samples. J Biol Chem 257:8569–8572

10. Heid CA, Stevens J, Livak KJ, Williams PM (1996) Real time quantitative PCR. Genome Res 6:986–994

11. Wong ML, Medrano JF (2005) Real-time PCR for mRNA quantitation. Biotechniques 39:75–85

12. Berggren WT, Takova T, Olson MC, Eis PS, Kwiatkowski RW, Smith LM (2002) Multiplexed gene expression analysis using the invader RNA assay with MALDI-TOF mass spectrometry detection. Anal Chem 74:1745–1750

13. Weidenhammer EM, Kahl BF, Wang L, Wang L, Duhon M, Jackson JA, Slater M, Xu X (2002) Multiplexed, targeted gene expression profiling and genetic analysis on electronic microarrays. Clin Chem 48:1873–1882

14. Ronaghi M (2001) Pyrosequencing sheds light on DNA sequencing. Genome Res 11:3–11

15. Ronaghi M, Uhlen M, Nyren P (1998) A sequencing method based on real-time pyrophosphate. Science 281:363–365

16. Schouten JP, McElgunn CJ, Waaijer R, Zwijnenburg D, Diepvens F, Pals G (2002) Relative quantification of 40 nucleic acid sequences by multiplex ligation-dependent probe amplification. Nucleic Acids Res 30:57

17. Elahi E, Ronaghi M (2004) Pyrosequencing: a tool for DNA sequencing analysis. Methods Mol Biol 255:211–219

18. Zhou GH, Kamahori M, Okano K, Harada K, Kambara H (2001) Miniaturized pyrosequencer for DNA analysis with capillaries to deliver deoxynucleotides. Electrophoresis 22:3497–3504

19. Zhou GH, Gotou M, Kajiyama T, Kambara H (2005) Multiplex SNP typing by bioluminometric assay coupled with terminator incorporation (BATI). Nucleic Acids Res 33:e133

20. Margulies M, Egholm M, Altman WE et al (2005) Genome sequencing in microfabricated high-density picolitre reactors. Nature 437:376–380

21. Hardenbol P, Baner J, Jain M, Nilsson M, Namsaraev EA, Karlin-Neumann GA, Fakhrai-Rad H, Ronaghi M, Willis TD, Landegren U, Davis RW (2003) Multiplexed genotyping with sequence-tagged molecular inversion probes. Nat Biotechnol 21:673–678

22. Wang WP, Ni KY, Zhou GH (2006) Multiplex single nucleotide polymorphism genotyping by adapter ligation-mediated allele-specific amplification. Anal Biochem 355:240–248

23. Langan JE, Rowbottom L, Liloglou T, Field JK, Risk JM (2002) Sequencing of difficult templates containing poly(A/T) tracts: closure of sequence gaps. Biotechniques 33(276):278–280

24. Rice JE, Sanchez JA, Pierce KE, Reis AH Jr, Osborne A, Wangh LJ (2007) Monoplex/multiplex linear-after-the-exponential-PCR assays combined with PrimeSafe and Dilute-'N'-Go sequencing. Nat Protoc 2:2429–2438

25. Pierce KE, Sanchez JA, Rice JE, Wangh LJ (2005) Linear-After-The-Exponential (LATE)-PCR: primer design criteria for high yields of specific single-stranded DNA and improved real-time detection. Proc Natl Acad Sci U S A 102:8609–8614

26. Sanchez JA, Pierce KE, Rice JE, Wangh LJ (2004) Linear-after-the-exponential (LATE)-PCR: an advanced method of asymmetric PCR and its uses in quantitative real-time analysis. Proc Natl Acad Sci U S A 101:1933–1938

27. Zhou GH, Kajiyama T, Gotou M, Kishimoto A, Suzuki S, Kambara H (2006) Enzyme system for improving the detection limit in pyrosequencing. Anal Chem 78:4482–4489

Chapter 20

Development of Pyrosequencing-Based Multiplex Bioassay by Designing Barcodes Encoded with Artificially Designed Sequences

Zhiyao Chen, Xiaodan Zhang, Xiqun Liu, Bingjie Zou, Haiping Wu, Qinxin Song, Hideki Kambara, and Guohua Zhou

Abstract

Multiplex analysis in a single tube is always preferable for genetic analysis. Here we propose a novel dye-free labeling method for multiplex bioassay. First, each of the targets was encoded by a short sequence-based barcode consisting of a report base and repeats of two stuffer bases; then, the barcodes were quantitatively decoded by a single pyrosequencing assay without any pre-separation. A barcode set is designed by sequentially inserting a reporter base into different locations of the repeats. Because the location of the reporter base is unique at a given barcode, each addition of dNTP complementary to the stuffer base results in the release of the reporter base corresponding to a unique barcoded target. The multiplex level based on the present barcoding method can be unlimitedly increased if long-read pyrosequencing is accurate enough. Using these barcodes, we have developed a barcoded adapter-based method for multiplex gene expression analysis; as a proof of concept, the 12-plex gene expression analysis of four different genes among 12 kinds of tissues of a mouse was successfully demonstrated. In comparison to conventional barcodes based on dyes or nanocrystals, our sequence-based barcodes do not need laser, gel, and electrophoresis. Most importantly, this barcode strategy significantly extends the scope of pyrosequencing capability.

Key words Sequence-based barcodes, Pyrosequencing, Gene expression analysis

---

1 Introduction

Multiplex detection allowing multiple discrete assays in a single tube at the same time is always preferable for genetic analysis. An efficient technique for achieving multiplex analysis is barcoding [1, 2]. Dyes with different emission profiles are conventionally used as barcodes to label multiple targets; however, the number of dye-based barcodes is greatly limited by the overlap of dye's broad emission spectra. DNA fragments with various base sequences can be informative barcodes if the encoded sequences could be uniquely decoded [3]. Pyrosequencingis based on the real-time monitoring of bioluminescence emitted from the primer extension

Guohua Zhou and Qinxin Song (eds.), *Advances and Clinical Practice in Pyrosequencing*, Springer Protocols Handbooks, DOI 10.1007/978-1-4939-3308-2_20, © Springer Science+Business Media New York 2016

reaction [4, 5], and is very suitable for sequencing several tens of bases; thus it could be used to decode the target-specific tags encoded in the PCR primers before amplification. However, it is difficult to pick up multiple barcodes by pyrosequencing the mixed amplicons in a single tube because all the extendable ends of barcodes contribute to the peaks in a pyrogram [6]. Here we have proposed a novel barcoding approach based on conventional pyrosequencing to decode barcodes only by peaks in a pyrogram. The logic for designing the barcodes is that there is no extension reaction occurring at all other barcodes when extending a target-specific reporter base, causing a unique target-specific peak in a pyrogram. For the illustration of the principle, assign "Y" and "Z" the stuffer bases, and "X" the reporter base. At first, design a 6-nt stuffer base sequence as "YZYZYZ," and then insert the reporter base "X" at each possible place of "YZYZYZ," resulting in the following six unique barcodes: "X_1YZYZYZ," "YX_2ZYZYZ," "YZX_3YZYZ," "YZYX_4ZYZ," "YZYZX_5YZ," and "YZYZYX_6Z." The bases "Y" and "Z" should be arranged by turns in the barcodes, so that the extension of a stuffer base ("Y" or "Z") only releases the end for extending a specific reporter base "X" in a unique barcode. To uniquely decode these barcodes, the dispensing order of dNTPs during pyrosequencing should be designed in the light of the encoding rule. For example (see Fig. 1a), only the barcode "X_1YZYZYZ" contributes the extension signal when dispensing a dNTP complementary to the base X_1; and the dispensing of a dNTP complementary to the base Y causes the extension of one base in all barcodes; only the barcode "Y$X2$ZYZYZ" gives a peak when dispensing a dNTP complementary to the base X_2; again, all barcodes extend one base when dispensing a dNTP complementary to the base Z, giving an extendable end to the next base X_3 in the barcode "YZX_3YZYZ." By repeatedly dispensing dNTPs in the above order, a 6-plex detection is achieved only by a single pyrosequencing assay. However this labeling efficiency is not so high because the decoding of six barcodes needs 11 times dNTP dispensing. Since two bases are available for reporters, the same 6-nt length of the sequence can yield 12 unique barcodes if two different reporter bases are used; thus 17 dNTP dispension could result in the decoding of 12 barcodes. A typical example of 12 barcodes using two different reporter bases in a 6-nt DNA fragment is illustrated in Fig. 1b. The multiplex level based on the present barcoding method can be unlimitedly increased if a long-read pyrosequencing is accurate enough; theoretically n-base length of the barcoded DNA fragments is able to produce $2n$ sample identifiers, and the minimum number of dNTP dispensing is $3n - 1$. Usually, a conventional pyrosequencing can give an accurate reading length of at least 20 bases; hence, the optimal value of n should be 7, which could yield 14 barcodes in a single pyrosequencing assay.

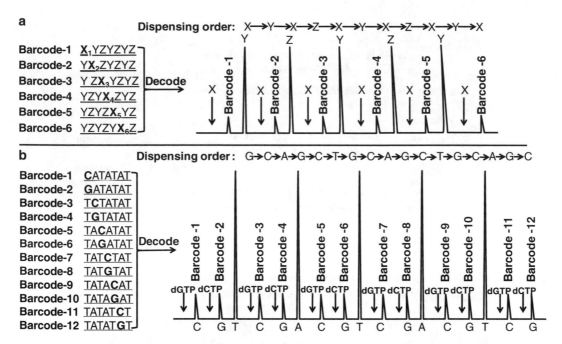

Fig. 1 Principle of barcode design (**a**) and a typical example of 12 barcodes constructing with 6-nt DNA fragments using base "g" and "C" as reporter bases. (**b**) Left side is the structure of barcodes, and right side is the corresponding pyrogram for decoding the barcodes. Base "X" represents a reporter base; and bases "Y" and "Z" represent stuffer bases

To use these barcodes for multiplex bioassays, we developed a method, termed barcoded adapter-based multiplex gene expression analysis ("BAMGA" for short). Barcodes specific to each different gene source were encoded in source-specific adapters. As seen in Fig. 2a, the assay consists of the following steps: (1) extracting total RNA from different tissues and followed by a reverse transcription into ds-cDNA; (2) digesting the ds-cDNA with restriction endonuclease *Mbo* I, which specifically cuts DNA strands to form a "GATC" cohesive end; (3) labeling the digested ds-cDNA fragments with adapters encoded with source-specific barcodes by ligation reaction; (4) amplifying the barcode-ligated fragments with a universal primer and a biotinylated gene-specific primer; and (5) quantitatively decoding the barcodes in amplicon mixtures by pyrosequencing. The sequence in the resulting pyrogram represents the source of the gene, and the intensity of the peak represents the relative expression levels of the gene; the signal ratio reflects the proportion of the amount of mRNAs among different sources. The key to the success of the method is the structure of source-selective adapters. We designed the adapter with a "GATC" 3′-overhang in one end for capturing the digested ds-cDNA, while the other end is "Y" shaped with one strand having a barcode together with an around 20-nt 5′-overhang for supplying a

234   Zhiyao Chen et al.

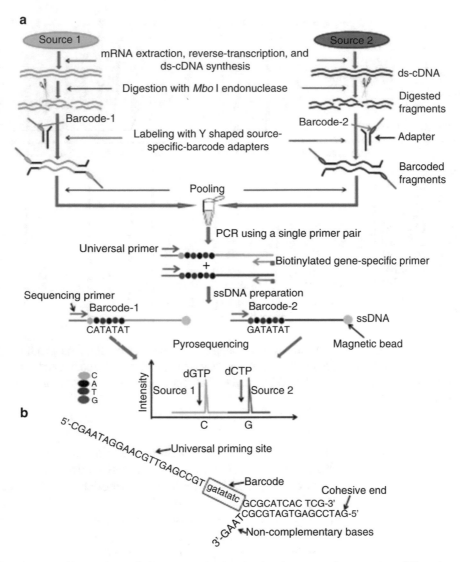

Fig. 2 Flowchart used to analyze relative expression levels of a given gene between two different sources (**a**) and the typical structure of "Y"-shaped source-specific barcode adapter (**b**). This figure illustrates the principle of BAMGA and the structure of "Y"-shaped source-specific barcode adapter

universal PCR-priming site, and the opposite strand having several non-complementary bases in the 3′-terminal to block nonspecific extension reaction. Each barcode sequence has the same base content but a different base order; thus the Tm values of barcode-ligated fragments are completely identical. By this design, unbiased amplification of all barcoded templates is achieved (Fig. 2b). The BAMGA assay of a different gene can be easily achieved only by changing a gene-specific primer.

2 Materials

1. TaKaRa M-MLV RTase cDNA synthesis kit, Mbo I endonuclease, T4 DNA ligase, SYBR Premix Ex TaqTM, TaKaRa M-MLV RTase cDNA Synthesis Kit, and rTaq DNA polymerase were purchased from TaKaRa (Dalian, China).

2. Exo-Klenow Fragment and QuantiLum recombinant luciferase were purchased from Promega (Madison, WI).

3. TRIzol reagent and Superscript II RNase H-Reverse Transcriptase were from Invitrogen Inc. (Faraday Avenue, Carlsbad, CA).

4. Dynabeads M-280 Streptavidin (2.8 μm) was from Dynal Biotech ASA (Oslo, Norway).

5. ATP sulfurylase, D-luciferin, bovine serum albumin (BSA), polyvinylpyrrolidone (PVP), adenosine 5′-phosphosulfate (APS), and apyrase were obtained from Sigma (St. Louis, MO).

6. 2′-Deoxyguanosine-5′-triphosphate(dGTP),2′-deoxythymidine-5′-triphosphate (dTTP), 2′-deoxycytidine-5′-triphosphate (dCTP), 2′, 3′-dideoxycytidine-5′-triphosphate (ddCTP), 2′, 3′-dideoxyguanosin e-5′-triphosphate (ddGTP), sodium 2′-deoxyadenosine-5′-O-(1-triphosphate) (dATPαS), and Sequenase 2.0 were purchased from Amersham Pharmacia Biotech (Amersham, UK).

7. BioSpin PCR purification kit was purchased from Bio Flux Corporation (Hangzhou, China).

3 Methods

3.1 RNA Extraction and ds-cDNA Synthesis

1. Total RNAs (see Note 1) from small intestines, right brain, large intestine, cerebellum, spleen, lung, left brain, bladder, heart, stomach, ear, and kidney tissues of a mouse were extracted using TRIzol reagent according to the manufacturer's instructions.

2. The purity and concentration of the extracted RNA were determined by a UV-Vis spectrophotometer (NaKa Instrument Co., ltd, Japan).

3. Then 1.5 μg of each total RNA from different tissues was used for first-strand cDNA synthesis by Superscript II RNase H-Reverse Transcriptase, respectively. First, total RNA in RNase-free water was heated to 65 °C for 5 min and cooled on ice for at least 1 min. Then a 10 μl of reaction mixture containing 0.5 mM of each dNTP, 1× RT buffer, 1 μM oligo (dT)$_{15}$ primer, 0.5 U/μl RNase inhibitor, and 0.2 U/μl Superscript II

RNase H-Reverse Transcriptase was added to each tube containing extracted RNA, and incubated at 42 °C for 60 min, followed by 93 °C for 5 min to terminate the reaction.

4. All of the first-strand cDNA was used to synthesize double-stranded cDNA (ds-cDNA) by TaKaRa M-MLV RTase cDNA Synthesis Kit according to the manufacturer's instructions. The 50 μl of ds-cDNA synthesis reactions containing 10 μl of first-strand cDNA solution, 10 μl of 5× ds-cDNA synthesis buffer (18.8 mM Tris–HCl, 90.6 mM KCl, 4.6 mM MgCl$_2$, 10 mM (NH4)$_2$SO4, pH 8.3), 0.15 mM NAD, 0.002 % BSA, 3.8 mM DTT, 0.1 mM dNTPs, 6 U of *E. coli* DNA ligase, 6 U of DNA polymerase I, 1 U of *E. coli* RNase H, and RNase-free water up to 50 μl was incubated at 16 °C for 1.5 h followed by 70 °C for 10 min to terminate the reaction.

3.2 Digestion and Ligation of ds-cDNA

1. Digestion and ligation reaction were performed on an O.T.P. Safety thermostat (PolyScience, USA). The 5 μl of digest ion mixture containing 2.5 μl of ds-cDNA solution, 0.5 μl of 10× K Buffer, 5 U of *Mbo* I endonuclease, and 1.5 μl of sterilized water was mixed gently and incubated at 37 °C for 2 h followed by 75 °C for 15 min to terminate the reaction. Then digested ds-cDNA was ligated to source-specific adapters, respectively.

2. The 20 μl of ligation reaction mixture containing 4 μl of the digested mixture, 2 μl of sterilized water, and 20 pmol of a source-specific adapter was incubated at 70 °C for 10 min, and then 2 μl of 10 U/μl T4 DNA ligase and 2 μl of 10× T4 DNA ligase buffer were added before the incubation at 16 °C for 2 h. The ligase was inactivated at 75 °C for 15 min. Finally, equal volume of the barcode-ligated fragments from different sources was pooled for PCR amplification.

3.3 PCR and Purification of PCR Product

1. PCR amplification was performed on the PTC-225 Thermal Cycler PCR system (MJ Research, Inc., USA). Fifty microliters of PCR reaction contains 1.5 mM MgCl$_2$, 0.2 mM of each dNTP, 1.2 μM of each gene-specific primer and the universal primer, 1 μl of equally mixed ligation products as templates, and 1.25 U of rTaq DNA polymerase. The PCR program is as follows: denatured at 94 °C for 3 min, followed by 35 thermal cycles (94 °C for 30 s; 55 °C for 30 s; 72 °C for 45 s). After the cycle reaction, the product was incubated at 72 °C for 10 min and held at 16 °C.

2. Then the PCR products were purified by BioSpin PCR purification kit to remove surplus biotinylated primers (*see* **Note 2**). Agarose gel electrophoresis can be used to verify the negative control. If a clear pattern is obtained, pyrosequencing is then performed on samples.

3.4 Template Preparation for Pyrosequencing

The biotinylated PCR products were immobilized onto streptavidin-coated Dynabeads, and DNA strands were separated by melting with 0.1 M NaOH. After washing with 1× annealing buffer (4 mM Tris–HCl, pH 7.5, 2 mM $MgCl_2$, 5 mM NaCl), the sequencing primer was added to the single-stranded DNA for annealing at 80 °C for 2 min.

3.5 Pyrosequencing Reaction

Pyrosequencing was carried out by the reported method [1–7]. The reaction volume was 100 µl, containing 0.1 M Tris–acetate (pH 7.7), 2 mM EDTA, 10 mM magnesium acetate, 0.1 % BSA, 1 mM dithiothreitol, 2 µM adenosine 5′-phosphosulfate 0.4 mg/ml PVP, 0.4 mM D-luciferin, 200 mU/ml ATP sulfurylase, 3 µg/ml luciferase, 18 U/ml Sequenase 2.0 or 18 U/ml Exo- Klenow Fragment, and 1.6 U/ml apyrase. Pyrosequencing can also be performed by using commercialized PyroMark GOLD reagent kit (Qiagen, Germany) at PyroMark ID instrument (Qiagen, Germany).

3.6 Real-Time PCR

Real-time PCR amplification was carried out with a DNA Engine Opticon 2 Thermal Cycler system (MJ Research, Inc., USA). Twenty-five microliters of reaction mixture contains 12.5 µl of SYBR Premix Ex Taq™ (2×), 0.4 µM each primer, 1 µl of diluted (1/30) ss-cDNA (synthesized from 1.5 µg of total RNA), and 9.5 µl of sterilized water. The program used was initial denaturation at 94 °C for 5 min followed by 40 cycles of 94 °C for 30 s, 55 °C for 30 s, 72 °C for 40 s, plate read at 81 °C for 0.01 s, followed by a final extension of 7 min at 72 °C.

4 Method Validation

4.1 The Effect of Coexisting Nontarget RNA on the Accuracy

It is necessary to investigate the effect of coexisting nontarget RNA on the accuracy of target RNA detection by BAMGA. Mouse-source double-stranded nontarget cDNA of 0.42 µg was, individually, spiked into 6.8, 27.2, 40.8, 54.4, and 68 ng of human-source target DNA which was artificially prepared by PCR, resulting in the samples –1, –2, –3, –4, and –5, respectively. After the digestion of each sample, sample –1 was ligated with the adaptor encoded with the barcode-2, and each of the other four samples was ligated with the adaptor encoded with the barcode-1. The ligated product of sample –1 was equally pooled with that of samples –2, –3, –4, and –5, respectively, yielding pools –1*2, –1*3, –1*4, and –1*5. After PCR on each pool, pyrosequencing was carried out for quantitatively decoding the barcodes. As seen in Fig. 3, the ratios of signal intensities between two barcode-specific peaks were measured as 4.1:1, 5.7:1, 7.9:1, 10.8:1, respectively, which are well consistent with the expected ratios of 4:1, 6:1, 8:1, and 10:1 (barcode-1:barcode-2). Therefore, nontarget RNA coexisting with target RNA less affects the accuracy of

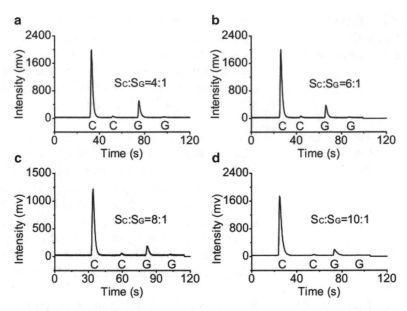

Fig. 3 Effect of coexisting DNA fragments on the accuracy of BAMGA. The theoretical ratios of the β-ACTIN gene between two artificially prepared sources, which contains extra 0.42 μg of mouse-source double-stranded nontarget cDNA, are 4:1 (**a**), 6:1 (**b**), 8:1 (**c**), and 10:1 (**d**), respectively. The expected ratios were directly marked in the pyrograms. The ratios were calculated with the peak intensities specific to barcodes encoded by adapter ligation reaction

BAMGA. The results also proved that barcodes encoded in each source-specific template did not cause any amplification bias in a single PCR tube.

4.2 Accuracy of BAMGA

To investigate the accuracy of BAMGA, a series of pooled samples were artificially prepared. For the illustration, the *GAPDH* gene expressed in mouse kidneys was used as an example. At first, the *Mbo* I-digested ds-cDNA reverse transcribed from the mouse kidney was divided into two aliquots, and each aliquot was used as a source of the *GAPDH* gene. The two aliquots were ligated with two source-specific adapters encoded with different barcodes, respectively, and then the two source-specific ds-cDNAs labeled with barcodes were mixed in the ratios of 10:0, 9:1, 8:2, 7:3, 6:4, 5:5, 4:6, 3:7, 2:8, 1:9, and 0:10, respectively. After PCR, pyrosequencing was performed on each pool. Ratios measured from signal intensities of peaks corresponding to two source-specific barcodes are 10:0.18, 8.1:1, 8.6:2, 6.4:3, 5.9:4, 4.9:5, 4:6.5, 3:7.3, 1:8.2, and 0.16:10, respectively, very close to the expected ratios. The correlation between the measured ratios and theoretical ratios was as high as 0.996 ($n = 3$), indicating that the ratio among barcode-specific peaks can accurately reflect the relative gene expression levels among different sources. The typical pyrograms are shown in Fig. 4.

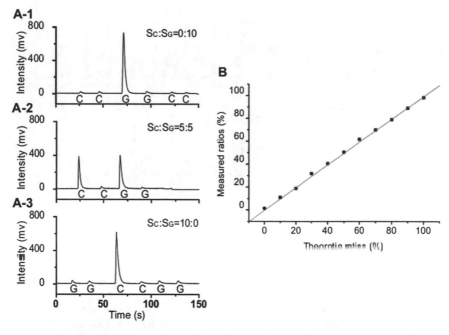

Fig. 4 Quantitative evaluation of the multiplex bioassay based on BAMGA. (**a**) Typical pyrograms of artificially prepared sources by mixing ds-cDNAs ligated with barcode-1 and barcode-2 at various ratios (0:10, 5:5, and 10:0). Each dNTP was dispensed twice for monitoring the background due to PPi impurity in dNTP solution. (**b**) Correlation between the expected ratios of the amounts of the GAPDH transcripts in two sources and the measured ratios by BAMGA. The ratios were calculated with the formula of "$G/(G+C) \times 100$" where G and C mean the peak intensity

4.3 Quantitaive Analysis

After detection by BAMGA, we found that the signal intensities of barcode-specific peaks from the sample at the ratio of 1:1:1:1:1:1:1:1:1:1:1:1 are unexpectedly increased in the later dNTP cycles (see arrows in Fig. 5). As each source-specific barcoded template was equal in concentration, nearly equal peak intensities should be expected in the pyrogram of this sample. To achieve a quantitative analysis, it is better to eliminate these unexpected signals. The best way to suppress these signals is to block the extended ends of barcodes. As it is unnecessary to extend the barcoded fragment if the reporter base is extended, we tried to employ ddNTPs instead of dNTPs to extend the reporter base. The false-positive signals in later dNTP cycles were thus effectively suppressed (Fig. 5b) by using ddNTPs. The problem of slow incorporation of ddNTPs by Klenow polymerase was successfully overcome by the use of Sequenase 2.0.

After the use of ddNTP for pyrosequencing, the relative expression levels of the given gene in 12 different sources were accurately quantified (Fig. 6a, b). To simply evaluate the accuracy of BAMGA, an intensity ratio of the two reporter peaks between two stuffer bases, i.e., peaks "C" and "G" in the pyrogram, was employed. Because the theoretical ratios between these two peaks are designed to be the same, each pooled sample should have six

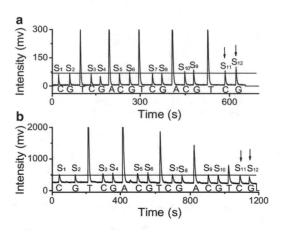

Fig. 5 Pyrograms for decoding barcodes by using dNTPs (**a**) and ddNTPs (**b**) in pyrosequencing reaction. The transcript concentration of the target gene (the CDK4 gene) in each of the 12 artificially prepared sources (from S1 to S12) is equal

different ratios of peaks "C" to "G"; thus, the average and RSD of these six ratios can be measured for each sample. The relationship between the expected ratios and measured ratios of pooled samples at various ratios (except for the ratio of 1:0:1:0:1:0:1:0:1:0:1:0) is shown in Fig. 6c, indicating that BAMGA is accurate enough in the comparative detection of a gene expressed among 12 sources.

4.4 Determination of Expression Levels of Four Genes

The utility of BAMGA was further investigated by using real biological samples. The relative expression levels of four genes (b-ACTIN, FAS, JUN, and RPL19) among the small intestine, right brain, large intestine, cerebellum, spleen, lung, left brain, bladder, heart, stomach, ear, and kidney tissues of a mouse were detected. The results (Figs. 7a and 8) indicate that all the four genes were expressed in the 12 organs of the mouse but with different expression levels. The accuracy of the results was confirmed by real-time qPCR (Fig. 7b). The comparison of the results between qPCR and BAMGA showed that BAMGA is accurate enough for gene expression analysis, suggesting that barcodes can well be used as source identifiers.

5 Technical Notes

1. To prevent the interference of the coexisting DNA in BAMGA, we have successfully employed DNase I for treating the RNA sample.

2. As pyrosequencing was used for decoding the barcodes in PCR products, cross-contamination from PCR products may occur. To prevent any possible false-positive results, it is necessary to perform PCR using filter tips at a qualified PCR lab. In addition, a negative control should be carried out in parallel from the beginning of the assay (enzyme digestion step).

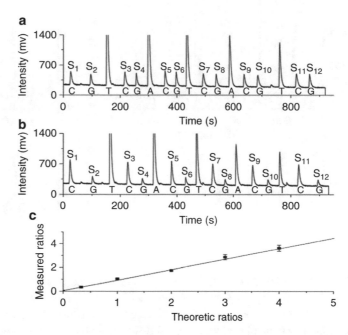

Fig. 6 Typical pyrograms for detecting the relative expression levels of the CDK4 gene among 12 artificially prepared sources (**a**, **b**). The ratio of the CDK4 gene spiked in 12 sources is 1:1:1:1:1:1:1:1:1:1:1:1 (**a**) and 4:1:4:1:4:1:4:1:4:1:4:1 (**b**), respectively. "S" means the source in which a gene of interest exists. (**c**) Relationship between expected ratios and measured ratios of peaks "C" to "G" of pooled samples at various ratios

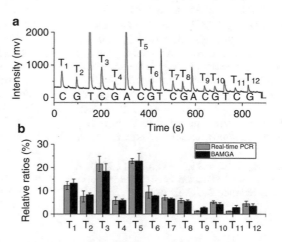

Fig. 7 Pyrograms for detecting the relative expression levels of the β-ACTIN gene among 12 organ tissues of a mouse. (**a**) The expression levels of the β-ACTIN gene among 12 organ tissues of a mouse by the proposed multiplex barcode assay based on BAMGA. "T" means the tissue in which a gene of interest exists. (**b**) Histograms for comparing the observed expression levels of the b-ACTIN gene by BAMGA and real-time PCR. Each dNTP was dispensed twice. The signal was measured by deducting the second peak intensity from the first one

242   Zhiyao Chen et al.

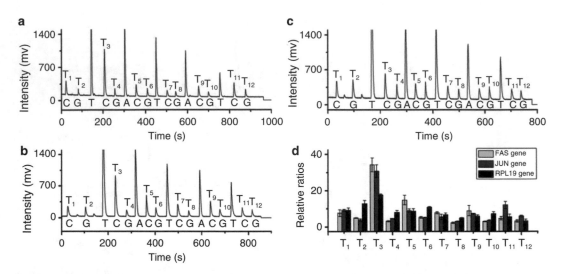

Fig. 8 Results of relative gene expression levels of the *JUN* gene (**a**), the *RPL19* gene (**b**), and the *FAS* gene (**c**) among 12 different organs (small intestines, right brain, large intestine, cerebellum, spleen, lung, left brain, bladder, heart, stomach, ear, and kidney) of a mouse by multiplex bioassay based on BAMGA. "T" means the tissue in which a gene of interest exists. (**d**) Histograms of relative gene expression levels of the three genes among 12 different organs of a mouse by pyrosequencing

References

1. Hamady M, Walker JJ, Harris JK, Gold NJ, Knight R (2008) Error-correcting barcoded primers for pyrosequencing hundreds of samples in multiplex. Nat Methods 5:235–237
2. Parameswaran P, Jalili R, Tao L, Shokralla S, Gharizadeh B, Ronaghi M, Fire AZ (2007) A pyrosequencing-tailored nucleotide barcode design unveils opportunities for large-scale sample multiplexing. Nucleic Acids Res 35, e130
3. Hoffmann C, Minkah N, Leipzig J, Wang G, Arens MQ, Tebas P, Bushman FD (2007) DNA barcoding and pyrosequencing to identify rare HIV drug resistance mutations. Nucleic Acids Res 35, e91
4. Ronaghi M, Uhlen M, Nyren P (1998) A sequencing method based on real-time pyrophosphate. Science 281:363–365
5. Wu H, Wu W, Chen Z, Wang W, Zhou G, Kajiyama T, Kambara H (2011) Highly sensitive pyrosequencing based on the capture of free adenosine 5′ phosphosulfate with adenosine triphosphate sulfurylase. Anal Chem 83:3600–3605
6. Zhang X, Wu H, Chen Z, Zhou G, Kajiyama T, Kambara H (2009) Dye-free gene expression detection by sequence-tagged reverse-transcription polymerase chain reaction coupled with pyrosequencing. Anal Chem 81:273–281
7. Schouten JP, McElgunn CJ, Waaijer R, Zwijnenburg D, Diepvens F, Pals G (2002) Relative quantification of 40 nucleic acid sequences by multiplex ligation-dependent probe amplification. Nucleic Acids Res 30:e57

Chapter 21

Quantitatively Discriminating Multiplexed LAMP Products with Pyrosequencing-Based Bio-Barcodes

Chao Liang, Yanan Chu, Sijia Cheng, Haiping Wu, Bingjie Zou, Qinxin Song, and Guohua Zhou

Abstract

The loop-mediated isothermal amplification (LAMP) is a well-developed method for replicating a targeted DNA sequence with a high specificity, but multiplex LAMP detection is difficult because LAMP amplicons are very complicated in structure. To allow simultaneous detection of multiple LAMP products, a series of target-specific barcodes were designed and tagged in LAMP amplicons by FIP primers. The targeted barcodes were decoded by pyrosequencing on nicked LAMP amplicons. To enable the nicking reaction to occur just near the barcode regions, the recognition sequence of the nicking endonuclease (NEase) was also introduced into the FIP primer. After the nicking reaction, pyrosequencing started at the nicked 3′ end when the added deoxyribonucleoside triphosphate (dNTP) was complementary to the non-nicked strand. To efficiently encode multiple targets, the barcodes were designed with a reporter base and two stuffer bases, so that the decoding of a target-specific barcode only required a single peak in a pyrogram. We have successfully detected the four kinds of pathogens including hepatitis B virus (HBV), hepatitis C virus (HCV), human immunodeficiency virus (HIV), and *Treponema pallidum* (TP), which are easily infected in blood, by a 4-plex LAMP in a single tube, indicating that barcoded LAMP coupled with NEase-mediated pyrosequencing is a simple, rapid, and reliable way in multiple target identification.

Key words Pyrosequencing, Multiplex loop-mediated isothermal amplification, Nicking endonuclease, Barcode, Pathogen detection

1 Introduction

Loop-mediated isothermal amplification (LAMP) is a well-developed method for rapidly detecting DNA and RNA [1]. Due to the high sensitivity, high specificity, and no need of thermocycler, LAMP has been widely used for analyzing various pathogens such as virus, bacteria, fungi, and parasite [2–7]. The identification of LAMP products is mainly based on a dsDNA-specific fluorescent dye, electrophoresis of amplicons, turbidity due to magnesium pyrophosphate, and the metal ion indicator [8]. However, all of these detection methods are not specific to template sequences;

Guohua Zhou and Qinxin Song (eds.), *Advances and Clinical Practice in Pyrosequencing*, Springer Protocols Handbooks, DOI 10.1007/978-1-4939-3308-2_21, © Springer Science+Business Media New York 2016

so the readout is identical for the amplicon of any sequence [4]. To achieve multiplex LAMP ("mLAMP" for short), it is necessary to develop a method which can discriminate target-specific amplicons from the mixture of LAMP products.

Unlike PCR, LAMP generates amplicons with various lengths, making the detection much complicated. To enable mLAMP, a conventional way is to introduce an endonuclease recognition site into the LAMP primers, and to make the length of endonuclease-digested amplicons specific to the target species [9, 10]. Usually, the enzymatic digestion of LAMP amplicons is incomplete due to the multiple types of structures of LAMP products. Thus, the electro-phoresis pattern of digested products usually contains more than one band for each target, which makes the multiplex detection dif-ficult [9]. An alternative way for mLAMP is the use of a fluoro-phore-labeled primer combined with an intercalator dye. As fluorescence resonance energy transfer (FRET) between the fluoro-phore (donor) and the intercalator dye (acceptor) occurs, a target-specific change in fluorescence appears in LAMP reaction [11, 12]. Although two different genes were simultaneously detected, the method cannot be used for discriminating the low copies of genes.

We have previously developed a dye-free method for multiplex gene expression analysis by sequence-tagged reverse-transcription PCR coupled with pyrosequencing [13, 14]. In this method, a short sequence was used as a target-specific barcode. After PCR, each barcode was decoded by pyrosequencing, which is a sequence-by-synthesis method for quantitatively sequencing a short target. The peak and its intensity in a pyrogram represent the target species and the relative abundance in the mixture, respectively. To apply the similar method for detecting dye-free mLAMP, a short sequence in the middle of an FIP primer for LAMP is used as a barcode to label each target. After LAMP, pyrosequencing is used to decode the barcodes. However, unlike PCR amplicons, LAMP amplicons are a mixture of multiple structures, so it is difficult to make single-stranded DNA for pyrosequencing. To enable pyrosequencing on LAMP products, we introduced a recognition site of nicking endo-nuclease (NEase) into the FIP primer. As NEases only cleave one specific strand of a duplex DNA, the 3′ end at the nick is extendable and can be extended by a polymerase with strand-displacement activity [15], such as Sequenase 2.0, Klenow exo⁻, phi-29, and Bst polymerases. Consequently, NEase-digested LAMP products can be directly pyrosequenced without the use of any primer annealing process. We have successfully used this method for 4-plex LAMP detection of hepatitis B virus (HBV), hepatitis C virus (HCV), human immunodeficiency virus (HIV), and *Treponema pallidum* (TP) in blood. The principle is shown in Fig. 1 for detail. In con-ventional LAMP, there is a poly (T) region in the FIP primer. For mLAMP detection, we replaced this region with a target-specific barcode as well as a NEase recognition sequence. As a proof of

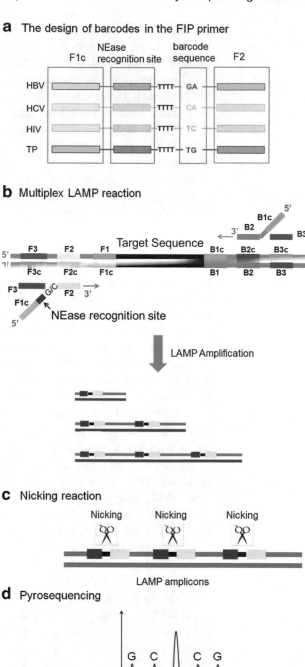

Fig. 1 Schematic of barcoded LAMP coupled with NEase-mediated pyrosequencing. (**a**) The structure of FIP primer which contains the NEase recognition site and target-specific barcodes. (**b**) Introduction of target-specific barcodes into LAMP amplicons by the FIP primer. (**c**) Nicking reaction of mLAMP amplicons by NEase. (**d**) Decoding of the barcodes by pyrosequencing the nicked LAMP amplicons

concept, four pathogens of HIV, HBV, HCV, and TP, which should be detected before blood transfusion [16], were employed as an example for illustrating the methodology.

The key point of the method is how to design the barcodes enabling each pathogen corresponding to a unique peak in a decoded pyrogram. Because only four kinds of bases (A, T, G, and C) are available for designing the barcodes, the maximum number of multiplex level is three if one base is used for labeling one target. This is because we should use one base as a stuffer to prevent the further extension from the extended end in the next dNTP addition. For example, the above three barcodes can be designed as "CA," "TA," and "GA," respectively; here base "A" is the stuffer. The peaks "C, T, and G" should hence appear in the pyrogram when dispensing dCTP, dTTP, and dGTP for pyrosequencing. As no dispensation of dATP, each barcode only has one-base extension, and can thus be the reporter of a target. We have successfully demonstrated the application of this simple dye-free labeling method in comparative analysis of gene expression profiling, but the number of barcodes is limited to three [13]. To overcome this limitation, a new barcode constructed by a report base and repeats of two stuffer bases was proposed to encode multiple targets. For example, we can design the barcodes of "GA," "CA," "TC," and "TG" to label HBV, HCV, HIV, and TP, respectively. Similarly, "GAT," "CAT," "TGT," "TCT," "TAG," and "TAC" can label six different targets. By constructing barcodes with a report base and repeats of two stuffer bases, a sequence of n bases can encode 2n different targets.

Instead of one type of FIP primer in conventional LAMP, four types of FIP primers specific to four different targets were added into LAMP reaction mixture for amplifying all the possible targets. After LAMP, the purified amplicons were nicked by the NEase (Nt. BstNBI). Although LAMP amplicon strands are complicated in structure, the NEase will recognize all of the specific sequences in each strand. The 3′-end of all the nicks will extend in pyrosequencing reaction when the dispensed dNTP is complementary to the non-nicked template sequence. To efficiently decode each target, the dNTP dispensing order should be designed in the light of barcode sequence; for example, the order of "G → C → T → C → G" should be dispensed for the barcodes of "GAT," "CAT," "TCA," and "TGA," which are used to label HBV, HCV, HIV, and TP, respectively. When dGTP is dispensed, only the HBV-specific amplicon gives a peak in the resulting pyrogram; likewise, peak "C" corresponds to HCV. Then, the dispensing of dTTP (a stuffer base) releases the reporter bases in the other two barcodes ("TC" and "TG"); and the sequential dispensing of dGTP and dCTP yields the peaks corresponding to HIV and TP, respectively. Therefore, the peaks in a pyrogram can be the reporter of targeted pathogens. The type of the possible pathogen existing in a sample is readily identified by the target-specific peak. If the sample contains more than one pathogen, multiple peaks should appear in the pyrogram.

2 Materials

1. Bst DNA polymerase and Nt.BstNBI were purchased from New England BioLabs (Beijing, China).

2. AMV reverse transcriptase was purchased from Promega (Madison, WI).

3. ATP sulfurylase and Klenow fragment were obtained by gene engineering in our lab.

4. DNA polymerase was purchased from TaKaRa (Dalian, China).

5. Polyvinylpyrrolidone (PVP) and QuantiLum recombinant luciferase were purchased from Promega (Madison, WI).

6. Bovine serum albumin (BSA), APS, and apyrase-VII were obtained from Sigma (St. Louis, MO).

7. Sodium 2′-deoxyadenosine-5′-O-(1-triphosphate)(dATPαS), 2′-deoxyguanosine-5′-triphosphate (dGTP), 2′-deoxy-thymidine-5′-triphosphate (dTTP), and 2′-deoxycytidine-5′-triphosphate (dCTP) were purchased from MyChem (San Diego, CA).

8. BioSpin PCR purification kit was purchased from TransGene (Beijing, China). QIAamp MinElute Virus Spin Kit was purchased from Qiagen (Hilden, Germany).

9. Four conservative segments in the HBV, HCV, HIV, and TP were selected as the target sequences for the method. All of the oligomers were synthesized and purified by Invitrogen (Shanghai, China).

10. The blood samples were provided by Jingling Hospital (Nanjing, China) and Jiangsu Provincial Center for Disease Prevention and Control (Nanjing, China). The nucleic acids of HBV, HCV, HIV, and TP were extracted by QIAamp MinElute Virus Spin Kit.

3 Methods

3.1 Multiplex LAMP Reaction

1. Each 25 μL of mLAMP mixture contained 8 U of Bst DNA polymerase, 16 U of AMV reverse transcriptase, 1.2 mM dNTPs, 20 mM Tris–HCl (pH 8.8), 10 mM KCl, 8.0 mM $MgCl_2$, 10 mM $(NH_4)_2SO_4$, 0.1 % (V/V) Tween-20, 0.01 % BSA, 0.8 mM betaine, 0.4 μM each F3 and B3 primer, 3.2 μM each FIP and BIP primer, 0.1 μM each LF and LB primer, and 2 μL of DNA or RNA template.

2. Amplification was performed on a water bath at 65 °C for an hour (*see* **Note 1**).

3.2 Nicking Reaction

1. After the purification (*see* **Note 2**), mLAMP products (*see* **Note 3**) were incubated at 55 °C with Nt.BstNBI in a 1× reaction buffer recommended by the supplier. Typically, the incubation was performed for 1 h with 5 U of nicking endonuclease (*see* **Note 4**).

2. After incubation, the reaction was heat-terminated at 80 °C for 20 min and stored at 4 °C until pyrosequencing. One microliter (1 μL) of the treated products was used for pyrosequencing.

3.3 Pyrosequencing

1. The reaction volume of pyrosequencing was 40 μL, containing 0.1 M Tris–acetate (pH 7.7), 2 mM EDTA, 10 mM magnesium acetate, 0.1 % BSA, 1 mM dithiothreitol (DTT), 2 μM adenosine 5′-phosphosulfate (APS), 0.4 mg/mL PVP, 0.4 mM D-luciferin, 200 mU/mL ATP sulfurylase, 3 μg/mL luciferase, 18 U/mL Klenow polymerase, and 1.6 U/mL apyrase. One microliter of purified mLAMP product was used for an assay.

2. Pyrosequencing was performed at 28 °C on a portable pyrosequencer (Hitachi, Ltd., Central Research Laboratory, Japan) according to the manufacturer's protocols. The sequencing signal (peak) was recorded via a stepwise elongation of the primer strand through sequentially dispensing deoxynucleotide triphosphates.

4 Method Validation

4.1 Specificity

In n-plex LAMP reaction, the number of primers is 6n, so there are 24 types of primers in one tube when 4-plex LAMP is performed for identifying four different pathogens (HBV, HCV, HIV, and TP). The main issue of the n-plex LAMP is the interaction among these primers. To evaluate the interaction, four different pathogens (HBV, HCV, HIV, and TP) were individually analyzed by 4-plex LAMP with four sets of primers for identifying all the four targets, and by 3-plex LAMP without the target-specific primers but with all other primers, respectively. Theoretically, no amplicon should be observed in any 3-plex LAMP as no target-specific primers exist in the LAMP reaction. As expected, all 4-plex LAMP gave positive results, but no positive result was observed in all 3-plex LAMPs (Fig. 2). Thus, the coexisting primers would not cause any false-positive result in mLAMP detection, indicating that it is possible to use LAMP for identifying multiple targets simultaneously.

4.2 Sensitivity

The other issue we should address is whether or not multiple primers in mLAMP interfere with the sensitivity of regular LAMP. A sample with ten copies of HBV templates was used as an example for the investigation. At first, we performed a conventional single-plex LAMP with only the HBV primers on the HBV-positive sample, and then we performed three sets of 2-plex LAMP with primers specific to HBV and one of the other three pathogens (HIV, HBV, and TP), three sets of 3-plex LAMP with primers specific to HBV and two of the other three pathogens (HIV, HBV, and TP), and one set of 4-plex LAMP with primers specific to all four pathogens (HIV, HBV, and TP), respectively. As shown in Fig. 3, all the 2-plex LAMPs, all the 3-plex LAMPs, and the 4-plex LAMP gave the same positive amplicons as the single-plex LAMP which is only specific to HBV. The detection limit of the regular LAMP was detected as ten copies of templates per reaction; thus, the sensitivity of mLAMP was not reduced by the presence of multiple primers coexisted.

4.3 Optimization of Nicking Reaction

According to the protocol of Nt.BstNBI, the efficiency of a nicking reaction depends on the buffer used. The recommended buffer for Nt.BstNBI is 100 mM NaCl, 50 mM Tris–HCl, 10 mM $MgCl_2$, and 1 mM DTT (pH 7.9), so it is quite different from LAMP buffer, which is 20 mM Tris–HCl (pH 8.8), 10 mM KCl, 8.0 mM $MgCl_2$, 10 mM $(NH_4)_2SO_4$, 0.1 % (V/V) Tween-20, 0.01 % BSA, and 0.8 mM betaine. To achieve a high nicking efficiency, it is

	3-plex	4-plex	3-plex	4-plex	3-plex	4-plex	3-plex	4-plex
HBV primer	-	+	+	+	+	+	+	+
HCV primer	+	+	-	+	+	+	+	+
HIV primer	+	+	+	+	-	+	+	+
TP primer	+	+	+	+	+	+	-	+
HBV template	+	+	-	-	-	-	-	-
HCV template	-	-	+	+	-	-	-	-
HIV template	-	-	-	-	+	+	-	-
TP template	-	-	-	-	-	-	+	+

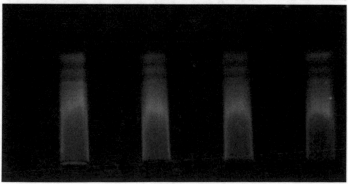

Fig. 2 The electropherograms for investigating the specificity in multiplex-LAMP reaction. The template type and primers used for LAMP reaction are listed in the top of the electropherogram. No positive result is found when no target-specific primers exist in the LAMP reaction

	1-plex		2-plex		2-plex		2-plex		3-plex		3-plex		3-plex		4-plex	
HBV primer	+	+	+	+	+	+	+	+	+	+	+	+	+	+	+	+
HCV primer	-	-	+	+	-	-	-	-	+	+	+	+	-	-	+	+
HIV primer	-	-	-	-	+	+	-	-	+	+	-	-	+	+	+	+
TP primer	-	-	-	-	-	-	+	+	-	-	+	+	+	+	+	+
HBV template	-	+	-	+	-	+	-	+	-	+	-	+	-	+	-	+

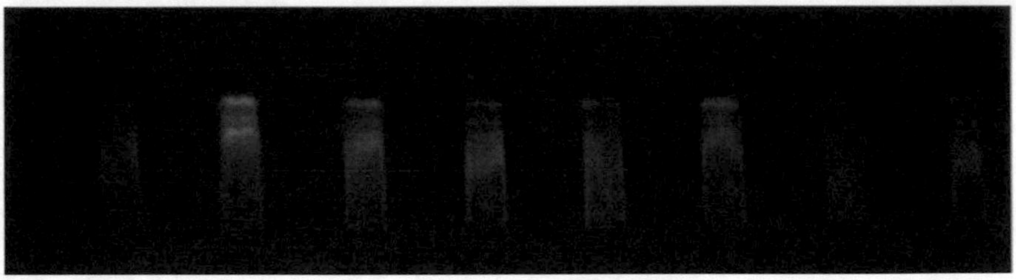

Fig. 3 The electropherograms for investigating the interference of multiple primers on the sensitivity of LAMP reaction of ten copies of HBV templates. The template type and primers used for LAMP reaction are listed in the top of the electropherogram. All multiplex LAMP reactions gave the same results as the single-plex LAMP

necessary to purify LAMP products before adding the buffer required by Nt.BstNBI.

In addition, the amount of substrates (LAMP products) and the NEase as well as the nicking time should be optimized. Pyrograms (Fig. 4) with nicked LAMP amplicons ranging from 200 to 1000 ng show that the signal intensity of each peak increases lineally with the amplicon amount when less than 600 ng of amplicon was used for the nicking reaction, while no obvious increase of signal intensity was observed when more than 600 ng of amplicon was used. Furthermore, the unexpected peaks (noise) in the pyrograms become high when a large amount of nicked LAMP products were used. It indicates that the optimum amount of nicking substrate is not more than 600 ng of LAMP amplicons, equivalent to 2.5 μL of LAMP raw products.

According to the protocol of Nt.BstNBI, the time for nicking reaction should be 1 h. To look for the optimum time for nicking LAMP products, various incubation times, ranging from 0.25 to 2 h, were investigated in the case of a fixed amount of 5 U of Nt.BstNBI. After incubation, the nicking endonuclease was deactivated at 80 °C for 20 min before pyrosequencing. 0.25 h is enough for completing nicking reaction, and it is not necessary to use a longer incubation time in the nicking step. In the similar way, the concentration of the NEase used for nicking reaction was optimized by using Nt.BstNBI with the amount from 5 to 10 U in 20 μL to nick about 600 ng of purified LAMP products. The results (signal intensity of the first peak in each pyrogram) in Fig. 5 indicate that 10 U of Nt.BstNBI is sufficient for nicking 600 ng of LAMP products within 0.25 h.

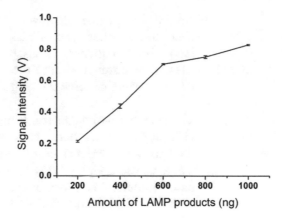

Fig. 4 Relationship between the amount of LAMP amplicons and the signal intensity of the first peak in a pyrogram

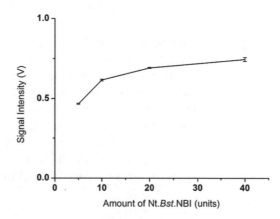

Fig. 5 Relationship between the amount of NEase used for nicking reaction and the signal intensity of the first peak in a pyrogram

4.4 Pyrosequencing on Nicked Single-Plex LAMP Products

To evaluate whether or not the nicked LAMP products can be the template of pyrosequencing, individual LAMP was performed on HBV, HCV, HIV, and TP, respectively. After nicking reaction of each LAMP product, pyrosequencing was carried out. As shown in Fig. 6, about ten bases can be accurately sequenced for all the four pathogens. The observed sequences and the expected sequences are indicated in each pyrogram, suggesting that pyrosequencing on nicked LAMP products is possible. Although there are some unexpected small peaks in the pyrograms, unequivocal sequences of 13, 13, 11, and 10 bp were obtained for HBV, HCV, HIV, and TP, respectively. This readable length is enough for decoding the 10-bp barcodes which can be used to label 20 different targets.

As nicking endonuclease Nt.BstNBI recognizes 5′-GAGTC-3′, a problem may occur if the sequence 5′-GAGTC-3′ is a part of the amplified sequence. However, the problem can be easily solved by changing another type of nicking endonuclease with a different recognition sequence. An alternative way to avoid the problem is to skip the amplification of the recognition sequence in the target if it is possible to reselect a targeted sequence.

4.5 Pyrosequencing on Nicked Multiplex LAMP Products

The possible pathogens infecting a blood sample are HBV, HCV, HIV, and TP. If a blood sample is positive to one of the pathogens, the pathogen carrier cannot be used as a blood donor. So it is preferable to use a 4-plex LAMP for screening the four pathogens in a blood sample. As a proof of concept, we used barcodes of "GAT," "CAT," "TCA," and "TGA" for labeling HBV, HCV, HIV, and TP, respectively. There are 15 possibilities for a pathogen-infected blood sample, including four types of a single-pathogen infection cases (Fig. 7a), six types of duplex-pathogen infection cases (Fig. 7b), four types of triplex-pathogen infection cases (Fig. 7c), and one type of quadruplex-pathogen infection cases (Fig. 7d). The peak "T" in each pyrogram is from a stuffer base. From the results in Fig. 7, it is readily to get accurate pathogen identification in a sample by the pathogen-specific peaks in a decoded pyrogram even if all of four pathogens coexist in one blood sample. Therefore, it is feasible to employ pyrosequencing to decode the barcodes encoded in mLAMP products by using a NEase to generate a nick in amplicons for polymerase extension reaction. Although each barcode consists of several bases, only one peak in a pyrogram is required to decode the barcode; thus, the barcoding efficiency is much higher. In the case of the identification of four pathogens in blood, pyrosequencing of five bases (plus a stuffer base) is sufficient.

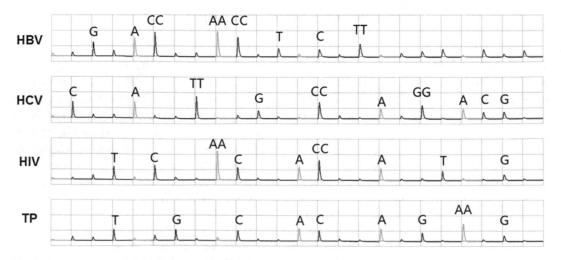

Fig. 6 The pyrograms of nicked single-plex LAMP amplicons of HBV, HCV, HIV, and TP, respectively. The detected sequences are directly marked above each peak

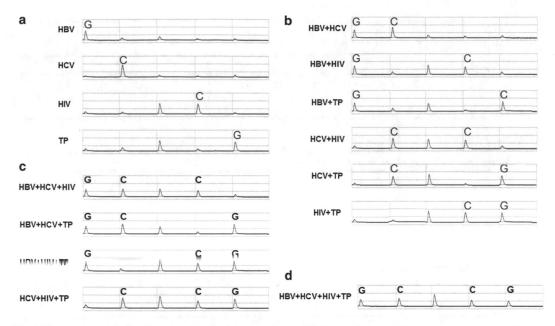

Fig. 7 The pyrograms of nicked amplicons from single-plex LAMP (**a**), 2-plex LAMP (**b**), 3-plex LAMP (**C**), and 4-plex LAMP (**d**). The pathogens in the sample for LAMP reactions are directly marked in each pyrogram. The *first peak* "G" corresponds to HBV; the *second peak* "C" corresponds to HCV. After the stuffer base "T" (*red peaks*), the peaks "C" and "G" correspond to HIV and TP, respectively

4.6 Determination of HBV, HCV, HIV, and TP

To further evaluate the feasibility of the barcoded LAMP coupled with NEase-mediated pyrosequencing, 60 blood samples which were detected to be pathogen positive by real-time PCR were measured by the method using a commercialized pyrosequencer for decoding the pathogen-specific barcodes uniquely tagged in LAMP products. After detection (*see* Fig. 8 for typical pyrograms) using a commercialized pyrosequencer (PyroMark ID System, Qiagen), we found that there are 20 HBV-infected, 20 HCV-infected, 10 HIV-infected, and 10 TP-infected blood samples in the samples. These results are fully consistent with that of real-time PCR, indicating that our method is very accurate, and can be used as a screening tool for blood safety.

5 Technical Notes

1. Coexisting targets with different concentrations can be individually amplified by mLAMP to reach a similar plateau concentration. Usually, 1 h is enough for LAMP to achieve a plateau, so we used 1 h for mLAMP amplification (Fig. 9).

2. To achieve a high nicking efficiency, it is necessary to purify LAMP products before adding the buffer required by Nt. BstNBI.

3. No obvious increase of signal intensity was observed when more than 600 ng of amplicon was used. Furthermore, the

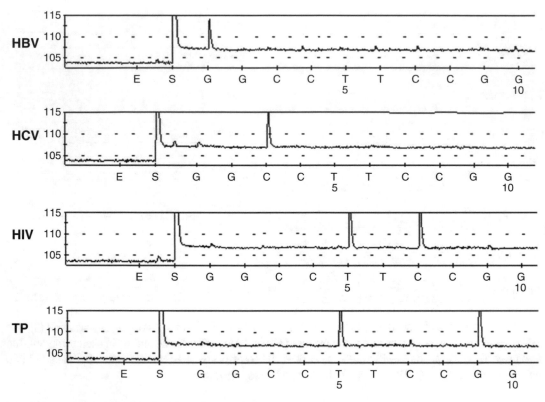

Fig. 8 The typical pyrograms of clinical blood samples detected by a commercialized pyrosequencer (PyroMark ID System, Qiagen, Germany)

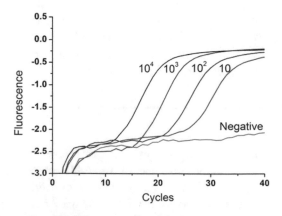

Fig. 9 The real-time LAMP results with different starting template amounts using SYBR Green I as indicator. This figure indicates that the amount of final amplicons of LAMP of a given target with 10, 100, 1000, and 10,000 copies is nearly equal

unexpected peaks (noise) in the pyrograms become high when a large amount of nicked LAMP products were used. It indicates that the optimum amount of nicking substrate is not more than 600 ng of LAMP amplicons, equivalent to 2.5 μL of LAMP raw products.

4. 0.25 h is enough for completing nicking reaction, and it is not necessary to use a longer incubation time in the nicking step.

References

1. Notomi T, Okayama H, Masubuchi H, Yonekawa T, Watanabe K, Amino N, Hase T (2000) Loop-mediated isothermal amplification of DNA. Nucleic Acids Res 28:E63

2. Dawood FS, Jain S, Finelli L, Shaw MW, Lindstrom S, Garten RJ, Gubareva LV, Xu X, Bridges CB, Uyeki TM (2009) Emergence of a novel swine-origin influenza A (H1N1) virus in humans. N Engl J Med 360:2605–2615

3. Jayawardena S, Cheung CY, Barr I, Chan KH, Chen H, Guan Y, Peiris JS, Poon LL (2007) Loop-mediated isothermal amplification for influenza A (H5N1) virus. Emerg Infect Dis 13:899–901

4. Mori Y, Notomi T (2009) Loop-mediated isothermal amplification (LAMP): a rapid, accurate, and cost-effective diagnostic method for infectious diseases. J Infect Chemother 15:62–69

5. Poon LL, Leung CS, Chan KH, Lee JH, Yuen KY, Guan Y, Peiris JS (2005) Detection of human influenza A viruses by loop-mediated isothermal amplification. J Clin Microbiol 43:427–430

6. Poon LL, Wong BW, Ma EH, Chan KH, Chow LM, Abeyewickrcme W, Tangpukdee N, Yuen KY, Guan Y, Looareesuwan S, Peiris JS (2006) Sensitive and inexpensive molecular test for falciparum malaria: detecting Plasmodium falciparum DNA directly from heat-treated blood by loop-mediated isothermal amplification. Clin Chem 52:303–306

7. Yoshikawa T, Ihira M, Akimoto S, Usui C, Miyake F, Suga S, Enomoto Y, Suzuki R, Nishiyama Y, Asano Y (2004) Detection of human herpesvirus 7 DNA by loop-mediated isothermal amplification. J Clin Microbiol 42:1348–1352

8. Tomita N, Mori Y, Kanda H, Notomi T (2008) Loop-mediated isothermal amplification (LAMP) of gene sequences and simple visual detection of products. Nat Protoc 3:877–882

9. Iseki H, Alhassan A, Ohta N, Thekisoe OM, Yokoyama N, Inoue N, Nambota A, Yasuda J, Igarashi I (2007) Development of a multiplex loop-mediated isothermal amplification (mLAMP) method for the simultaneous detection of bovine Babesia parasites. J Microbiol Methods 71:281–287

10. Shao Y, Zhu S, Jin C, Chen F (2011) Development of multiplex loop-mediated isothermal amplification-RFLP (mLAMP-RFLP) to detect Salmonella spp. and Shigella spp. in milk. Int J Food Microbiol 148:75–79

11. Aonuma H, Yoshimura A, Kobayashi T, Okado K, Badolo A, Nelson B, Kanuka H, Fukumoto S (2010) A single fluorescence-based LAMP reaction for identifying multiple parasites in mosquitoes. Exp Parasitol 125:179–183

12. Kouguchi Y, Fujiwara T, Teramoto M, Kuramoto M (2010) Homogenous, real-time duplex loop-mediated isothermal amplification using a single fluorophore-labeled primer and an intercalator dye: Its application to the simultaneous detection of Shiga toxin genes 1 and 2 in Shiga toxigenic Escherichia coli isolates. Mol Cell Probes 24:190–195

13. Zhang X, Wu H, Chen Z, Zhou G, Kajiyama T, Kambara H (2009) Dye-free gene expression detection by sequence-tagged reverse-transcription polymerase chain reaction coupled with pyrosequencing. Anal Chem 81:273–281

14. Song Q, Jing H, Wu H, Zhou G, Kajiyama T, Kambara H (2010) Gene expression analysis on a photodiode array-based bioluminescence analyzer by using sensitivity-improved SRPP. Analyst 135:1315–1319

15. Song Q, Wu H, Feng F, Zhou G, Kajiyama T, Kambara H (2010) Pyrosequencing on nicked dsDNA generated by nicking endonucleases. Anal Chem 82:2074–2081

16. Stramer SL, Wend U, Candotti D, Foster GA, Hollinger FB, Dodd RY, Allain JP, Gerlich W (2011) Nucleic acid testing to detect HBV infection in blood donors. N Engl J Med 364:236–247

Chapter 22

Multiplex Ligation-Dependent Sequence-Tag Amplification Coupled with Pyrosequencing for Copy Number Variation (CNV) Analysis

Haiping Wu, Bingjie Zou, Qinxin Song, and Guohua Zhou

Abstract

We describe a novel dye-free labeling method for multiplex copy number variation analysis, called multiplex ligation-dependent sequence-tag amplification (MLSA). In MLSA, not target DNA but probes added to the samples are amplified and quantified. Amplification of probes by PCR depends on the presence of target sequence in the sample. Each probe consists of two oligonucleotides that hybridize to the target sequence. Such hybridized oligonucleotides are ligated and will be used as a template for subsequent amplification. Each probe has two tag sequences, one for coding the sample sources, and another for the targets. Using pyrosequencing to analyze the probe amplicons, the detection and quantitative analysis of the copy number variations can be achieved by decoding the tag sequences. Relative quantification of copy number variations in chromosome X or Y is described in the applications. Results show that MLSA is accurate enough for the quantitative analysis of copy number variations in sex chromosomal sequences in both male and female samples.

Key words Multiplex ligation-dependent amplification, Sequence-tag, Pyrosequencing, Copy number variation

1 Introduction

Copy number variations (CNVs) are widely distributed in human genome [1, 2]. They have greatly enriched the diversity of genetic variation with the much higher frequency than the chromosome structural variations as well as the higher coverage of nucleotides than the single-nucleotide polymorphisms (SNPs) [3]. More and more evidence shows that CNVs are closely related to human diseases. Down's syndrome is caused by an extra copy of complete chromosome 21 [4], and sex chromosome abnormalities are also owing to the changes in copy number of complete chromosome X or Y [5–7].

Different from the SNP typing, only several techniques are available for quantitative analysis of CNVs, including fluorescence

Guohua Zhou and Qinxin Song (eds.), *Advances and Clinical Practice in Pyrosequencing*, Springer Protocols Handbooks, DOI 10.1007/978-1-4939-3308-2_22, © Springer Science+Business Media New York 2016

in situ hybridization (FISH) [8], array-based comparative genomic hybridization (array-CGH) [9], loss of heterozygosity (LOH) [10], bacterial artificial chromosomes array (BAC array) [11], and Southern blots. These techniques are time consuming (FISH, LOH) or require large amounts of sample DNA (Southern blots). Above all, most of these techniques are difficult to perform as multiplex assays.

Recently, there are two relative quantitative techniques reported to be sensitive, reproducible, and sequence specific for multiplex analysis of CNVs, called multiplex ligation-dependent probe amplification (MLPA) and multiplex ligation-dependent genome amplification (MLGA) [12–14]. In MLPA, each probe consists one short synthetic oligonucleotide and one, phage M13-derived, long-probe oligonucleotide; the two oligonucleotides can be ligated to each other when hybridized to a target sequence. All the probes are amplified with a pair of universal primers, and the products of different sizes are then detected by capillary electrophoresis. Contrast with MLPA, MLGA uses only the single short synthetic probe for each target, and the genomic DNA is amplified rather than the probe molecules. Although MLGA avoids a tedious biosynthesis of the long-probe oligonucleotide, a restriction digestion of genomic DNA is needed. For both MLPA and MLGA, a complicated and costly laser-induced fluorescence capillary electrophoresis is needed to analyze the amplification products.

Here, we introduce an accurate and sensitive approach based on the sequence barcode with no need of fluorescence labeling, called multiplex ligation-dependent sequence-tag amplification (MLSA). MLSA is based on the ligation of target-specific probes with different sequence tags of same length, while MLPA distinguishes targets by probes with different lengths. We use the pyrosequencing to decode the sequence tags instead of the laser-induced fluorescence capillary electrophoresis [15–18].

The principle of MLSA is shown in Fig. 1; each probe includes two oligonucleotides (P1 and P2). The P1 contains a universal primer sequence for PCR amplification and a target-specific sequence for hybridization. The P2 contains two more sequence tags than P1, tag X for coding sample sources and tag Y for different targets. The MLSA probes can be ligated to each other when hybridized to a target sequence. All ligated probes are simultaneously amplified using a pair of universal primers and then the tag sequences will be decoded by pyrosequencing. In Fig. 1, we focus on two targets in each of the two samples. There are four different amplicons resulted from the four groups of probes. When detecting the targets in sample 1, we use the sequencing primer 1 which is complementary to the tag X for sample 1, and then the target is quantitatively analyzed according to the signal intensity of tag Y ("ATC" for target A, "CTG" for target B). Sample 2 can be detected in the same way by using the sequencing primer 2.

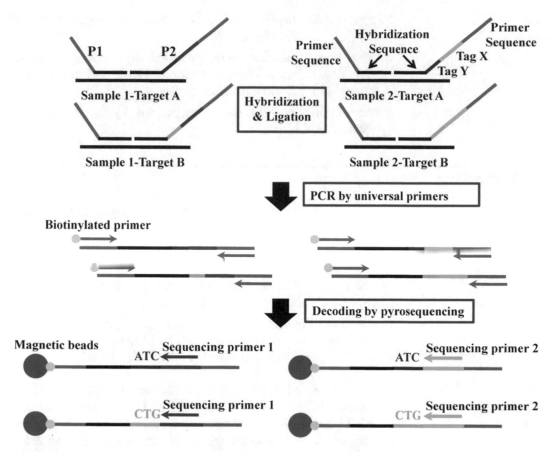

Fig. 1 Schematic of multiplex ligation-dependent sequence-tag amplification for detecting two targets in each of the two samples

2 Materials

1. Ligase-65 and SALSA MLPA reagents were purchased from MRC-Holland (Amsterdam, The Netherlands).

2. T4 polynucleotide kinase and *Taq* DNA polymerase were purchased from TaKaRa (Dalian, China).

3. Bovine serum albumin (BSA), D-luciferin, adenosine 5′-phosphosulfate (APS) and apyrase VII were purchased from Sigma (St. Louis, USA).

4. ATP sulfurylase and the Klenow fragment were obtained by gene engineering in our lab.

5. Polyvinylpyrrolidone (PVP) and QuantiLum Recombinant luciferase were purchased from Promega (Madison, USA).

6. 2′-Deoxyadenosine-5′-O-(1-thiotriphosphate) sodium salt (dATPαS), dGTP, dTTP, and dCTP were purchased from MyChem (San Diego, USA).

7. Streptavidin Sepharose™ beads were purchased from GE Healthcare (New Jersey, USA).

8. The blood samples were provided by Jingling Hospital (Nanjing, China). Purified genomic DNA was extracted by phenol-chloroform extraction protocol.

9. All oligonucleotides were synthesized by Invitrogen Inc. (Shanghai, China).

3 Methods

3.1 Ligation Reaction

1. Genomic DNA (50–100 ng) samples were diluted with TE to 5 µL, heated at 98 °C for 5 min, and then placed on ice immediately.

2. After addition of 5 fmol of each probe, 1.5 µL MLPA buffer, and 8 µL 1×TE, samples were heated at 95 °C for 1 min and then incubated at 60 °C for 12–16 h.

3. Ligation of annealed oligonucleotides was performed by adding 3 µL buffer A, 3 µL buffer B, 1 U Ligase-65, and H_2O up to 25 µL, and then incubating at 54 °C for 15 min.

3.2 PCR Amplification

1. A 50 µL reaction contained 1× *Taq* buffer, 200 mmol/L for each of dATP, dCTP, dGTP, and dTTP, 1.5 mmol/L $MgCl_2$, 1.5 U *Taq* DNA polymerase, 0.4 mmol/L of each universal primer, 10 µL Ligase-65 ligation products, and H_2O added up to 50 µL.

2. The reaction was initiated at 94 °C for 5 min, followed by 35 cycles of 94 °C for 30 s, 55 °C for 30 s, 72 °C for 30 s, and a final extension at 72 °C for 7 min.

3.3 Single-Stranded DNA Preparation

1. Streptavidin-coated sepharose beads were used to capture biotinylated PCR products.

2. The preparation of single-stranded DNA (ssDNA) was performed in our in-house-designed instrument. After sedimentation and washing steps, purified double-stranded DNA were denatured by alkali to yield ssDNA.

3. The immobilized biotinylated strand was then annealed with a sequencing primer under the condition of 85 °C for 2 min and 25 °C for 10 min before being used as a sequencing template.

3.4 Pyrosequencing Reaction

1. The reaction volume of pyrosequencing was 40 µL, containing 0.1 mol/L Tris–acetate (pH 7.7), 2 mmol/L EDTA, 10 mmol/L magnesium acetate, 0.1 % BSA, 1 mmol/L dithiothreitol (DTT), 2 µmol/L adenosine 5′-phosphosulfate (APS), 0.4 mg/mL PVP, 0.4 mmol/L D-luciferin, 200 mU/mL ATP sulfurylase, 3 µg/mL luciferase, 18 U/mL Klenow polymerase, and 1.6 U/mL apyrase.

2. Pyrosequencing was performed at 28 °C on a portable pyrosequencer (Hitachi, Ltd., Central Research Laboratory, Japan) according to the manufacturer's protocols.

3. Each of the dNTPs was added according to the barcode sequence, and the peak value was calculated as signal intensity.

4 Typical Examples

4.1 Analysis of Copy Number Variation in Chromosome X or Y

Changes in copy number of sex chromosomal sequences are frequently implicated in the cause of human diseases and syndromes. Such changes include the presence of an extra copy of a complete chromosome X as in Klinefelter syndrome, the deficiency of a complete chromosome X or in Turner syndrome, and other trisomic sex chromosome.

For the analysis of copy number variation in chromosome X or Y in male or female, we prepared a pair of MLSA probe for *SRY* gene in chromosome Y, three pairs of probes for *FMR2* gene, *PQBP1* gene, and *GDI1* gene in chromosome X, respectively. For relative quantification, we chose the *GAPDH* gene in chromosome 12 and the *ACTB* gene in chromosome 7 as reference gene. We used the 3-base sequence tags for coding the six targets, "CAT" for *GAPDH* gene, "GAT" for *ACTB* gene, "TCT" for *SRY* gene, "TGT" for *FMR2* gene, "TAC" for *PQBP1* gene, and "TAG" for *GDI1* gene. The pyrosequencing was chosen to carry out the decoding of the six targets, and the dNTP adding order is recommended to be "CGTCGACG," according to the tag sequence. The pyrograms of MLSA products for female and male are shown in Fig. 2; the three "C" signal peaks represent the *GAPDH* gene, *SRY* gene, and *PQBP1* gene, respectively; the three "G" signal

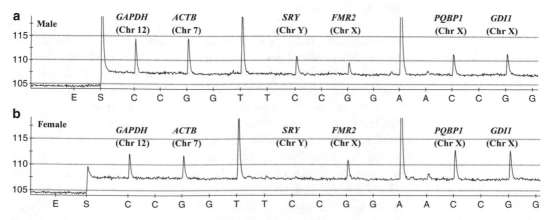

Fig. 2 Pyrograms of MLSA products for male and female samples

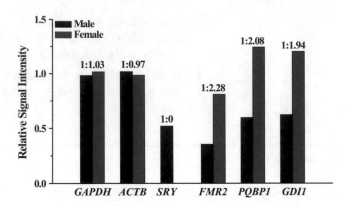

Fig. 3 Relative signal intensity of the six targets in female and male samples

peaks represent the *ACTB* gene, *FMR2* gene, and *GDI1* gene, respectively. Based on the mechanism of pyrosequencing, the intensity of the signal peak corresponds to the quantity of targets.

For relative quantification, we divided each signal intensity of the target gene by the mean intensity of the two reference genes, *GAPDH* and *ACTB* gene. The relative signal intensity of the targets is shown in Fig. 3. The relative signal intensity of *SRY* gene is very close to the expected values which are 0.5 in male samples and 0 in female samples. In some target genes, there are deviations between the observed results and the expected values, slightly lower relative signal intensity in *FMR2* gene, and slightly higher relative signal intensity in *PQBP1* and *GDI1* genes. We believe that the bias was caused by discriminative efficiency in the ligation reaction. To eliminate the bias among the targets, we calculate the ratios of each relative signal intensity between female and male samples. The relative ratios measured from the samples are shown in Fig. 3 and are very close to the expected values, indicating that the ratios can accurately reflect the relative gene copy numbers among different sources.

To validate the accuracy of MLSA method, we analyzed ten samples, five male and five female, and failed to obtain sex chromosome abnormality samples. As mentioned above, the relative signal intensity of each target is normalized to that obtained from a male control sample (Fig. 4). Results show that MLSA is accurate enough for quantitative analysis of the gene copy number variations in chromosomes X and Y in male or female samples. The relative ratio of the *GAPDH* gene and the *ACTB* gene in autosomes is approximately equal to 1 in all ten samples. In female samples, lacking SRY gene, the relative ratio of the *FMR2* gene, *PQBP1* gene, and *GDI1* gene in chromosome X is approximately equal to 2. In male samples, all the normalized relative ratios are approximately equal to 1.

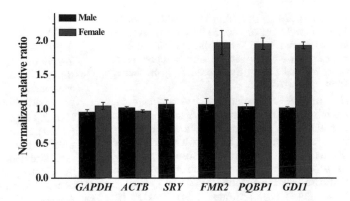

Fig. 4 Normalized relative ratios of each target in male and female samples

5   Technical Notes

1. The 5′ end of the oligonucleotide P2, which is complementary to the target gene in 5′ end, should be phosphorylated for the ligation reaction.

2. The sequence in target gene which is complementary to the hybridization sequence in probe must be continuous sequence without gap. The sequence is suggested to be 20–30 nt at length, with Tm value higher than 70 °C and GC bases within 45–60 %.

3. A thermostable ligase should be avoided in MLSA, or the residual ligase activity in PCR reaction would affect the quantitative analysis, resulting in approximately equal ligation products.

Acknowledgement

This work was supported by the National Natural Science Foundation of China (21405176); the China Postdoctoral Science Special Foundation (2014 T71011); the China Postdoctoral Science Foundation (2013 M542575); and the Postdoctoral Science Foundation of Jiangsu Province (1302035B).

References

1. Hayes JL, Tzika A, Thygesen H, Berri S, Wood HM, Hewitt S et al (2013) Diagnosis of copy number variation by Illumina next generation sequencing is comparable in performance to oligonucleotide array comparative genomic hybridisation. Genomics 3:174–181

2. Binder V, Bartenhagen C, Okpanyi V, Gombert M, Moehlendick B, Behrens B et al (2014) A new workflow for whole-genome sequencing of single human cells. Hum Mutat 10:1260–1270

3. Wheeler E, Huang N, Bochukova EG, Keogh JM, Lindsay S, Garg S et al (2013) Genome-wide SNP and CNV analysis identifies common and low-frequency variants associated with severe early-onset obesity. Nat Genet 5: 513–517

4. Hunter JE, Allen EG, Shin M, Bean LJ, Correa A, Druschel C et al (2013) The association of low socioeconomic status and the risk of having a child with Down syndrome: a report from the National Down Syndrome Project. Genet Med 9:698–705

5. van Rijn S, Stockmann L, Borghgraef M, Bruining H, van Ravenswaaij-Arts C, Govaerts L et al (2014) The social behavioral phenotype in boys and girls with an extra X chromosome (Klinefelter syndrome and Trisomy X): a comparison with autism spectrum disorder. J Autism Dev Disord 2:310–320

6. Hong DS, Hoeft F, Marzelli MJ, Lepage JF, Roeltgen D, Ross J et al (2014) Influence of the X-chromosome on neuroanatomy: evidence from Turner and Klinefelter syndromes. J Neurosci 10:3509–3516

7. Li X (2011) Sex chromosomes and sex chromosome abnormalities. Clin Lab Med 4(463–479):vii

8. Suzuki M, Nagura K, Igarashi H, Tao H, Midorikawa Y, Kitayama Y et al (2009) Copy number estimation algorithms and fluorescence in situ hybridization to describe copy number alterations in human tumors. Pathol Int 4:218–228

9. Guo Y, Sheng Q, Samuels DC, Lehmann B, Bauer JA, Pietenpol J et al (2013) Comparative study of exome copy number variation estimation tools using array comparative genomic hybridization as control. Biomed Res Int 915636

10. Devilee P, Cleton-Jansen AM, Cornelisse CJ (2001) Ever since Knudson. Trends Genet 10:569–573

11. Snijders AM, Nowak N, Segraves R, Blackwood S, Brown N, Conroy J et al (2001) Assembly of microarrays for genome-wide measurement of DNA copy number. Nat Genet 3:263–264

12. Schouten JP, McElgunn CJ, Waaijer R, Zwijnenburg D, Diepvens F, Pals G (2002) Relative quantification of 40 nucleic acid sequences by multiplex ligation-dependent probe amplification. Nucleic Acids Res 12:e57

13. Garcia-Canas V, Mondello M, Cifuentes A (2010) Simultaneous detection of genetically modified organisms by multiplex ligation-dependent genome amplification and capillary gel electrophoresis with laser-induced fluorescence. Electrophoresis 13:2249–2259

14. Isaksson M, Stenberg J, Dahl F, Thuresson AC, Bondeson ML, Nilsson M (2007) MLGA – a rapid and cost-efficient assay for gene copy-number analysis. Nucleic Acids Res 17:e115

15. Jing H, Song Q, Chen Z, Zou B, Chen C, Zhu M et al (2011) Dye-free microRNA quantification by using pyrosequencing with a sequence-tagged stem-loop RT primer. Chembiochem 6:845–849

16. Wu H, Wu W, Chen Z, Wang W, Zhou G, Kajiyama T et al (2011) Highly sensitive pyrosequencing based on the capture of free adenosine 5′ phosphosulfate with adenosine triphosphate sulfurylase. Anal Chem 9:3600–3605

17. Chen Z, Fu X, Zhang X, Liu X, Zou B, Wu H et al (2012) Pyrosequencing-based barcodes for a dye-free multiplex bioassay. Chem Commun (Camb) 18:2445–2447

18. Liang C, Chu Y, Cheng S, Wu H, Kajiyama T, Kambara H et al (2012) Multiplex loop-mediated isothermal amplification detection by sequence-based barcodes coupled with nicking endonuclease-mediated pyrosequencing. Anal Chem 8:3758–3763

Part V

Instrumentation

Chapter 23

Pyrosequencer Miniaturized with Capillaries to Deliver Deoxynucleotides

Guohua Zhou, Masao Kamahori, Kazunori Okano, Kunio Harada, and Hideki Kambara

Abstract

As the human genome project proceeds, various types of DNA analysis tools are required for life sciences and medical sciences including DNA diagnostics. For example, a small DNA sequencer for sequencing a short DNA is required for bedside DNA testing as well as DNA analysis in a small laboratory. Here, a new handy DNA sequencing system (pyrosequencer) based on the detection of inorganic pyrophosphate (PPi) released by polymerase incorporation is demonstrated. The system uses the bioluminescence detection system. The key point for the miniaturized DNA sequencer is to make a deoxynucleotide triphosphate (dNTP) delivery system small and inexpensive. It has been realized by using narrow capillaries to connect a reaction chamber and four dNTP reservoirs. Each dNTP is introduced into the reaction chamber by applying a pressure to the reservoir. Compared with other microdispensers, it is much cheaper and easier. By optimizing the conditions, an excellent sequencing ability is achieved while it is a simple and inexpensive system. In most cases, more than 40 bases can be successfully sequenced. A homopolymeric region, which cannot be easily sequenced by a conventional gel-based DNA sequencer, is readily sequenced with this system. The new system is successfully applied to sequence a GC-rich region or a region close to a priming region where misreading frequently occurs. A rapid analysis for a short DNA was easily achieved with this small instrument.

Key words Pyrosequencing, DNA analysis, DNA sequencing, Microdispenser

1 Introduction

The human genome project has been accelerated by the development of high-throughput sequencing instruments such as gel-based capillary-array DNA sequencers [1]. The draft sequence of human genome has been reported [2]. The next subjects are to clarify the functions of genes and to apply the genome sequence as well as genome function information to various fields. In the post-genome era, new analytical tools are required for gene expression profiling, DNA diagnostics, and genome comparative analysis including single-nucleotide polymorphism (SNP) analysis. It is not

Guohua Zhou and Qinxin Song (eds.), *Advances and Clinical Practice in Pyrosequencing*, Springer Protocols Handbooks, DOI 10.1007/978-1-4939-3308-2_23, © Springer Science+Business Media New York 2016

necessary to sequence long DNAs for those. Although an automated DNA sequencer, which uses gel electrophoresis coupled with a laser-induced fluorescence detector, is powerful and popular nowadays, it still has several drawbacks. Misreading of the base sequence or a gap occurs frequently for DNAs having GC-rich regions due to self-hybridization. Base sequences in a region close to a primer are not easily sequenced because of big mobility differences among the fragments due to labeled dyes. There are many DNA samples for diagnostic applications that do not require long base reading. It is desirable to develop a simple and inexpensive instrument for sequencing short DNAs, which is complementary to the conventional gel-based DNA sequencer. Besides, the new instrument should also be applied for a massive parallel analysis of DNAs because a comparative DNA sequencing analysis for a large number of short DNAs is becoming important. Various new technologies have been reported in this direction, including a DNA probe array on a chip [3, 4], a time-of-flight mass spectrometer coupled with laser desorption [5], bead technologies [6], and other PCR-related approaches [7, 8]. However, any good method to accurately sequence several tens of bases for identifying the DNA fragments has not yet been developed. Recently Nyren's group [9] reported a new technology called pyrosequencing that used the detection of DNA polymerase reaction by bioluminescence. DNA sequencing based on pyrophosphate detection was first developed by Hyman [10] in 1988 and then greatly improved by Nyren's group [9, 11] through the use of an enzyme-degrading dNTP and ATP as well as the use of 2′-deoxyadenosine 5′-O-(1-triphosphate) (dATPαS) instead of dATP which is a weak substrate of luciferase. It seems promising as a massive parallel method to sequence short DNA fragments, which can overcome the drawbacks in conventional gel-based electrophoresis. The purpose of present research is to develop a handy and inexpensive DNA minisequencer employing the pyrosequencing technology. The optimization of various conditions necessary for realizing and designing the system was carried out. It was successfully applied to sequence DNAs that were difficult to be sequenced by a conventional gel-based DNA sequencer.

In pyrosequencing, four enzymes are used. These are DNA polymerase for incorporating nucleotides, ATP sulfurylase for catalyzing inorganic pyrophosphate (PPi) to energy source ATP, luciferase for generating light (signals) from ATP, and apyrase for degrading ATP and extra nucleotides. When adding a dNTP species complementary to the template, the above cascade reactions occur in a short time. All the reagents are put in the chamber except for dNTPs. In each reaction step, only one of the four dNTPs is added to extend the complementary DNA strand. When dNTP is incorporated into the extended DNA strand, pyrophosphate is produced and therefore light emission is observed. Four dNTPs are added to the reaction mixture in turn (for example: dATPαS → dCTP → dTTP → dGTP). By detecting luminescence, the base species and its order in the template can be readily determined from the incorporated base species and the signal intensity. The excess dNTP and accumulated ATP in the reaction mixture are degraded by apyrase soon after the polymerization and before the addition of the next dNTP. The instrument based on this principle was commercialized recently [12]. As it uses a piezo dispenser to deliver dNTPs for the reaction, it is expensive and the size of the whole instrument is rather big.

2   Materials

1. Polyvinylpyrrolidone (PVP), deoxynucleotides (dNTPs), DNA polymerase I Klenow fragment (exo⁻), and QuantiLum™ recombinant luciferase (95 %) were purchased from Promega (Madison, WI, USA).

2. ATP disodium trihydrate salt was from Wako Pure Chemical Industries (Osaka, Japan), ATP sulfurylase, apyrase (type V, VI and VII), bovine serum albumin (BSA), D-luciferin, inorganic pyrophosphatase (PPase), and adenosine 5′-phosphosulfate (APS) from Sigma (St. Louis, MO, USA).

3. Dynabeads M-280 streptavidin (2.8 μm ID) was from Dynal A.C. (Oslo, Norway).

4. Sodium 2′-deoxyadenosine 5′-O-(1-triphosphate) (dATPαS) from Amersham Pharmacia Biotech (Amersham, UK).

5. Other chemicals were commercially extra pure. All solutions were prepared in deionized and sterilized water.

3   Methods

3.1 Degradation of Endogenous Pyrophosphate in dNTPs

1. Fifty microliters of 10 mM dNTPs containing 25 mM magnesium acetate and 5 mM Tris, pH 7.7, was incubated with 0.4 U of PPase for 60 min at room temperature.

2. The extra enzyme PPase was removed by ultrafiltration through a centrifugal filter tube with the nominal molecular weight cutoff of 10,000 (Millipore, Japan).

3.2 Oligonucleotides and DNA Template

1. The oligonucleotides (5′-biotin-TGTAAAACGACGGCC AGT-3′ and 5′-ACAGGAAACAGCTAT-3′) were used as forward and reverse primers, respectively, which were synthesized by Amersham Pharmacia Biotech (Hokkaido, Japan).

2. The DNA224 (224 bp) was used as a template in the condition optimization study, which was a gift from Professor Sakaki (Tokyo University).

3. Target DNA 278 was made by cloning a human cDNA fragment with 2260 bp into vector plasmids pUC19FL3 in our laboratory.

4. A 146 bp fragment was prepared by PCR using 5′-biotin-TAGTTTTAAGAGGGTTGTTGT-3′ and 5′-AAACACCCTTCACATACCCT-3′ as forward and reverse primers, respectively. For both templates, the forward primers were used for pyrosequencing.

3.3 Preparation of PCR-Amplified Template

1. DNA224 fragment was amplified by PCR with a PTC-225 thermocycler PCR System (MJ Research, Watertown, MA, USA) according to the following procedure: denatured at 94 °C for 2 min, followed by 35 thermal reaction cycles (94 °C for 30 s; 57 °C for 60 s; 72 °C for 1 min), and a final incubation at 72 °C for another 3 min.

2. The PCR products were purified by a QIAquick PCR purification kit (Qiagen, Hilden, Germany).

3. After purification and quantification, the PCR product was immobilized on streptavidin-coated magnetic Dynabeads M280 which can bind biotinylated DNA fragments (*see* **Note 1**).

4. After the beads with double-stranded template were washed completely, 0.1 M freshly diluted NaOH was added to resuspend the beads to denature the double-stranded template.

5. The mixture was then incubated at room temperature for 5 min, and the supernatant was collected.

6. The beads were washed again with a little amount of 0.1 M NaOH, and the supernatant was combined with that from the first wash.

7. Finally the solution was neutralized by adding 0.1 M HCl.

8. Both the immobilized (biotinylated) and nonimmobilized (nonbiotinylated) single-stranded DNA fragments were obtained and then hybridized with the primers described above at 65 °C for 5 min in 40 mM Tris–HCl (pH 7.5), 20 mM MgCl$_2$, and 50 mM NaCl, and then cooled to room temperature (*see* **Note 2**).

3.4 Gel-Based DNA Sequencing

1. The thermal cycling reaction was performed on a PTC225 instrument (*see* **Note 3**).

2. The product was recovered by ethanol precipitation, and then analyzed by an ABI373 DNA sequencer (Perkin-Elmer Palo Alto, CA, USA).

3.5 Pyrosequencing

1. The extra dNTPs were degraded by apyrase containing ATPase and ADPase (*see* **Note 4**).

2. The volume of standard assay mixture was 100 μL which contains the following components: 0.1 M Tris–acetate (pH 7.7), 2 mM EDTA, 10 m M magnesium acetate, 0.1 % BSA, 1 mM dithiothreitol (DTT), 3 μM APS, 0.4 mg/mL PVP, 0.4 mM D-luciferin, 200 mU/mL ATP sulfurylase, luciferase in an amount giving an appropriate sensitivity, 2 U apyrase VII, 150 fmol template, and 1–2 U DNA polymerase I Klenow fragment (exo$^-$).

3. The sequencing reactions started by adding complementary dNTP, one of dATPαS, dCTP, dTTP, and dGTP.

4 Method Validation

DNA polymerase reactions consist of two steps. The first step is the formation of an enzyme-DNA complex. The second step is the strand extension reaction. Assuming that the targets are the conjugate of DNA and enzyme, we just consider the second step a nucleotide incorporation reaction. The enzymatic reaction consists of an equilibrium reaction to produce the target-dNTP complex and a nucleotide incorporation reaction. Assuming that the concentration of the enzyme-target complex is constant, the overall reaction is characterized by the Michaelis-Menten constant Km. It is 0.18 μM for dTTP incorporation by Klenow polymerase. The concentration of dNTP should be higher than Km for a rapid polymerase reaction. As the amount of template DNA in 100 μL of reaction mixture was 0.15 pmol, 0.15 μM of each dNTP for one reaction step, which was two orders of magnitude larger than the amount consumed in the polymerase reaction, seemed enough. However, it was smaller than Km (0.18 μM), and a several times higher concentration of dNTP than the Km (for example 1 μM) should be used. For determining the optimum amount of dNTP, the dNTP degradation by apyrase should also be considered. As one unit apyrase can liberate 1.0 μmol of inorganic phosphate per minute at pH 6.5 at 30 °C, the amount of apyrase required for degrading 100 pmol dNTP (1 μM) in 1 s was about 10 mU at the same condition. In pyrosequencing, the condition was not ideal for apyrase activity and it was thought that a slightly bit larger amount of apyrase than 10 mU would be required. After several trials, 200 mU of apyrase VII was used for degrading dNTPs. With the fixed amount of apyrase, the pyrosequencing spectra at various dNTP concentrations are shown in Fig. 1. It suggests that 0.3 μM of dNTP was not sufficient because the signal intensity was small and not proportional to the identical base number in the homopolymeric region. On the other hand, the background signals caused by unincorporated dNTP became large with the increase of the dNTP concentration as shown in Fig. 1d. The results in Fig. 1c

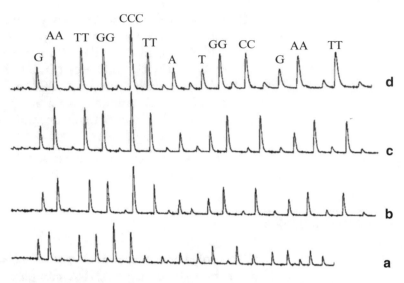

Fig. 1 Pyrosequencing at various dNTP concentrations: (**a**) 0.3; (**b**) 0.7; (**c**) 1.0; (**d**) 1.5 *μ*M. The reaction volume and sample amount were 100 *μ*L and 150 fmol, respectively

indicated that the best dNTP concentration was 1 μM in the present condition, which gave a good relationship between signal intensity and identical base number in one peak.

Unlike gel-based electrophoresis, the pyrosequencing is based on the step-by-step polymerase reactions and the bioluminometric detection. The number of bases in a homopolymeric region is determined by comparing the signal intensities of adjacent peaks in a pyrosequencing spectrum. Therefore, a quantitative relationship between signal intensities and the corresponding base numbers in a homopolymeric region should be clarified. The linear relationship between the signal intensity and the number of PPi in the presence of apyrase was observed in a concentration range from 0.833 to 167 nM ($R^2 = 0.9992$). Actually the linearity was confirmed ($R^2 = 0.9988$) between the light response and the number of nucleotides at a region of 1–3 identical nucleotides in DNA224. To investigate the linear relationship between the signal intensity and the number of homopolymeric nucleotides in a wide range, plural of nucleotide species are added simultaneously to make a large pseudo-homopolymeric region in a spectrum. For example, when dGTP, dATPαS + dTTP, dGTP + dCTP + dTTP, dATPαS + dTTP, dGTP + dCTP + dTTP, or dATPαS + dTTP were successively added to the reaction chamber containing the DNA224 template, the peaks obtained by the corresponding dNTP addition were associated with the base number of 1, 4, 7, 2, 5, and 4, respectively. The results are illustrated in Fig. 2, indicating that it was possible to determine the identical base number in one peak up to nine from the observed signal intensity.

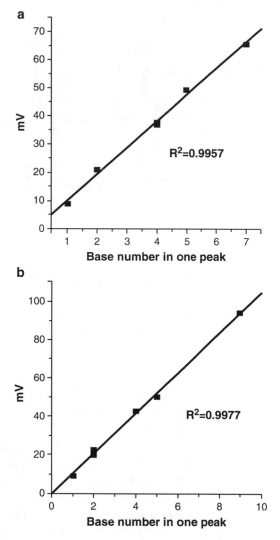

Fig. 2 Relationship between signal intensity and the corresponding incorporated base numbers in one peak. Pseudo-homopolymeric peaks in DNA224 were created by using the specific dNTP mixture instead of one dNTP. They produced big signals due to multiple dNTP incorporation. The dNTP mixture and its addition order were (**a**) dGTP, dATPαS + dTTP, dGTP + dCTP + dTTP, dATPαS + dTTP, dGTP + dCTP + dTTP, and dATPαS + dTTP; (**b**) dGTP, dATPαS, dGTP + dCTP + dTTP, dATPαS + dTTP, dGTP + dCTP + dTTP, and dATPαS + dTTP

The detecting sensitivity was determined by the background signal intensity due to impurities in the reaction mixture. It was 0.5 mV for 100 µL ATP detecting solution containing luciferin, luciferase, and apyrase, while it increased to 8.5 mV for 100 µL of PPi detecting solution containing luciferin, luciferase, ATP sulfurylase, APS, and apyrase. This is because APS is a substrate for the bioluminescence reaction with luciferin and luciferase. In addition to

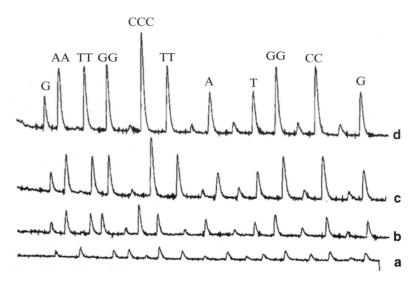

Fig. 3 Pyrosequencing spectra at different amounts of template DNA224. (**a**) 50 fmol, (**b**) 75 fmol, (**c**) 150 fmol, (**d**) 300 fmol in 100 μL reaction mixture. The injection volume and time were 0.2 μL and 3 s, respectively, by syringe. Adding sequence of dNTP is dATPαS, dCTP, dTTP, and dGTP

the signal produced by APS, the PPi contamination in dNTP produced a big background signal that could be reduced to 0.1–0.5 mV by adding small amounts of Ppase to each dNTP reservoir before sequencing. As the signal intensities for one base extension were about 0.7, 1.3, 2.1, and 4.1 mV for 50, 75, 150, and 300 fmol of DNA224 samples, respectively, the detection limit was estimated to be about 23 fmol. The pyrosequencing results of different amounts of templates are shown in Fig. 3 that shows that 150 fmol of sample was enough for a routine analysis.

It is frequently difficult to determine a base order of GC-rich DNAs from an electropherogram, because the fragments make secondary structures in both gel electrophoresis and polymerase reactions [14, 15]. Therefore, it is very difficult and time consuming to sequence GC-rich DNAs by the gel-based electrophoresis method. However, it is possible for the pyrosequencing method to sequence GC-rich DNAs or DNAs having stable secondary structures, as it uses nonthermal polymerase, Klenow that has stronger strand displacement activity than that of Tag DNA polymerase [16]. For example, the sequencing process was stopped when Thermo Sequenase was used to sequence a GC-rich (64.5 %) DNA fragment, which is presented in Fig. 4a. With this electropherogram, it is difficult to read the base order in the region. However, its sequence could be read by the pyrosequencing with a primer hybridized to the portion just before the terminated region. The sequencing reaction was successfully carried out with exo⁻ Klenow as shown in Fig. 4b. It was found that this short template

a

b

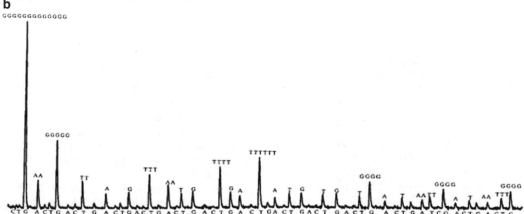

Fig. 4 Comparison of DNA sequencing spectra for a fragment 278 of genome DNA obtained with (**a**) gel-based electrophoresis using Thermo Sequenase; and (**b**) with pyrosequencing using exo⁻ Klenow

contained 13 identical Gs in homopolymeric region, and the total number of base G in the first 20 bases is 18. A good correlation between the signal intensity and the base number in homopolymeric regions in Fig. 4b is obtained for the first 31 bases ($R^2 = 0.9997$). The successful base order determination including 13 identical bases in a homopolymeric region further proved the usefulness of pyrosequencing. The result indicates that the pyrosequencing is a good tool to sequence DNA gaps including GC-rich fragments even if containing a homopolymeric region with many identical Gs or Cs.

5 Technical Notes

1. The immobilization was carried out according to the Dynabeads protocol.

2. In this presentation, we only show the results obtained with the single-stranded DNAs in the liquid phase.

3. Conventional Sanger's sequencing reaction was carried out using a Thermo Sequenase sequencing kit (RPN 2440, Amersham) and the universal primers described above.

4. We used the approach developed by Nyren and Lund [13] to monitor the PPi formed in the DNA polymerase reaction.

References

1. Kheterpal I, Mathies RA (1999) Capillary array electrophoresis DNA sequencing. Anal Chem 71:31A–37A

2. Venter JC et al (2001) The sequence of the human genome. Science 291:1304–1313

3. Ramsay G (1998) DNA chips: state-of-the art. Biotechnology 16:40–44

4. Fan JB, Chen X, Halushka MK, Berno A, Huang X, Ryder T, Lipshutz RJ, Lockhart DJ, Chakravarti A (2000) Parallel genotyping of human SNPs using generic high-density oligonucleotide tag arrays. Genome Res 10:853–860

5. Kirpekar F, Nordhoff E, Larsen LK, Kristiansen K, Roepstorff P, Hillenkamp F (1998) DNA sequence analysis by MALDI mass spectrometry. Nucleic Acids Res 26:2554–2559

6. Chen J, Iannone MA, Li MS, Taylor JD, Rivers P, Nelsen AJ, Slentz-Kesler KA, Roses A, Weiner MP (2000) A microsphere-based assay for multiplexed single nucleotide polymorphism analysis using single base chain extension. Genome Res 10:549–557

7. Landegren U, Nilsson M, Kwok PY (1998) Reading bits of genetic information: methods for single-nucleotide polymorphism analysis. Genome Res 8:769–776

8. Nollau P, Wagener C (1997) Methods for detection of point mutations: performance and quality assessment. Clin Chem 43:1114–1128

9. Ronaghi M, Uhlen M, Nyren P (1998) A sequencing method based on real-time pyrophosphate. Science 281:363–365

10. Hyman ED (1988) A new method of sequencing DNA. Anal Biochem 174:423–436

11. Ronaghi M, Karamohamed S, Pettersson B, Uhlén M, Nyrén P (1996) Real-time DNA sequencing using detection of pyrophosphate release. Anal Biochem 242:84–89

12. http://www.pyrosequencing.com

13. Nyrén P, Lundin A (1985) Enzymatic method for continuous monitoring of inorganic pyrophosphate synthesis. Anal Biochem 151:504–509

14. Szita N, Sutter R, Dual J, Buser R (2000) Proceedings of MEMS2000, Miyazaki Japan, January 23–27, 2000. pp 409–413

15. http://www.tecan.com/index_tecan.htm

16. Ronaghi M, Nygren M, Lundeberg J, Nyren P (1999) Analyses of secondary structures in DNA by pyrosequencing. Anal Biochem 267:65–71

Chapter 24

Pyrosequencing on Acryl-Modified Glass Chip

Huan Huang, Haiping Wu, Pengfeng Xiao, Bingjie Zou,
Qinxin Song, and Guohua Zhou

Abstract

A new method (termed as "chip-BAMPER" (bioluminometric assay coupled with modified primer extension reactions)) for single-nucleotide polymorphism (SNP) genotyping was developed by pyrosequencing chemistry coupled with hydrogel chip immobilized with single-stranded target DNAs. The method is based on allele-specific extension reaction, which is switched by the base type in the 3′ end of allele-specific primers. A genotype is determined by comparing the light intensity from a pair of gel pads, and the specificity is improved by introducing an artificially mismatched base at the third position upstream from the 3′ end of the allele-specific primer. The big problem of chip-BAMPER is the ultrahigh background of the detection mixture because apyrase could not be used. Here, we successfully prepared and used beaded apyrase, which can be removed from the detection mixture before sample typing, to decrease the high background due to adenosine 5′-triphosphate and inorganic pyrophosphate or sodium pyrophosphate decahydrate contamination. Unlike gel-based pyrosequencing, chip-BAMPER is highly sensitive because many bases are extended at a time in one extension reaction. Usually, less than 0.25 mL of PCR products can give a successful genotyping. To evaluate the method, four SNPs, OLR1-C15577T, OLR1-C14417G, PPARG-Pro12Ala, and PPARG-C2821T, were detected. To avoid the cross talk between two adjacent spots in a gel-chip, mineral oil was dispensed to coat the gel-chip for physically separating two spots. It is shown that this new strategy of SNP typing based on the acryl-modified glass chip is highly sensitive, simple, inexpensive, and easy to be automated. It can be used for various applications of DNA analysis at a relatively high throughput.

Key words Acryl-modified glass chip, Allele-specific extension reaction, Genotyping, Pyrosequencing chemistry

1 Introduction

Single-nucleotide polymorphisms (SNPs) are DNA sequence variations that occur when a single nucleotide in the genome sequence is altered. Although more than 99 % of human DNA sequences are the same across the population, variations in DNA sequence can predispose people to disease or influence their responses to a drug [1]. It is important to develop a simple, inexpensive, and especially high-throughput method allowing an efficient, sensitive, and

Guohua Zhou and Qinxin Song (eds.), *Advances and Clinical Practice in Pyrosequencing*, Springer Protocols Handbooks,
DOI 10.1007/978-1-4939-3308-2_24, © Springer Science+Business Media New York 2016

reproducible genotyping of SNPs. Up to now, there are many methods developed for this purpose, such as oligonucleotide microarray [2], bead-based "liquid microarray"[3], and optical fiber array [4]. Pyrosequencing [5–8] is a newly developed technology, and SNP typing is carried out by pyrosequencing a short amplicon containing an SNP with an interest. To perform pyrosequencing on a glass slide, we have developed a hydrogel-based chip platform to immobilize ssDNA for pyrosequencing [9]. However, we found that it is difficult to use this gel-based pyrosequencing for an accurate genotyping because the linear relationship between signal intensities of peaks and the number of incorporated deoxynucleoside triphosphates (dNTPs) is not always satisfied. This problem especially occurs when the polymorphism is located in a homogeneous region of the target sequence. Moreover, we found that the sensitivity of pyrosequencing on gel-immobilized slide is much low although a polyacrylamide gel with three-dimensional structure has a high binding capacity of template DNAs, and thus a large amount of PCR products (410 mL) is required.

In order to use our well-developed hydrogel-chip platform for sensitive SNP typing, bioluminometric assay coupled with modified primer extension reactions (BAMPER) method [10], which is highly sensitive due to many bases extended at a time in one allele-specific extension reaction, was applied instead of pyrosequencing. The specificity of BAMPER is high enough for an accurate SNP typing due to the artificial introduction of mismatched base in the 3′ end of allele-specific primer. Since apyrase was not allowed in BAMPER detection mixture, the big problem of BAMPER is the ultrahigh background signal caused by adenosine 5′-triphosphate (ATP) and PPi contaminated in the detection mixture. This background is the key to the assay sensitivity. To overcome this problem, beaded apyrase, having been used to improve detection limits in bioluminometric ATP monitoring [11] and to remove adenosine dephosphate from the rigor muscle solutions [12], was prepared by our new method and employed to decrease the high background. Successful genotyping of four SNPs (PPARG-Pro12Ala [13], OLR1-C15577T [14], OLR1-C14417G [15], and PPARG-C2821T [16]) demonstrated that the gel-based BAMPER (termed as chip-BAMPER) is sensitive, accurate, simple, and straightforward.

Schematic illustration of chip-BAMPER for SNP typing is shown in Fig. 1. At first, PCR is performed using a primer with an acrylamide group at the 5′ end; then the raw amplicons are immobilized with polyacrylamide gel on an acryl-modified glass chip by copolymerization. The ssDNA is prepared by electrophoresing the chip at an alkali condition [17]. After allele-specific primers anneal to the ssDNAs immobilized on the gel, a detection mixture containing four dNTPs and reagents for extension reaction, PPi

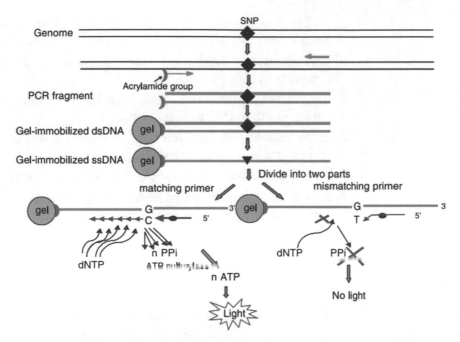

Fig. 1 Schematic illustration of chip-BAMPER for SNP typing

conversion, and light production is dispensed onto the chip surface. If the 3′ end of a primer is complementary to the template, extension reaction occurs and a large amount of by-product PPi is released. On the other hand, if the 3′ end of the primer does not perfectly match the template, almost no extension reaction occurs. To improve the specificity of allele-specific extension, an artificially mismatched base is introduced into the third position upstream from the 3′ end of the allele-specific primer [10]. The allele type is identified by comparing the signal intensities from two gel pads corresponding to a pair of allele-specific primers on the chip. As the signal intensity is proportional to the number of bases incorporated by DNA polymerase at a time, the extension of many bases in the BAMPER gives a very high sensitivity [18–20].

2   Materials

1. Luciferase and Exo⁻ Klenow were purchased from Promega (Madison, USA).

2. ATP sulfurylase, adenosine 5′-phospho-sulfate, inorganic pyrophosphate or sodium pyrophosphate decahydrate (PPi), apyrase, inorganic pyrophosphatase, BSA, and D-luciferin were purchased from Sigma (St Louis, MO).

3. 2′-Deoxyadenosine-5′-O-(1-thiotriphosphate) was purchased from Biolog Life Science Institute (Bremen, Germany).

4. dNTPs were purchased from Amersham Biosciences (Piscataway, NJ).

5. Taq DNA polymerase was purchased from TaKaRa Biotechnology (Dalian, P. R. China).

6. Dynabeads M-280 Tosylactivated (2.8 mm id) was purchased from Dynal AC (Oslo, Norway).

7. ATP was obtained from Oriental Yeast (Osaka, Japan).

8. All solutions were prepared in deionized and sterilized water. Other chemicals were analytical pure grade or molecule biology grade.

3   Methods

3.1   Primers and Template DNA

1. The oligonucleotides modified with acrylamide group at the 5′ end were purchased from TaKaRa Biotechnology and were purified by HPLC.

2. Other oligonucleotides were purchased from Invitrogen Biotechnology (Shanghai, P. R. China) and were PAGE purified.

3.2   Immobilization of the Acrylamide-Modified PCR Products and ssDNA Preparation

1. The samples were amplified with an unmodified primer and an acrylamide-modified primer.

2. PCR was carried out in a final volume of 50 mL containing 0.2 mM dNTP, 200 nM of each primer, 2 U of Taq DNA polymerase, 10× buffer, 1.5 mM $MgCl_2$, and DNA template.

3. The thermocycling conditions were at an initial denaturation at 95 °C for 3 min, then 35 cycles of 94 °C, 50 s, and 72 °C for 30 s, 45 °C for 45 s each, followed by 72 °C for 7 min.

4. The resulting DNA fragments were resolved by electrophoresis in a 2 % agarose gel and stained with ethidium bromide.

5. Gel images were captured on a Bio Imaging System (Syngene, UK).

6. The raw PCR products combined with acrylamide monomers were co-polymerized on the glass chip [9]. After polymerizations, glass chips were subjected to an electrophoresis in 0.1 M NaOH solutions (100 mA, 5 min), followed by an electrophoresis in 1× TBE (40 V/cm, 5 min). The gel-immobilized ssDNAs on the slide were prepared for BAMPER analysis.

3.3   The Preparation of Beaded Apyrase and Beaded Ppase

1. Dynabeads M-280 Tosylactivated was resuspended well by pipetting or vortexing for approximately 1 min and then the volume of beads to be used were pipetted into a test tube.

2. After the tube was placed on a magnet until the beads have migrated to the side of the tube, the supernatant was pipetted off carefully.

3. The tube was then removed from the magnet and the beads were resuspended carefully in an ample volume of buffer A (0.1 M Na-phosphate buffer, pH 7.4).

4. After applying the magnet and pipetting off the supernatant, the washed beads were resuspended in the same volume of buffer A.

5. The washing step was repeated again.

6. Then the protein (apyrase or inorganic pyrophosphatase (PPase)) dissolved in buffer A was added into the Dynabeads and the mixture was incubated for 4 h at 37 °C with slow tilt rotation.

7. After incubation, the tube was placed on the magnet for 2 min, and then the supernatant was removed.

8. Finally the coated beads were washed with buffer C (phosphate-buffered saline, pH 7.4) for 5 min at 41 °C twice, treated with buffer D (0.2 M Tris, 0.1 % BSA, pH 8.5) (37 °C, 1 h), and stored in buffer C at 41 °C for use.

3.4 Degradation of Endogenous Pyrophosphate in dNTPs

1. As the proposed method is based on the detection of PPi released from primer extension, any contaminated PPi existing in the dNTPs will give a spurious signal.

2. An aliquot of 1 mM dNTPs containing 5 mM Tris (pH 7.5) and 25 mM of magnesium acetate was incubated with beaded PPase (about 10 mU) for 10 min at room temperature (*see* **Note 1**).

3. Then beaded PPase was removed from the dNTP solution. The desired concentration of dNTP solution was diluted directly before the incorporation reaction.

3.5 Degradation of Contaminated PPi and ATP in BAMPER Detection Mixture

1. As the BAMPER detection mixture contaminates PPi and ATP, beaded apyrase was prepared and added into the reaction buffer instead of free apyrase.

2. The prepared buffer was incubated with beaded apyrase for less than 5 min, which is enough for degrading contamination producing high spurious signal in the detection mixture.

3. After applying the magnet and pipetting off the supernatant of the treated detection mixture, the treated detection mixture was gathered for genotyping.

4. Finally, the beaded apyrase was washed with buffer C and stored in buffer C for the repeated use.

1. Allele-specific extension and PPi detection were performed in a mixture similar to pyrosequencing at room temperature (*see* **Note 2**).

2. The detection mixture (5 mL for each sample) containing 0.1 M Tris–acetate (pH 7.7), 2 mM EDTA, 10 mM magnesium acetate, 0.02 % BSA, 1 mM DTT, 1 mM adenosine 5′-phosphosulfate, 0.4 M PVP, 0.4 mM luciferin, 0.2 U/mL ATP sulfurylase, 14.6 mM luciferase, and 18 U/mL DNA polymerase I Klenow fragment (exo⁻) was added on the surface of the glass slides (*see* **Note 3**).

3. The detection started just after adding dNTPs (200 mM).

4 Method Validation

To degrade the ATP, there are two ways: one is to add apyrase directly into the mixture and the other is to add PPase for degrading the PPi in the light production step [21]. As shown in curve 2 in Fig. 2, the background signal decreased by the addition of PPase, but is still very high, suggesting that PPase is not effective to reduce the background. Therefore, we have to use apyrase for lowering the background signal. As shown in curve 3 in Fig. 2, the background significantly decreased when a small amount of apyrase (0.032 U) was added for 5-min incubation. Since apyrase degrades dNTPs, a method that does not allow the residual apyrase existing in the solution is recommended. As apyrase fixed on

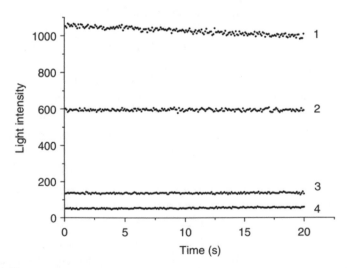

Fig. 2 Time courses of background signals from the detection mixture without any treatment (*1*) and with the treatment by PPase (*2*), by a small amount of free apyrase (*3*), and by beaded apyrase (*4*)

magnetic beads can be easily removed by a magnet, beaded apyrase was prepared for reducing the background [22, 23]. As shown
in curve 4, the background signal was greatly reduced by the
beaded apyrase (6 mL).

To increase the throughput of BAMPER, amplicons modified
with an acrylamide group at the 5' end of one strand were immobilized with polyacrylamide gel on a glass chip by copolymerization initiated by the evaporation of TEMED [24]. In order to
prepare ssDNAs for allele-specific reaction, electrophoresis was
performed on the gel-chip immobilized with dsDNAs under 0.1 M
NaOH, which can dissociate the dsDNAs. Any non-acrylamidated
oligos or PCR components that may cause the spurious signal flow
out of the gel, leaving only the ssDNA template in the gel spot. We
found that electrophoresis is very effective to remove the free DNA
strand and impurities in the gel [9]. A raw PCR product could thus
be directly immobilized on the gel without any prior purification.
The electrophoresis-treated chip is much clear, and gives a very low
background signal.

To demonstrate the specificity of chip-BAMPER, four SNPs
(PPARG-Pro12Ala, OLR1-C15577T, OLR1-C14417G, and
PPARG-C2821T) were analyzed. As shown in Fig. 3a, allele-C of
OLR1-C14417G gave a very high false-positive signal when
detecting "GG" genotype, indicating that one mismatched base in
the 3' end cannot effectively block the extension reaction. To
decrease the probability of spurious extension reaction, an artificially mismatched base at the third position upstream from the 3'
end of the allele-specific primer was thus introduced. As shown in
Fig. 3b, the spurious extension signals decreased significantly, so
that accurate genotypes of OLR1-C14417G were obtained. By
this modified allele-specific extension reaction on polyacrylamide-
gel chip, three SNPs (OLR1-C15577T, OLR1-C14417G, and
PPARG-C2821T) were successfully typed, but the specificity for
typing PPARG-Pro12Ala is still not perfect although the modified
strategy was used. It was observed that the extension signal of
allele-C was much stronger than that of allele-G in Fig. 3c, so that
a high spurious signal from allele-C-specific extension reaction
occurred when typing GG genotype. To decrease the high spurious signal, we tried to change the type of the artificially mismatched
base in the allele-C-specific primer from A to G, and the spurious
signal disappeared (see Fig. 3d). This example indicates that we can
try another type of the artificially mismatched base in case the specificity is not satisfied (see **Note 4**).

In order to type SNPs in a way of a high throughput, the CCD
camera (Cascade 1 K, Photometrics, USA) is a preferable detector
for getting a total image of a chip in a short time. One SNP
(PPARG-C2821T) was selected as an example for the investigation, and three different samples with known genotypes were analyzed. As shown in Fig. 4, the signal intensities from the extension

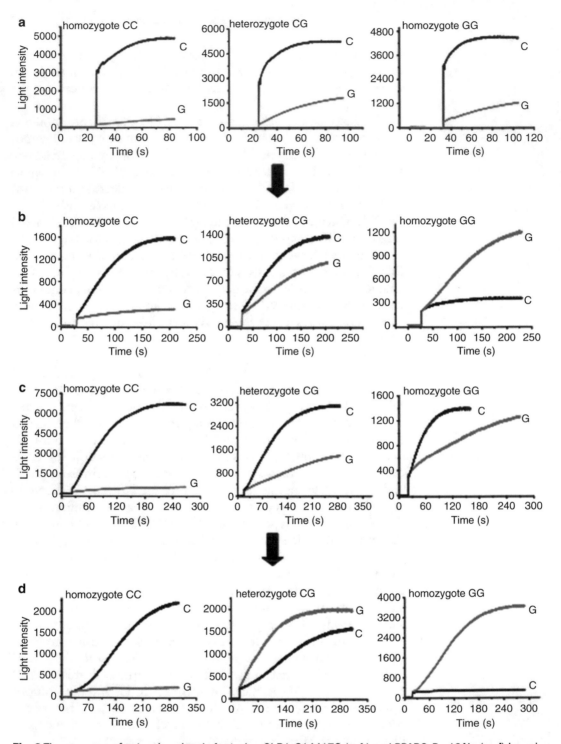

Fig. 3 Time courses of extension signals for typing OLR1-C14417G (**a**, **b**) and PPARG-Pro12Ala (**c**, **d**) by using a pair of allele-specific primers without any artificially mismatched base (**a**), each with an artificially mismatched base (**b**, **c**), and one with an artificially mismatched base (**d**). The type of the artificially mismatched base in the allele-C-specific primer was changed from A (**c**) to G (**d**), while the artificially mismatched base in the allele-G-specific primer (**c**) was changed back to the matched one (**d**). The paired allele-specific primers used in panels (**a**)–(**d**) are 14417-C and 14417-G, 14417-C-3 and 14417-G-3, Pro12Ala-G-3 and Pro12Ala-C-3, and Pro12Ala-G and Pro12Ala-C-3-2

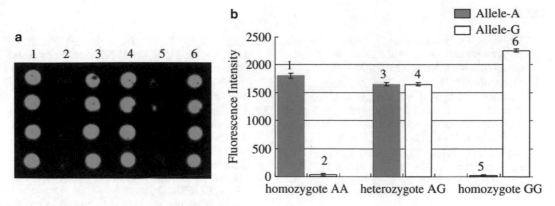

Fig. 4 Readout of gel-chip-based genotyping system by CCD (**a**) and a column graph of the signal intensities (**b**) for typing Promoter-C2821T. Three typical samples, homozygote AA (*columns* 1 and 2), heterozygote AG (*columns* 3 and 4), and homozygote GG (*columns* 5 and 6), were detected by allele specific primers C28211-A-3 (*columns* 1, 3, and 5) and C2821T-G-3 (*columns* 2, 4, and 6)

reactions by two allele-specific primers hybridized on gel-immobilized ssDNA are quite different for three typical genotypes; thus the genotype of a given sample was easily discriminated. For example, homozygotes AA and GG yielded strong signals at the allele-A specific-spots (column 1 in Fig. 4a) and at allele-G-specific spots (column 6 in Fig. 4a), respectively. On the other hand, the heterozygote AG gave strong signals at both allele-specific spots (columns 3 and 4 in Fig. 4a). To make the typing results more straightforward, a column graph was made based on the signal intensities, which was read by the software of QCapture-Pro5.1. As shown in Fig. 4b, the specificity of genotype discrimination is quite good.

5 Technical Notes

1. It is necessary to degrade the endogenous PPi in dNTPs before the dNTP incorporation reaction.

2. The ssDNA templates attached on gel pads were annealed with an allele-specific primer.

3. BAMPER-based genotyping system does not use any apyrase; so the background signal in the BAMPER detection mixture is very high because both PPi and ATP are contaminated in the mixture. In the BAMPER detection mixture, the contaminated PPi is converted into ATP; so the final contribution of the background signal is due to ATP [25].

4. It was found that the artificially mismatched base in allele-G-specific primer greatly slowed down the rate of extension reaction, and this affects the accurate discrimination of a heterozygote.

References

1. Sripichai O, Fucharoen SJ (2007) Genetic polymorphisms and implications for human diseases. J Med Assoc Thai 90:394–398

2. Hardenbol P, Baner J, Jain M, Nilsson M, Namsaraev EA, Karlin-Neumann GA, Fakhrai-Rad H et al (2003) Multiplexed genotyping with sequence-tagged molecular inversion probes. Nat Biotechnol 21:673–678

3. Taylor JD, Briley D, Nguyen Q, Long K, Iannone MA, Li MS, Ye F et al (2001) Flow cytometric platform for high-throughput single nucleotide polymorphism analysis. Biotechniques 30(661–666):668–669

4. Ferguson JA, Steemers FJ, Walt DR (2000) High-density fiber-optic DNA random microsphere array. Anal Chem 72: 5618–5624

5. Ahmadian A, Gharizadeh B, Gustafsson AC, Sterky F, Nyren P, Uhlen M, Lundeberg J (2000) Single-nucleotide polymorphism analysis by pyrosequencing. Anal Biochem 280:103–110

6. Lavebratt C, Sengul S, Jansson M, Schalling M (2004) Pyrosequencing-based SNP allele frequency estimation in DNA pools. Hum Mutat 23:92–97

7. Sun YQ, Monstein HJ, Ryberg A, Borch K (2007) Multiple strand displacement amplification of DNA isolated from human archival plasma/serum: identification of cytokine polymorphism by pyrosequencing analysis. Clin Chim Acta 377:108–113

8. Zackrisson AL, Lindblom B (2003) Identification of CYP2D6 alleles by single nucleotide polymorphism analysis using pyrosequencing. Eur J Clin Pharmacol 59: 521–526

9. Xiao P, Huang H, Zhou G, Lu Z (2007) Gel immobilization of acrylamide-modified single-stranded DNA template for pyrosequencing. Electrophoresis 28:1903–1912

10. Zhou GH, Shirakura H, Kamahori M, Okano K, Nagai K, Kambara H (2004) A gel-free SNP genotyping method: bioluminometric assay coupled with modified primer extension reactions (BAMPER) directly from double-stranded PCR products. Hum Mutat 24: 155–163

11. Nyren P (1994) Apyrase immobilized on paramagnetic beads used to improve detection limits in bioluminometric ATP monitoring. J Biolumin Chemilumin 9:29–34

12. Thirlwell H, Corrie JE, Reid GP, Trentham DR, Ferenczi MA (1994) Kinetics of relaxation from rigor of permeabilized fast-twitch skeletal fibers from the rabbit using a novel caged ATP and apyrase. Biophys J 67:2436–2447

13. Cardona F, Morcillo S, Gonzalo-Marin L, Garrido-Sanchez M, Macias-Gonzalez M, Tinahonesz FJ (2006) Pro12Ala sequence variant of the PPARG gene is associated with post-prandial hypertriglyceridemia in non-E3/E3 patients with the metabolic syndrome. Clin Chem 52:1920–1925

14. Trabetti E, Biscuola M, Cavallari U, Malerba G, Girelli D, Olivieri O, Martinelli N et al (2006) On the association of the oxidised LDL receptor 1 (OLR1) gene in patients with acute myocardial infarction or coronary artery disease. Eur J Hum Genet 14:127–130

15. Yamada Y, Kato K, Kameyama T, Yokoi K, Matsuo H, Segawa T, Watanabe S et al (2006) Genetic factors for obesity. Int J Mol Med 18:843–851

16. Doney AS, Fischer B, Cecil JE, Boylan K, McGui-gan FE, Ralston SH, Morris AD, Palmer CN (2004) Association of the Pro12Ala and C1431T variants of PPARG and their haplotypes with susceptibility to Type 2 diabetes. Diabetologia 47:555–558

17. Gharizadeh B, Eriksson J, Nourizad N, Nordstrom T, Nyren P (2004) Improvements in Pyrosequencing technology by employing Sequenase polymerase. Anal Biochem 330: 272–280

18. Pettersson M, Bylund M, Alderborn A (2003) Molecular haplotype determination using allele-specific PCR and pyrosequencing technology. Genomics 82:390–396

19. Alderborn A, Kristofferson A, Hammerling U (2000) Determination of single-nucleotide polymorphisms by real-time pyrophosphate DNA sequencing. Genome Res 10:1249–1258

20. Pacey-Miller T, Henry R (2003) Single-nucleotide polymorphism detection in plants using a single-stranded pyrosequencing protocol with a universal biotinylated primer. Anal Biochem 317:166–170

21. Verri A, Focher F, Tettamanti G, Grazioli V (2005) Two-step genetic screening of thrombophilia by pyrosequencing. Clin Chem 51: 1282–1284

22. Palmieri O, Toth S, Ferraris A, Andriulli A, Latiano A, Annese V, Dallapiccola B et al

(2003) CARD15 genotyping in inflammatory bowel disease patients by multiplex pyrosequencing. Clin Chem 49:1675–1679

23. Syed AA, Irving JA, Redfern CP, Hall AG, Unwin NC, White M, Bhopal RS et al (2004) Low prevalence of the N363S polymorphism of the glucocorticoid receptor in South Asians living in the United Kingdom. J Clin Endocrinol Metab 89:232–235

24. Xiao PF, Cheng L, Wan Y, Sun BL, Chen ZZ, Zhang SY, Zhang CZ et al (2006) An improved gel-based DNA microarray method for detecting single nucleotide mismatch. Electrophoresis 27:3904–3915

25. Ramon D, Braden M, Adams S, Marincola FM, Wang L (2003) Pyrosequencing trade mark: a one-step method for high resolution HLA typing. J Transl Med 1:9–18

Chapter 25

Pyrosequencing On-Chip Based on a Gel-Based Solid-Phase Amplification

Huan Huang, Pengfeng Xiao, Zongtai Qi, Bingjie Zou, Qinxin Song, and Guohua Zhou

Abstract

As conventional solid-phase amplification (SPA) on a two-dimensional slide has a low amplification capacity due to a limited amount of immobilized primers, we propose a three-dimensional SPA by immobilizing primers in hydrogel attached to a slide. One of the PCR primers, modified with an acrylamide group at the 5′-terminal, was copolymerized with both polyacrylamide gel and an acryl-modified glass slide, resulting in a high amplification capacity. The immobilization process was carried out by adding the catalysis reagent N,N,N',N'-tetramethylethylenediamine (TEMED) volatilized in vacuum, with uniform sample concentration and gel viscosity in the course of one-step nucleic acid immobilization. The porous structure of polyacrylamide gel, which allows PCR reagents such as Taq DNA polymerase, primers, dNTPs, and DNA templates to freely enter the gel matrix, provides a homogeneous solution-mimicking environment for SPA on the interface or the inside of gel pads. Based on gel-based SPA, genotypes of different samples were accurately discriminated by either dual-color fluorescence hybridization or BAMPER (Bioluminometric Assay coupled with Modified Primer Extension Reactions). Pyrosequencing was also successfully carried out on SPA products. As the linkage between DNA molecules and gel is very strong, SPA products immobilized on gel pads could be reused several times if extended strands were removed by electrophoresis. Thus, the gel-based SPA provides a powerful tool for directly using on-chip amplicons for parallel detection.

Key words Gel-based solid-phase amplification, SNP typing, On-chip amplicons

1 Introduction

SNP typing and sequencing are widely used in molecular diagnosis and large-scale genetic association studies. If there is a limited amount of target, most approaches for SNP typing and DNA sequencing need polymerase chain reaction (PCR), which can generate millions of DNA copies from the amplification of a single or several copies of DNA [1–4]. For a high-throughput detection format such as a DNA chip, PCR in parallel is required. Solid-phase amplification (SPA), which is an improved PCR technique for an

Guohua Zhou and Qinxin Song (eds.), *Advances and Clinical Practice in Pyrosequencing*, Springer Protocols Handbooks,
DOI 10.1007/978-1-4939-3308-2_25, © Springer Science+Business Media New York 2016

efficient high-throughput assay on a chip, has been proposed for molecular diagnosis [5, 6]. As SPA has the advantage of easy purification of amplicons on slides, it has been widely used for various applications [7–9]. Immobilized primers in SPA should meet the requirements of a high surface density and a strong linkage between primers and substrates [5]; thus the selection of supporting matrix and an immobilization method is very important for SPA on a chip. In the case of rigid supports on a flat surface, such as glass and microwell used in conventional SPA [5, 7, 9, 10], the binding capacity is very limited due to a small surface area. Therefore three-dimensional (3-D) hydrophilic gel (e.g., polyacrylamide) has been employed as a substrate to improve the surface area in SPA [11], but DNA attachment still requires the following steps: preparation of polyacrylamide gel pads, activation of the gel to produce aldehyde groups, and immobilization of 5′-terminal amino-modified primers. These steps are tedious and labile. Although the copolymerization step and the polymerization-mediated immobilization step were further improved [12], the whole process is still complex and time consuming. Thus, a simple (ideally one-step) and rapid method for immobilization is preferable for controlling the quality of immobilization.

A simple process was developed for immobilizing oligonucleotides bearing an acrylamide group at the 5′-terminal onto a solid support by using acrylamide monomers for copolymerization, and the gel activation step was skipped [13]. However, the direct addition of the ammonium persulfate and N,N,N',N'-tetramethylethylenediamine (TEMED) into prepolymers would cause the polymerization to be uncontrollable, so that it becomes very difficult to spot the mixed prepolymers homogeneously onto a large-scale microarray. To get a uniform sample concentration and gel viscosity in the course of nucleic acid immobilization, we proposed a novel method to control the polymerization process by adding the catalysis reagent TEMED separately, and the copolymerization was catalyzed after volatilized TEMED molecules in vacuum reached onto the spotted prepolymers [14]. This method enables the spotting time to be controlled, and the attachment of gel to slides is extremely stable. In contrast to flat surfaces, polyacrylamide gel can provide a 3-D surface with a very high probe density (200 fmol/mm^2) [14]. We have successfully used this method to bind PCR products for SNP typing and DNA sequencing [15]. However the whole process is tedious as a regular amplification reaction is still needed to supply amplicons for gel immobilization. To simplify the process, we tried to perform PCR amplification directly on a previously well-developed 3-D gel-chip to produce gel-immobilized amplicons for downstream genotyping and pyrosequencing.

2   Materials

1. Model 391 DNA Synthesizer (Applied Biosystems).

2. Microarray (Capital Biochip Corporation, China).

3. Frame seal chamber (ABgene, Surrey, UK).

4. 16×16 twin tower block thermocycler (PTC 200, MJ Research).

5. Scanner (ScanArray Lite, Packard BioScience Company, USA).

3   Methods

3.1   Oligonucleotides and DNA Templates

1. Primers modified with acrylamide groups at the 5′ terminal were synthesized on Model 391 DNA Synthesizer using a commercially available acrylamide phosphoramidite (Acrydite ™; Matrix Technologies).

2. A 135 bp fragment including the 14417 SNP locus of Ox-LDL receptor 1 (OLR-1) gene was selected for SPA. The forward primer was 5′-TACTATCCTTCCCAGCTCCT-3′, and the acrylamide group-modified reverse primer was 5′-acrylamide-TTTTCAGCAACTTGG   CAT-3′.   14417C   (5′-Cy3-GGAAAACAGCCAA-3′) and 14417G (5′-Cy5-GGAAAAGAG CCAA-3′) were labeled with Cy3 and Cy5 fluorescent dyes, respectively, as hybridization reporters.

3. 14417C-2 (5′-GGCTACTTTAACTGGGAAcAC-3′)   and 14417G-2 (5′-GGCTACTTTAAC TGGGAAcAG-3′) were used for bioluminometric assays coupled with modified primer extension   reactions   (BAMPER)   [16].   The   small   characters represent the artificially mismatched bases.

4. 14417C (or 14417C-2) and 14417G (or 14417G-2) were matched with homozygote 14417C/C and homozygote 14417G/G of 14417 locus, respectively. The forward primer of SPA was also used as a sequencing primer for pyrosequencing.

3.2   Attachment of Modified Oligonucleotides to Acryl-Modified Slide Surface

1. The spotting solution, acrylamide-modified oligonucleotide mixture containing 3 % w/w acrylamide monomer (29:1 w/w acrylamide:bis-acrylamide), 30 % w/w glycerol, and 1 % w/v ammonium persulfate, was prepared at the desired concentration of 2 mM.

2. The solution was spotted on the acryl-modified slide by an ink-jet using a microarray or by manual operation.

3. After spotting, the slide was placed into a humid airtight chamber which was vacuumed to about 1000 Pascal (Pa), and the

chamber was kept at room temperature for about 20 min to vaporize TEMED in a water glass pre-placed in the chamber.

4. Copolymerization started when the vaporized TEMED molecules reached onto the slide surface.

3.3 Gel-Based SPA

1. The glass slide on which oligonucleotides were covalently bonded to the gel was subjected to electrophoresis at 10 V/cm for 5 min in 1×TBE to remove the non-immobilized oligonucleotides and other impurities.

2. Then PCR mix was added into a frame seal chamber on the slide, and then the glass slide was put into a 16×16 twin tower block thermocycler.

3. Amplification was carried out in a volume of 25 mL containing 0.2 mM dNTPs, 16 nM reverse primers, 400 nM forward primers, 1.8 U of promega Taq DNA polymerase, 1.5 mM $MgCl_2$, and genomic DNA.

4. Thermocycling condition was as follows: 94 °C for 5 min, then 40 cycles of 94 °C for 45 s, 58 °C for 60 s, and 72 °C for 90 s, followed by 72 °C for 7 min (see **Notes 1** and **2**).

3.4 Detection of the Gel-Based SPA Products

1. After SPA, glass slides attached with amplicons were subjected to electrophoresis in 0.1 M NaOH (100 mA) for 5 min, followed by electrophoresis at 40 V/cm for 5 min in 1×TBE to remove free single-stranded DNA (ssDNA) and impurities.

2. Three methods were adapted for detection: Dual-color fluorescence hybridization. The labeled-reporters solution was applied to the chip and the hybridization was performed in a humid glass chamber at 40 °C for 2 h. After hybridization, the slide was subjected to electrophoresis under 10 V/cm for 8 min in 1×TBE at room temperature to remove the free reporters and the mismatched reporters. After the electrophoresis was completed, the slide was rinsed with water and dried under a stream of nitrogen. Finally images of the slides were captured by a scanner;

3. BAMPER: Pyrosequencing mixture containing 0.1 M Tris–acetate (pH 7.7), 2 mM ethylenediaminetetraacetic acid (EDTA), 10 mM magnesium acetate, 0.2 % bovine serum albumin (BSA), 1 mM dithiothreitol (DTT), 2.5 mM adenosine 5′-phospho-sulfate, 0.4 mg/mL polyvinylpyrrolidone (PVP), 0.4 mM D-luciferin, 200 mU/mL ATP sulfurylase, luciferase in an amount determined to give appropriate sensitivity, and 18 U/mL DNA polymerase I Klenow fragment (exo⁻) was added on the chip, where ssDNA templates immobilized in the gel were annealed with the primers of 14417C-2 and 14417G-2, respectively. The extension reaction started with the addition of the mixture of all four dNTPs (see **Note 3**).

4. Pyrosequencing: Apyrase VII (1.6 U/mL) was added into the above pyrosequencing mixture. The prepared reaction solution was used to detect the sequence of ssDNA templates which were immobilized in the gel and annealed with the sequencing primer. Sequencing reactions were initiated by individually dispensing dATP αS, dCTP, dTTP, and dGTP.

4 Method Validation

4.1 Development of Gel-Based SPA Approach

The process of gel-based SPA was illustrated briefly in Fig. 1a. At first, reverse primers modified with a 5′-terminal acrylamide group and acrylamide monomers were copolymerized to form polyacrylamide gel pads attached to the acryl-modified slides. During the copolymerization, ammonium persulfate was used to catalyze the polymerization reaction; we didn't find any obvious effect of ammonium persulfate on the oligonucleotides although ammonium persulfate is a strong oxidant. After removing the non-immobilized primers by electrophoresis [15], a mixture required for SPA was added into a reaction chamber containing a gel pad. Finally SPA was performed in an airproof environment. During the early cycles, solution-phase exponential amplification was predominant; with the consumption of reverse primers, linear amplification became dominant in the later cycles (several tens), generating large amounts of ssDNA from the extension of forward primes. Reverse primers immobilized on gel captured the free ssDNA, and then extended. The linkage between the acrylamide-modified primers and the gel was strong enough to tolerate the stringent temperature variation in SPA. The amplicons immobilized on gel can be directly used for downstream detection.

To achieve a highly efficient SPA, the selection of a thermal-stable linkage type is considered as the most important factor. We tried to use oligonucleotides modified with four different chemical groups (amino, phosphate, biotin, and acrylamide) as immobilized primers for SPA. The thermal stability and the binding capacity of the four oligonucleotides were evaluated by subjecting each kind of immobilized oligonucleotide to an identical PCR cycling condition (94 °C for 5 min; then 35 cycles of 94 °C for 30 s, 48 °C for 40 s, and 72 °C for 40 s, followed by 72 °C for 7 min). As can be seen in Fig. 2, the total amount of the immobilized oligonucleotides modified with an amino group, phosphate group, and biotin group greatly decreased after PCR thermal cycling, and only 37 % (Fig. 2a), 58 % (Fig. 2b), and 63 % (Fig. 2c) of the immobilized oligonucleotides remain on the support. Therefore, the primers modified with these three groups are not good enough for SPA. In the case of acrylamide-modified

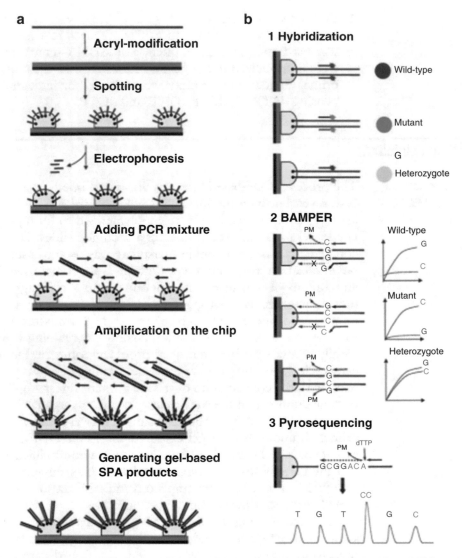

Fig. 1 A schematic overview of gel-based SPA (**a**) and the methods for detecting the gel-based SPA products (**b**)

oligonucleotides, 75 % (*see* Fig. 2d) of the immobilized oligonu-cleotides remain on the support after PCR. These results indicate that the thermal stability of acrylamide-modified oligonucleotides is the most suitable for SPA.

4.2 Evaluation of Polyacrylamide Gel Used as the Substrate to Immobilize PCR Primers

To evaluate whether gel-immobilized primers and other PCR reagents can effectively perform SPA in gel pads, Cy3-modified dUTP, which should be incorporated into amplicons during SPA, was employed as a reporter. After gel-based SPA, electrophoresis (20 V/cm, 10 min) was used to remove excess Cy3-modified dUTP. As the amplicons were fixed on gel support, a signal should not be observed if SPA does not occur. The SPA results from the polyacrylamide gel copolymerized with or without

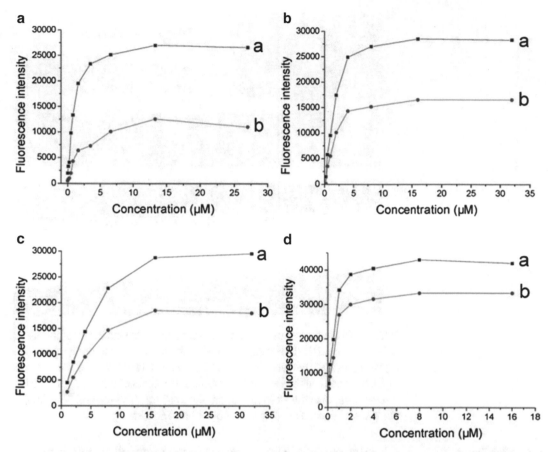

Fig. 2 Hybridization results of four kinds of immobilized oligonucleotides with the chemical modifications of amino (**a**), phosphate (**b**), biotin (**c**), and acrylamide (**d**) at different concentrations. After immobilization, the modified oligonucleotides were hybridized with fluorescence probes directly (*a*) or after PCR thermal cycling (*b*)

acrylamide-modified primers showed that acrylamide-modified primers attached to gel could successfully extend in SPA (*see* Fig. 3a), and that electrophoresis is effective for removing excess Cy3-modified dUTP. Therefore, the SPA can be performed on the substrate of polyacrylamide gel.

4.3 Optimization of Gel-Based SPA Conditions

In SPA, forward primers were free in solution, but reverse primers were in two forms: one was immobilized to gel for generating SPA products, and the other was free in solution for producing free amplicons to activate the extension reaction of the immobilized primers. However, too many free reverse primers would compete with the immobilized primers, causing a lower SPA efficiency; thus the amount of the free reverse primers should be optimized. The results of SPA with various concentration ratios of the free reverse primers to the forward primers indicated an optimal ratio of 1/25 (*see* Fig. 3b–d).

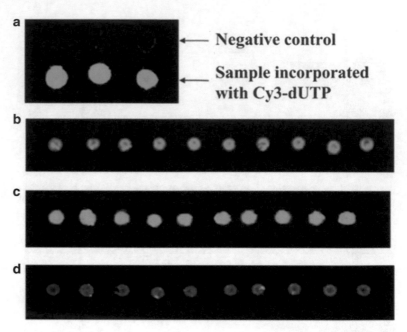

Fig. 3 (**a**) The fluorescence scan image of SPA products with the incorporation of Cy3-modified dUTP. *Row 1*: controls (gel without immobilized primers) and *row 2*: gel-immobilized primers. (**b–d**) Hybridization results of SPA products amplified by different amounts of free reverse primers. The concentration ratios of the free reverse primers to the forward primers are 1/10 (**b**), 1/25 (**c**), and 1/50 (**d**). The slides were scanned at 75 % laser power and 75 % PMT gain

4.4 SNP Typing of Gel-Based SPA Products by Dual-Color Fluorescence Hybridization

After the gel-based SPA, electrophoresis under alkali conditions was applied to repress DNA templates for probe hybridization. As illustrated in Fig. 1, a pair of dual-color allele-specific fluorescence robes differing by one base in the middle of the sequence was used as the hybridization reporters for genotyping. Genotypes can be determined by observing fluorescent signals from probe hybridization. The genotyping results of three typical samples are shown in Fig. 4. For the 14417C/C homozygote, only the Cy3 fluorescent signal (green fluorescence) from the 14417C reporter was obtained, because the Cy5-labeled 14417G reporter, having one mismatched base in the middle, was removed by electrophoresis (*see* Fig. 4a). In the same way, only the Cy5 fluorescence signal (red fluorescence) appeared for the 14417G/G homozygote (*see* Fig. 4b); both Cy3 and Cy5 fluorescent signals (green and red fluorescence) were detected for the 14417C/G heterozygote, causing a "yellow" signal in Fig. 4c. The results completely coincided with those obtained by Sanger's sequencing method (*see* Fig. 4e), demonstrating that genotyping using gel-based SPA amplicons is possible.

4.5 SNP Typing of Gel-Based SPA Products by BAMPER

The genotypes were identified by comparing signal intensities from the extension of two allele-specific primers hybridized on the ssDNA templates. Further study showed that the products of SPA on gel pads can be reused after removing the extended strands by

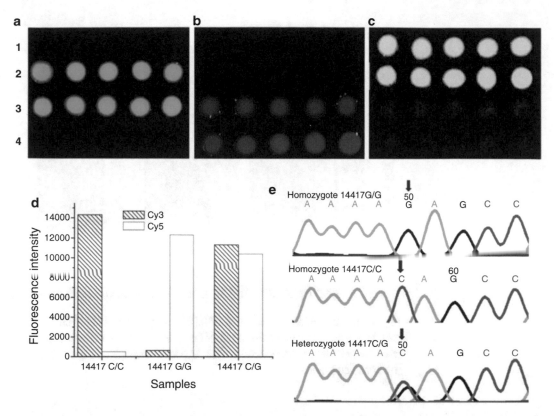

Fig. 4 Hybridization results of samples with three genotypes at 14417 locus in the OLR-1 gene. (**a**) Homozygote 14417 C/C. *Rows 2* and *3*: acrylamide-modified primers, and *rows 1* and *4*: controls (gel without immobilized primers); (**b**) homozygote 14417 G/G. *Rows 3* and *4*: acrylamide-modified primers, and *rows 1* and *2*: controls; (**c**) heterozygote 14417C/G. *Rows 1* and *2*: acrylamide-modified primers, and *rows 3* and *4*: controls; (**d**) plot of the relative fluorescence intensities of three typical samples; (**e**) sequencing results of the samples with Sanger's method. The *arrows* indicate the tested SNP locus

electrophoresis. As shown in Fig. 5, the same gel pad was detected three times, and we did not find an obvious decrease of signal intensities from the used pads; therefore, the same SPA products immobilized on a gel pad can be used for multiple purposes, such as the typing of other SNPs, or pyrosequencing. Figure 6a–c shows the SNP typing results of gel-based SPA products by BAMPER. For the homozygotes 14417C/C and 14417G/G, photoemission profiles from matched primers were at least ten times higher than those from mismatched primers (Fig. 6a, b); for the heterozygote 14417C/G, two approximate photoemission profiles were obtained from both the primers (Fig. 6c). Therefore genotypes can be accurately detected only by comparing the pair of real-time photoemission profiles.

4.6 Sequencing of SPA Products by Pyrosequencing

Pyrosequencing is a sequence-by-synthesis technology, and needs ssDNA as a template for the extension reaction. As it is easy to prepare ssDNA from SPA products, we tried to adapt pyrosequencing to gel-based SPA. After the annealing of a pyrosequencing

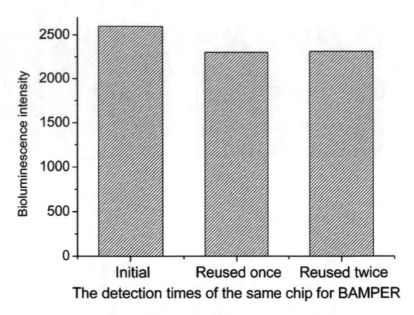

Fig. 5 The light emission profiles of BAMPER for typing the 14417C/C homozy-gote by reusing the same gel-chip at different times. Before reusing the chip for BAMPER detection, electrophoresis was used to remove the extended ssDNA and the annealed primers

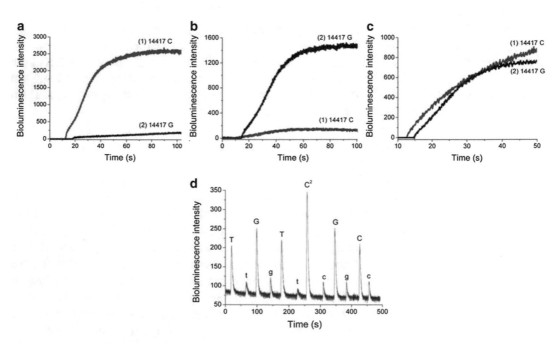

Fig. 6 Application of gel-based SPA products for BAMPER (**a–c**) and pyrosequencing (**d**). Light emission profiles of BAMPER for genotyping homozygote 14417C/C (**a**), homozygote 14417G/G (**b**), and heterozygote 14417C/G (**C**). (**d**) Pyrogram of the gel-based SPA products by pyrosequencing. Each dNTP was dispensed twice for detecting the background due to PPi impurity in the dNTP solution

primer to ssDNA immobilized on the gel, the sequence of the sample can be obtained by the individual addition of dATPαS, dCTP, dTTP, and dGTP into the gel pads where components required for the pyrosequencing reaction are added in advance. As shown in Fig. 6d, we have successfully detected the sequence of SPA products by pyrosequencing, demonstrating that gel-based SPA products are a suitable template for pyrosequencing.

5   Technical Notes

1. As SPA needs a stringent temperature variation for denaturing, annealing, and extension steps, the linkage between the 5′-terminal of a primer and a solid-phase support should be strong.

2. The thermal stability of acrylamide-modified oligonucleotides is the most suitable for SPA.

3. In BAMPER, the 3′-terminals of two allele-specific primers are at the SNP locus for controlling the extension reaction. Detection sensitivity of BAMPER is much higher due to the extension of many bases at a time, and specificity is greatly improved by introducing an artificially mismatched base into the third position upstream from the 3′-terminal of allele-specific primers [17–18].

References

1. Goossens D, Moens LN, Nelis E, Lenaerts AS, Glassee W, Kalbe A, Frey B, Kopal G, De Jonghe P, De Rijk P, Del-Favero J (2009) Simultaneous mutation and copy number variation (CNV) detection by multiplex PCR-based GS-FLX sequencing. Hum Mutat 30:472–476

2. Elenis DS, Ioannou PC, Christopoulos TK (2009) Quadruple-allele chemiluminometric assay for simultaneous genotyping of two single-nucleotide polymorphisms. Analyst 134:725–730

3. Hosono N, Kubo M, Tsuchiya Y, Sato H, Kitamoto T, Saito S, Ohnishi Y, Nakamura Y (2008) Multiplex PCR-based real-time invader assay (mPCR-RETINA): a novel SNP-based method for detecting allelic asymmetries within copy number variation regions. Hum Mutat 29:182–189

4. Hashimoto M, Barany F, Xu F, Soper SA (2007) Serial processing of biological reactions using flow-through microfluidic devices: coupled PCR/LDR for the detection of low-abundant DNA point mutations. Analyst 132:913–921

5. Adessi C, Matton G, Ayala G, Turcatti G, Mermod JJ, Mayer P, Kawashima E (2000) Solid phase DNA amplification: characterisation of primer attachment and amplification mechanisms. Nucleic Acids Res 28:E87

6. Mitra RD, Church GM (1999) In situ localized amplification and contact replication of many individual DNA molecules. Nucleic Acids Res 27:e34

7. Mitterer G, Huber M, Leidinger E, Kirisits C, Lubitz W, Mueller MW, Schmidt WM (2004) Microarray-based identification of bacteria in clinical samples by solid-phase PCR amplification of 23S ribosomal DNA sequences. J Clin Microbiol 42:1048–1057

8. Shapero MH, Leuther KK, Nguyen A, Scott M, Jones KW (2001) SNP genotyping by multiplexed solid-phase amplification and fluorescent minisequencing. Genome Res 11:1926–1934

9. Turner MS, Penning S, Sharp A, Hyland VJ, Harris R, Morris CP, van Daal A (2001) Solid-phase amplification for detection of C282y and H63D hemochromatosis (HFE) gene mutations. Clin Chem 47:1384–1389

10. Oroskar AA, Rasmussen SE, Rasmussen HN, Rasmussen SR, Sullivan BM, Johansson A (1996) Detection of immobilized amplicons by ELISA-like techniques. Clin Chem 42:1547–1555

11. Strizhkov BN, Drobyshev AL, Mikhailovich VM, Mirzabekov AD (2000) PCR amplification on a microarray of gel-immobilized oligonucleotides: detection of bacterial toxin- and drug-resistant genes and their mutations. BioTechniques 29: 844-848, 850-852, 854 passim

12. Rubina AY, Pan'kov SV, Dementieva EI, Pen'kov DN, Butygin AV, Vasiliskov VA, Chudinov AV, Mikheikin AL, Mikhailovich VM, Mirzabekov AD (2004) Hydrogel drop microchips with immobilized DNA: properties and methods for large-scale production. Anal Biochem 325:92–106

13. Rehman FN, Audeh M, Abrams ES, Hammond PW, Kenney M, Boles TC (1999) Immobilization of acrylamide-modified oligonucleotides by co-polymerization. Nucleic Acids Res 27:649–655

14. Xiao PF, Cheng L, Wan Y, Sun BL, Chen ZZ, Zhang SY, Zhang CZ, Zhou GH, Lu ZH (2006) An improved gel-based DNA microarray method for detecting single nucleotide mismatch. Electrophoresis 27:3904–3915

15. Xiao P, Huang H, Zhou G, Lu Z (2007) Gel immobilization of acrylamide-modified single-stranded DNA template for pyrosequencing. Electrophoresis 28:1903–1912

16. Zhou GH, Shirakura H, Kamahori M, Okano K, Nagai K, Kambara H (2004) A gel-free SNP genotyping method: bioluminometric assay coupled with modified primer extension reactions (BAMPER) directly from double-stranded PCR products. Hum Mutat 24:155–163

17. Huang H, Wu H, Xiao P, Zhou G (2009) Single-nucleotide polymorphism typing based on pyrosequencing chemistry and acryl-modified glass chip. Electrophoresis 30:991–998

18. Leamon JH, Lee WL, Tartaro KR, Lanza JR, Sarkis GJ, deWinter AD, Berka J, Weiner M, Rothberg JM, Lohman KL (2003) A massively parallel PicoTiterPlate based platform for discrete picoliter-scale polymerase chain reactions. Electrophoresis 24:3769–3777

Part VI

Clinical Practice

Chapter 26

Prenatal Diagnosis of Trisomy 21 by Quantitatively Pyrosequencing Heterozygotes Using Amniotic Fluid as Starting Material of PCR

Hui Ye, Haiping Wu, Huan Huang, Yunlong Liu, Bingjie Zou, Qinxin Song, and Guohua Zhou

Abstract

Allelic ratio of an SNP has been used for prenatal diagnosis of fetal trisomy 21 by MALDI-TOF mass spectrometry (MS). Because MALDI-TOF MS is challenging in quantification performance, pyrosequencing was proposed to replace MS for better quantification of allelic ratios. To achieve a simple and a rapid clinical diagnosis, PCR with a high-pH buffer (HpH buffer) was developed to directly amplify amniotic fluid without any step of genomic DNA extraction. By the established assay, 114 samples of amniotic fluid were directly amplified and individually analyzed by the pyrosequencing of five SNPs of each sample; the allelic ratios of euploid heterozygotes were thus calculated to determine the cutoff values of prenatal diagnosis of trisomy 21. The panel of five SNPs is much high in heterozygosity, and at least one heterozygote was found in each of the 114 samples, and 86 % of the samples have at least two heterozygotes in the panel, giving a nearly 100 % sensitivity of the assay. By using the cutoff values of each SNP, 20 pre-diagnosed clinical samples were detected as trisomy 21 carriers with the confidence level over 99 %, indicating that our method and karyotyping analysis are consistent in results. In conclusion, this pyrosequencing-based approach, coupled with the direct amplification of amniotic fluid, is accurate in quantitative genotyping and is simple in operation. We believe that the approach could be a promising alternative to karyotyping analysis in prenatal diagnosis.

Key words Pyrosequencing, Amniotic fluid, Heterozygote, Trisomy 21, SNP

1 Introduction

One of the major contents of prenatal diagnosis is to detect fetal chromosomal aneuploidies. Currently, karyotyping is the preferred test method for fetal trisomy; however, it involves lengthy procedures for culturing amniotic fluid and chorionic villus cells before analysis, increasing parental stress during the wait for a culture result. With a PCR-based method, a rapid prenatal diagnosis can be achieved by using a small amount of specimens as a detection target [1–3].

Guohua Zhou and Qinxin Song (eds.), *Advances and Clinical Practice in Pyrosequencing*, Springer Protocols Handbooks, DOI 10.1007/978-1-4939-3308-2_26, © Springer Science+Business Media New York 2016

As a normal fetus is different from a trisomy 21 fetus in genomic copy number of chromosome 21, a method enabling the prenatal diagnosis should be able to quantify the copy number of chromosomes. Since each chromosome is from a parent, paired chromosomes should have many polymorphisms; thus, the allelic ratio of a euploid heterozygote should be 1:1, while the allelic ratio will be 2:1 or 1:2 for a trisomy 21 fetus. Consequently, a heterozygous SNP on chromosome 21 can be a diagnostic biomarker of a trisomy 21 patient. Quantitative detection of allelic ratios was thus proposed by Lo's research group [4, 5]. The detection was based on a single base-extension assay coupled with MALDI-TOF mass spectrometry (MS), and the quantification was achieved by calculating the relative yield of each allele peak in an MS tracing of an SNP [6–8]. However, it was found that the data from MALDI-TOF MS was not so quantitative [7]. Although the quantitative performance of MALDI-TOF MS was improved by using the peak height ratio in MS tracings [9], unlike ESI-MS, MALDI-TOF MS is still challenging in quantification. In addition, a mass spectrometer used for the assay should be specific to the determination of DNA molecules; for the moment, only iPLEX Gold MALDI-TOF MS system is available in the market, limiting the wide application of this strategy to the clinical screening of Down's syndrome.

Pyrosequencing is a sequencing-by-synthesis method which is based on the bioluminometric detection of inorganic pyrophosphate (PPi) coupled with multiple enzymatic reactions. In a pyrogram, the relative intensity of each peak is proportional to the number of incorporated nucleotides. As only one base species is extended at a time, the intensity of each peak is proportional to the template amounts incorporated with the dispensed dNTP; hence, two peaks with the equal height should appear in a pyrogram for an SNP if no homogenous region is adjacent to the SNP. Consequently, two peaks with the ratio of 1:2 or 2:1 would be observed for a trisomy 21 fetus when the SNP of interest is located on chromosome 21.

Like most molecule diagnostic methods, pyrosequencing still requires a PCR step to supply enough templates for sequencing [10–12]. Conventionally, a purification process is necessary to extract target DNAs from biological samples before amplification. However, DNA extraction is costly and laborious and most importantly increases the risk of cross-contamination; hence, it is preferred to develop an amplification method directly using raw samples (e.g., blood or amniotic fluid). Although amnio-PCR has been successfully developed for amplifying small tandem repeat markers on chromosome 21 from uncultured amniotic fluid, pretreatment steps involving cell lysis and pH adjustment are still required before amplification [13, 14]. To avoid complex pretreatment, a novel "HpH buffer"-based PCR, which was previously developed to directly amplify target DNA from whole blood, was proposed for replacing amnio-PCR. It was found that amniotic fluid could be used as starting material of "HpH buffer"-based PCR. Based on the simplified amplification, prenatal diagnosis of trisomy 21 was successfully achieved by calculating the peak height ratio of two alleles.

2   Materials

1. *Taq* polymerase was purchased from TaKaRa (Dalian, China).

2. Bovine serum albumin (BSA), D-luciferin and adenosine 5′-phosphosulfate (APS), and apyrase VII were obtained from Sigma (St. Louis, MO).

3. ATP sulfurylase and *exo–* Klenow fragment were obtained by gene engineering in our lab.

4. Polyvinylpyrrolidone (PVP) and QuantiLum recombinant luciferase were purchased from Promega (Madison, WI).

5. 2′-Deoxyadenosine-5′-O-(1-thiotriphosphate) sodium salt (dATPαS), dGTP, dTTP, and dCTP were purchased from Mychem (San Diego, CA).

6. Streptavidin sepharose beads was from GE Healthcare (Piscataway, NJ).

7. PCR primers were designed by PyroMark Assay 2.0 and synthesized by Invitrogen Inc., Shanghai, China.

3   Methods

3.1 Sample Collection and Processing

1. A set of 114 samples was collected from patients who came for an amniocentesis after the combination test indicated high risk for Down's syndrome. Samples were obtained with informed consent and approval of the Ethics Committee.

2. One milliliter of amniotic fluid was centrifuged at $10,000 \times g$ for 10 min (*see* **Note 1**). Remove the supernatant and mix the remainder evenly. The concentrated amniotic fluid was moved to a 200-µL tube and heated at 94 °C for 15 min. Three microliter of the treated amniotic fluid (*see* **Note 2**) was used in a 50-µL reaction.

3.2 SNP Selection and Genotyping

The SNP information of chromosome 21 was obtained from NCBI database. In this study, we selected six SNP loci with a reported high heterozygosity in Chinese population: rs464783, rs767055, rs914195, rs914232, rs2254522, and rs243609. We also used another panel of six SNPs previously reported by our group: rs1053315, rs818219, rs2839110, rs1042917, rs35548026, and rs8130833 [15](*see* **Note 3**).

3.3 PCR Amplification

1. A 50-µL reaction contained 5.35 µL of "HpH buffer" (*see* **Note 4**); 200 µmol/L each of dATP, dCTP, dGTP, and dTTP; 0.4 µmol/L of each primer; and 2.5 U of *Taq* polymerase.

2. We initiated the reaction at 94 °C for 5 min, followed by 35 cycles of 94 °C for 30 s, 72 °C for 30 s, 55–60 °C for 30 s, and a final extension at 72 °C for 7 min.

3.4 Single-Stranded DNA (ssDNA) Preparation

1. Streptavidin-coated sepharose beads were used to capture biotinylated PCR products. After sedimentation and washing steps, purified double-stranded DNA was denatured by alkali to yield ssDNA.

2. The immobilized biotinylated strand was then annealed with a sequencing primer under the condition of 80 °C for 5 min and 25 °C for 10 min before used as a sequencing template.

3.5 Pyrosequencing Reaction

1. A 100 µL of pyrosequencing mixture contained 0.1 M Tris–HAc (pH 7.7), 2 mM EDTA, 10 mM $Mg(Ac)_2$, 0.1 % BSA, 1 mM DTT, 2 µmol/L APS, 0.4 g/L PVP, 0.4 mM D-luciferin, 2 µmol/L ATP sulfurylase, 1.6 U/mL apyrase VII, 18 U/mL *exo*–Klenow fragment, and an appropriate amount of luciferase.

2. Pyrosequencing was performed in a portable bioluminescence analyzer (Hitachi, Ltd., Japan) as we previously described [16, 17].

4 Method Validation

4.1 Investigation of "HpH Buffer" for PCR

An approach that amplified DNA directly from whole blood was developed by using "HpH buffer" [18]. To investigate whether or not this buffer could be used to amplify DNA from amniotic fluid directly, PCR with conventional PCR buffer (Fig. 1, lane 1) and HpH buffer (Fig. 1, lane 2) were individually performed using amniotic fluid as starting material. As shown in Fig. 1, the amount of amplicons from "HpH buffer" (lane 2) is much larger than that from conventional PCR buffer (lane 1), indicating that the PCR suppression from components in amniotic fluid was greatly blocked by "HpH buffer." Although the amount of amplicons in lane 1 could be used for pyrosequencing, the intensity of peaks in a pyrogram was low. A higher peak intensity is preferred for better quantification performance; hence, it is better to concentrate amniotic fluid by centrifugation so as to improve PCR yield by increasing the initial template amount. After centrifugation at $10,000 \times g$ for 10 min, 90 % of supernatant was removed, and the remaining was used for PCR. As shown in Fig. 1 (lane 3), the amount of

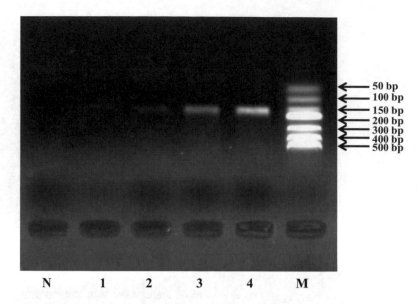

Fig. 1 Gel electropherograms of amplicons using conventional PCR buffer (*lane 1*) and "HpH buffer" (*lanes 2–4*) *lane N*: Blank control; *lane 1*: PCR with conventional PCR buffer by using raw amniotic fluid; *lane 2*: PCR with "HpH buffer" by using raw amniotic fluid; *lane 3*: PCR with "HpH buffer" by using concentrated amniotic fluid; *lane 4*: PCR with "HpH buffer" by using concentrated and preheated amniotic fluid; *lane M*: DNA markers

amplicons was significantly increased, indicating that centrifugation could efficiently increase the amount of initial genomic DNA for PCR. Conventionally a process that lyses cells at a higher temperature could increase the amount of PCR templates. Lane 4 in Fig. 1 further indicated that the PCR yield was remarkably increased after a preheating step in addition to the centrifugation of amniotic fluid. Therefore, "HpH buffer" could be used for efficiently amplifying target DNA sequence from amniotic fluid directly.

4.2 Investigation of the Effect of Template Amounts on PCR Yield

As the concentration of fetus cells varies greatly among different amniotic fluid samples, it is necessary to investigate the effect of template amounts on PCR yields. As shown in Fig. 2, the amount of amplicons that was sufficient for pyrosequencing could be obtained from the amplification of different volumes (ranging from 0.5 to 5 µL) of tenfold concentrated amniotic fluid. To get a reproducible result, a higher volume is preferred; thus, 3 µL of concentrated amniotic fluid in a 50-µL PCR reaction was used routinely. This means that a PCR assay needs 30 µL of raw amniotic fluid. If a triple detection is performed, around 0.1 mL of raw amniotic fluid will be required for an SNP assay; hence, 1 mL of raw amniotic fluid is enough for an assay with a panel of ten SNPs. Usually, 10 mL of raw amniotic fluid is needed for karyotyping. Therefore, our method requires only one-tenth of the amount of raw amniotic fluid in a karyotyping assay.

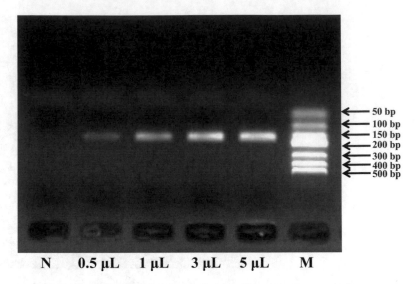

50 bp
100 bp
150 bp
200 bp
300 bp
400 bp
500 bp

N   0.5 μL   1 μL   3 μL   5 μL   M

Fig. 2 Gel electropherograms of amplicons using different template amounts. *Lane N*: Blank control; *lane M*: DNA markers

4.3 Selection of SNP Markers for Prenatal Diagnosis of Trisomy 21

As the proposed method is based on the allelic ratio of an SNP in a pyrogram, the heterozygosity of an SNP should be high in the population. At first, we selected six SNPs from the NCBI database with a heterozygosity over 40 % in the Chinese population and a panel of six SNPs from reported information with a population coverage of 92.9 % in Chinese. After 20 individual blood samples were genotyped by pyrosequencing, five SNPs with the highest heterozygosity were selected out of 12 SNPs for further study. Before being used as markers for prenatal diagnosis of trisomy 21, this panel of five SNPs was typed for 114 samples of amniotic fluid by using "HpH buffer"-based PCR and pyrosequencing. As shown in Table 1, the heterozygosities were between 0.421 and 0.589. In these 114 samples, it was found that at least one heterozygote appeared in each sample, and 86 % of samples had at least two heterozygotes, giving a 100 % heterozygote coverage; thus, the selected panel of SNPs can be a marker for prenatal diagnosis of trisomy 21. Although the allele frequency of SNP 4 is the lowest one in the five according to Table 2, the sensitivity (population coverage) will be decreased without SNP 4. For example, 99.1 % (113/114) of samples were covered by at least one heterozygote without SNP 4 in the panel. In addition, the number of samples with at least two heterozygotes decreased from 98 to 83 without the use of SNP 4. Therefore, SNP 4 should be included in the panel.

4.4 Cutoff Values of Allelic Ratios for Prenatal Diagnosis of Trisomy 21

In a pyrogram, the allelic ratio of an SNP should be close to 1 if no homogenous sequence exists around the SNP locus. However, this ratio may fluctuate with a target sequence; it is not a problem for SNP typing, but it may be problematic for the accurate

Table 1

Allele frequency of the five SNPs from 114 samples

SNP	Allele	Genotype frequency	Allele frequency	Heterozygosity
SNP 1	T/C	TT: 0.351 C/T: 0.526 CC: 0.123	T: 0.614 C: 0.386	0.526
SNP 2	T/C	TT: 0.333 C/T: 0.518 CC: 0.149	T: 0.592 C: 0.408	0.518
SNP 3	T/C	TT: 0.219 C/T: 0.588 CC: 0.193	T: 0.513 C: 0.487	0.589
SNP 4	G/A	GG: 0.421 G/A: 0.421 AA: 0.158	G: 0.632 A: 0.368	0.421
SNP 5	A/G	AA: 0.377 G/A: 0.448 GG: 0.175	A: 0.601 G: 0.399	0.447

Table 2

Cutoff values of each SNP assay in euploid heterozygous samples

SNP	Expected allelic ratio	Observed allelic ratio (mean value ± SD, n^a)	Cutoff values (mean value ± 1.96 SD)
SNP 1	1 (T:C)	1.06 ± 0.09, 50	0.88 ≤ cutoff value ≤ 1.23
SNP 2	3 (C:T)	2.91 ± 0.19, 43	2.54 ≤ cutoff value ≤ 3.28
SNP 3	3 (T:C)	2.98 ± 0.18, 53	2.63 ≤ cutoff value ≤ 3.33
SNP 4	1 (G:A)	0.86 ± 0.11, 42	0.64 ≤ cutoff value ≤ 1.08
SNP 5	1 (G:A)	0.82 ± 0.06, 36	0.70 ≤ cutoff value ≤ 0.94

[a]n is the number of heterozygotes in 94 samples

determination of an allelic ratio, particularly for an SNP close to a homogenous region. In the selected five SNPs, the expected allelic ratios are 1, 3, 3, 1, and 1 for SNP 1, SNP 2, SNP 3, SNP 4, and SNP 5, respectively. To investigate whether the observed values of each allelic ratio were close to the expected values, the five SNPs in 94 euploid samples were detected by pyrosequencing, and the corresponding allelic ratio of every heterozygote was calculated for each SNP. As a small amount of PPi (due to the decomposition of dNTPs) may exist in dNTPs, each dNTP was dispensed twice, and a peak height was then calculated by subtracting the noise at the second dNTP dispensation from the signal at the first dNTP dispensation. The allelic ratio was the height ratio of two allele-specific peaks in a pyrogram. As shown in Table 2, the average observed allelic ratios of each SNP were 1.06, 2.91, 2.98, 0.86, and 0.82 for SNP 1, SNP 2, SNP 3, SNP 4, and SNP 5, respectively. As described in Ref. [7], the cutoff value of each SNP was calculated as the mean heterozygote allelic ratio $\pm [1.96 \times SD]$. The intervals of cutoff value were [0.88, 1.23], [2.54, 3.28], [2.63, 3.33], [0.64, 1.08], and [0.70, 0.94], respectively, and it was found that 95.5 % of detected allelic ratios fell within these intervals. Therefore, it is possible to employ these cutoff values for the discrimination of trisomy 21 fetus.

4.5 Genotyping Trisomy 21 Samples

With the cutoff values of each SNP, 20 samples, which were diagnosed as trisomy 21 carriers, were detected by pyrosequencing. The typical pyrograms of the five SNP loci for a euploid heterozygote and two types of trisomic heterozygotes are shown in Fig. 3. It was found that at least two heterozygotes were detected for each trisomic sample. The detected allelic ratios of all heterozygotes for 20 samples were out of the cutoff value intervals in Fig. 4, indicating that these samples were significantly different from euploidies. To further investigate the confidence level of detected results, Z-scores were employed and calculated by the formula of "Z-score = (the detected allelic ratio of a sample – the mean allelic ratio of euploid heterozygotes)/SD of the mean allelic ratio of heterozygotes." The larger the Z-score is, the higher the degree of confidence level is. Further study showed that the low Z-score of sample no. 20 was due to its low signal intensity in the pyrogram, and this was overcome by increasing the template amount of pyrosequencing. Conventionally, there was more than one heterozygote in a sample; therefore, the accuracy of trisomy 21 discrimination would not be affected if the Z-score of only one heterozygote was not desirably high. The coherence between karyotyping analysis and our proposed method indicated that our method could be a promising alternative to karyotyping analysis in prenatal diagnosis.

5 Technical Notes

1. Conventionally, a process that lyses cells at a higher temperature could increase the amount of PCR templates [19, 20]. Our result obtained from real-time PCR showed that preheating at 94 °C for 15 min gave a 100-fold increase of starting template amount.

2. To get a reproducible result, a higher volume is preferred; thus, 3 μL of concentrated amniotic fluid in a 50 μL PCR reaction was used routinely. This means that a PCR assay needs 30 μL of raw amniotic fluid. If a triple detection is performed,

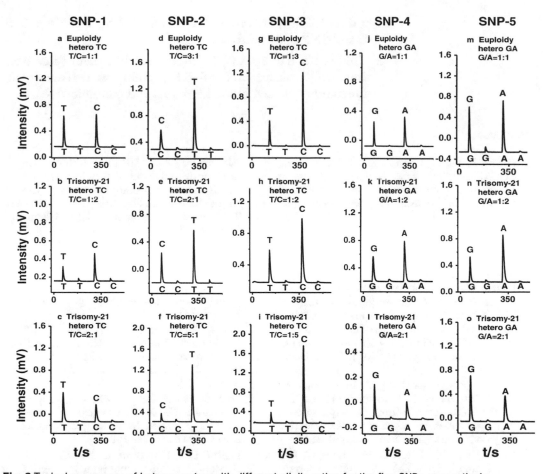

Fig. 3 Typical pyrograms of heterozygotes with different allelic ratios for the five SNPs, respectively

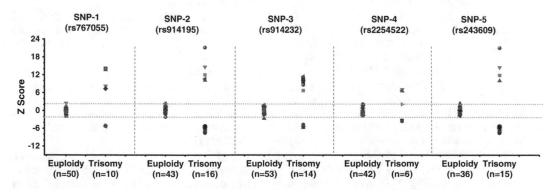

Fig. 4 Distribution of Z-scores for the five SNPs. The *gray dash lines* indicate that the Z-score is 1.96 or −1.96, which refer to the cutoff values of allelic ratios for each SNP

around 0.1 mL of raw amniotic fluid will be required for an SNP assay.

3. PCR primers were designed by PyroMark Assay 2.0 and synthesized by Invitrogen Inc., Shanghai. To simplify the name of each selected SNP, rs767055, rs914195, rs914232, rs2254522,

and rs243609 were referred to as SNP 1, SNP 2, SNP 3, SNP 4, and SNP 5, respectively.

4. HpH buffer had a pH (9.1–9.6) higher than that of a conventional PCR buffer (pH 8.5–8.8), aiming at weakening the interaction between blood inhibitors and genomic DNA.

References

1. Zhang Y, Liu H, Chen X, Xie X, Liu S, Wang H (2012) Noninvasive prenatal diagnosis of Down syndrome in samples from Southwest Chinese gravidas using pregnant plasma placental RNA allelic ratio. Genet Test Mol Biomarkers 16:1051–1057

2. Dutta UR, Pidugu VK, Goud VA, Dalal AB (2012) Mosaic Down syndrome with a marker: molecular cytogenetic characterization of the marker chromosome. Gene 495:199–204

3. Ghosh D, Sinha S, Chatterjee A, Nandagopal K (2012) Discerning non-disjunction in Down syndrome patients by means of GluK1-(AGAT)(n) and D21S2055-(GATA)(n) microsatellites on chromosome 21. Indian J Hum Genet 18:204–216

4. Tsui NB, Chiu RW, Ding C, El-Sheikhah A, Leung TN, Lau TK, Nicolaides KH, Lo YM (2005) Detection of trisomy 21 by quantitative mass spectrometric analysis of single-nucleotide polymorphisms. Clin Chem 51:2358–2362

5. Chow KC, Chiu RW, Tsui NB, Ding C, Lau TK, Leung TN, Lo YM (2007) Mass spectrometric detection of an SNP panel as an internal positive control for fetal DNA analysis in maternal plasma. Clin Chem 53:141–142

6. Huang DJ, Nelson MR, Zimmermann B, Dudarewicz L, Wenzel L, Spiegel R, Nagy B, Holzgreve W, Hahn S (2006) Reliable detection of trisomy 21 using MALDI-TOF mass spectrometry. Genet Med 8:728–734

7. Lo YM, Tsui NB, Chiu RW, Lau TK, Leung TN, Heung MM, Gerovassili A, Jin Y, Nicolaides KH, Cantor CR, Ding C (2007) Plasma placental RNA allelic ratio permits noninvasive prenatal chromosomal aneuploidy detection. Nat Med 13:218–223

8. Tsui NB, Wong BC, Leung TY, Lau TK, Chiu RW, Lo YM (2009) Non-invasive prenatal detection of fetal trisomy 18 by RNA-SNP allelic ratio analysis using maternal plasma SERPINB2 mRNA: a feasibility study. Prenat Diagn 29:1031–1037

9. Trewick AL, Moustafa JS, de Smith AJ, Froguel P, Greve G, Njolstad PR, Coin LJ, Blakemore AI (2011) Accurate single-nucleotide polymorphism allele assignment in trisomic or duplicated regions by using a single base-extension assay with MALDI-TOF mass spectrometry. Clin Chem 57:1188–1195

10. Zhang X, Wu H, Chen Z, Zhou G, Kajiyama T, Kambara H (2009) Dye-free gene expression detection by sequence-tagged reverse-transcription polymerase chain reaction coupled with pyrosequencing. Anal Chem 81:273–281

11. Huang H, Wu H, Xiao P, Zhou G (2009) Single-nucleotide polymorphism typing based on pyrosequencing chemistry and acryl-modified glass chip. Electrophoresis 30:991–998

12. Song Q, Wu H, Feng F, Zhou G, Kajiyama T, Kambara H (2010) Pyrosequencing on nicked dsDNA generated by nicking endonucleases. Anal Chem 82:2074–2081

13. Ogilvie CM, Donaghue C, Fox SP, Docherty Z, Mann K (2005) Rapid prenatal diagnosis of aneuploidy using quantitative fluorescence-PCR (QF-PCR). J Histochem Cytochem 53:285–288

14. Levett LJ, Liddle S, Meredith R (2001) A large-scale evaluation of amnio-PCR for the rapid prenatal diagnosis of fetal trisomy. Ultrasound Obstet Gynecol 17:115–118

15. Liu XQ, Wu HP, Bu Y, Zou BJ, Chen ZY, Zhou GH (2009) Quantitative pyrosequencing of heterozygous single nucleotide polymorphisms for rapid diagnosis of Down's syndrome. Zhonghua Yi Xue Yi Chuan Xue Za Zhi 26:331–335

16. Wu H, Wu W, Chen Z, Wang Z, Zhou G, Kajiyama T, Kambara H (2011) Highly sensitive pyrosequencing based on the capture of free adenosine 5′ phosphosulfate with adenosine triphosphate sulfurylase. Anal Chem 83:3600–3605

17. Chen Z, Fu X, Zhang X, Liu X, Zou B, Wu H, Song Q, Li J, Kajiyama T, Kambara H, Zhou G (2012) Pyrosequencing-based barcodes for a

dye-free multiplex bioassay. Chem Commun (Camb) 48:2445–2447

18. Bu Y, Huang H, Zhou G (2008) Direct polymerase chain reaction (PCR) from human whole blood and filter-paper-dried blood by using a PCR buffer with a higher pH. Anal Biochem 375:370–372

19. Heung MM, Jin S, Tsui NB, Ding C, Leung TY, Lau TK, Chiu RW, Lo YM (2009) Placenta-derived fetal specific mRNA is more readily detectable in maternal plasma than in whole blood. PLoS One 4, e5858

20. Deng YH, Yin AH, He Q, Chen JC, He YS, Wang HQ, Li M, Chen HY (2011) Non-invasive prenatal diagnosis of trisomy 21 by reverse transcriptase multiplex ligation-dependent probe amplification. Clin Chem Lab Med 49:641–646

Chapter 27

Comparative Gene Expression Analysis of Breast Cancer-Related Genes by Multiplex Pyrosequencing Coupled with Sequence Barcodes

Qinxin Song, Hua Jing, Haiping Wu, Bingjie Zou, Guohua Zhou, and Hideki Kambara

Abstract

Most methods used for gene expression analysis are based on dye labeling, which requires costly instruments. Recently, a dye-free gene expression analysis method-SRPP (sequence-tagged reverse-transcription polymerase chain reaction coupled with pyrosequencing) was developed to compare relative gene expression levels in different tissues, but the throughput of the SRPP assay is very limited due to the use of a photomultiplier tube (PMT)-based pyrosequencer for the detection. To increase the throughput of the SRPP assay, an inexpensive photodiode (PD) array-based bioluminescence analyzer (termed as "PD-based pyrosequencer") was coupled to SRPP; however, the low sensitivity of PD limited the wide application of SRPP. To enable SRPP analyzing low abundance genes in clinical samples, sequence-tagged gene-specific primers instead of sequence-tagged poly $(T)_n$ primers were used for reverse transcription, and the SRPP sensitivity was thus improved more than ten times. This improvement compensates the sensitivity loss due to the use of PD in a pyrosequencer. The accurate determination of the expression levels of ten prognostic marker genes (AL080059, MMP9, EXT1, ORC6L, AF052162, C9orf30, FBXO31, IGFBP5, ESM1, and RUNDC1) differing between normal tissues and tumor tissues of breast cancer patients demonstrated that SRPP using gene-specific RT primers coupled with the PD array-based bioluminescence analyzer is reliable, inexpensive, and sensitive in gene expression analysis.

Key words Gene expression profiling, Breast cancer, Prognostic diagnosis, SRPP, Pyrosequencing, Portable bioluminescence analyzer

1 Introduction

Clinical studies have shown that the expression levels of some genes are closely related to the carcinogenesis, progress, and prognosis of various cancers [1]; thus, the comparative detection of these genes in normal tissue and tumor tissue can help doctors to make clinical decisions. Up to now, various techniques were developed for quantifying gene expression levels [2]. The most popular methods used now are DNA microarrays and real-time PCR.

Guohua Zhou and Qinxin Song (eds.), *Advances and Clinical Practice in Pyrosequencing*, Springer Protocols Handbooks, DOI 10.1007/978-1-4939-3308-2_27, © Springer Science+Business Media New York 2016

Although microarrays are regularly used for gene expression profiling on a large scale, problems appear when the detected genes are expressed at low levels [3].

Real-time PCR is highly sensitive and quantitative, but TaqMan probes are expensive, and standard curve construction is labor intensive [4]. Recently, we have developed a sensitive and inexpensive method, SRPP (sequence-tagged reverse-transcription PCR coupled with pyrosequencing) [5], to quantitatively detect gene expression levels. In comparison to real-time PCR, this assay does not require any dye labeling and standard curve preparation [5]. There are three main steps in SRPP: reverse transcription of mRNA with RT primers that contain a source-specific sequence in the middle, PCR of the templates produced by pooling equal amounts of sequence-labeled cDNAs from different sources, and quantitative decoding of the source-specific sequence tags in the amplicons by pyrosequencing. The signal is obtained by observing bioluminescence, and differential gene expression detection is achieved by the comparison of the signal intensities between peaks in a pyrogram. The pyrogram's sequence represents the gene source, and peak intensities represent the relative expression levels in corresponding sources. The gene expression analysis has been realized on a homemade pyrosequencer based on photomultiplier tube (PMT). However, it is difficult to scale up the sensor number due to the size of PMT. Recently, we developed an inexpensive bioluminescence analyzer by using a photodiode (PD) array; pyrosequencing with this instrument was successfully performed [6]. However, the PD-based pyrosequencer is less sensitive than PMT, and this causes a difficulty of SRPP in analyzing low abundance genes. To increase SRPP sensitivity, we employed a sequence-tagged gene-specific primer for reverse transcription [7, 8], and the flowchart of the improved SRPP is showed in Fig. 1. This improvement compensates the sensitivity loss due to the use of PD in a pyrosequencer. The accurate determination of the expression levels of ten breast cancer-related genes by the improved SRPP was successfully demonstrated.

2 Materials

1. HotStarTaq DNA polymerase (Qiagen GmbH, Hilden, Germany).

2. SuperScript II Reverse Transcriptase and TRIzol reagent (Invitrogen Inc., Faraday Avenue, Carlsbad, CA).

3. Exo⁻ Klenow fragment, polyvinylpyrrolidone (PPV), and QuantiLum recombinant luciferase (Promega, Madison, WI).

4. Dynabeads M-280 Streptavidin (2.8 μm) (Dynal Biotech ASA, Oslo, Norway).

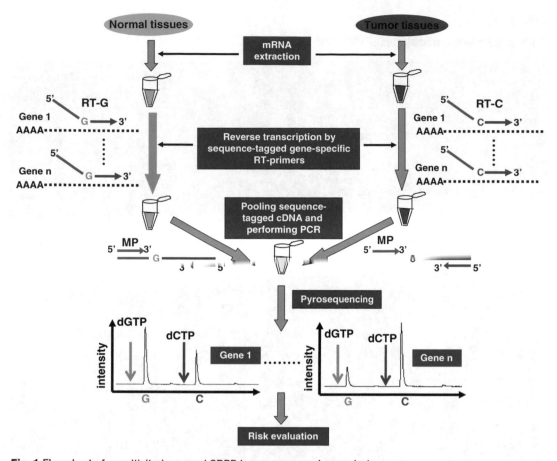

Fig. 1 Flowchart of sensitivity-improved SRPP in gene expression analysis

5. ATP sulfurylase, apyrase, D-luciferin, bovine serum albumin (BSA), and adenosine 5′-phosphosulfate (APS) were obtained from Sigma (St. Louis, MO).

6. 2′-Deoxyadenosine-5′–O–(1-thiotriphosphate) sodium salt (dATP-α-S) was purchased from Amersham Pharmacia Biotech (Amersham, UK).

7. dGTP, dTTP, and dCTP were purchased from Amersham Pharmacia Biotech (Piscataway, NJ).

8. For the evaluation, ten genes (AL080059, MMP9, EXT1, ORC6L, AF052162, C9orf30, FBXO31, IGFBP5, ESM1, and RUNDC1) selected from the prognostic markers of breast cancer used in MammaPrint™ kit were used as examples [1].

9. The sequences of reverse-transcription (RT) primers, gene-specific primers, and a biotinylated common primer (bio-MP) used in SRPP, as well as real-time PCR primers used to evaluate accuracy, are listed in Table 1. All of the oligomers were synthesized and purified by Invitrogen (Shanghai, China).

Table 1

Primers for reverse transcription, SRPP, and real-time PCR

Symbol	Sequence (5′-3′)	Amplicon size (bp)
Universal primers for reverse transcription		
RT-G	CCATCTGTTCCCTCCCTGTC g *atc* tttttttttttttt VN	
RT-C	CCATCTGTTCCCTCCCTGTC c *atg* tttttttttttttt VN	
Gene-specific primers for reverse transcription		
MMP9-G	CCATCTGTTCCCTCCCTGTC g *atc* GCAAGTCTTCCGAGTAGTTT	328
AF052162-G	CCATCTGTTCCCTCCCTGTC g *atc* ACATCCTCATCACCCTCC	306
ESM1-G	CCATCTGTTCCCTCCCTGTC g *atc* CCTGAGACTGTGCGGTAG	244
MMP9-C	CCATCTGTTCCCTCCCTGTC c *atg* GCAAGTCTTCCGAGTAGTTT	328
AF052162-C	CCATCTGTTCCCTCCCTGTC c *atg* ACATCCTCATCACCCTCC	306
ESM1-C	CCATCTGTTCCCTCCCTGTC c *atg* CCTGAGACTGTGCGGTAG	244
Common primer and sequencing primer		
bio-MP	bio-CCATCTGTTCCCTCCCTGTC	
Gene-specific primers for PCR		
AL080059	GTTCTGTGAAAATAACCTCCCC	194
MMP9	GGGCTCCCGTCCTGCTTT	228
EXT1	GCTCCAAACTCACCTCACT	191
ORC6L	AATGGCAGTCCCTTGTCT	183
AF052162	GCCTGCAAATGGCCAATG	197
C9orf30	CTGCACCCTCTGTACCCC	148
FBXO31	CCCGAGCCTCGCTCTAAG	140
IGFBP5	GGCTCCCGTTTAGCATTTTG	211
ESM1	AGTCATCTTCCCTACCCA	235
RUNDC1	TTCATGTCTTAAAATTGCCACC	345
Primers for real-time PCR		
AL080059	Fw:CTGTTCTTCCCTACCTTC Rv:CCTCCCATACTCTATCACT	224
MMP9	Fw:CCTGGAGACCTGAGAACC Rv:GCAAGTCTTCCGAGTAGTTT	304
EXT1	Fw:AGGAAGAAATACCGAGACAT Rv:GGAGCCAGGAGTTGAGTT	205
ORC6L	Fw:CCCCAGCAAAGGAAAT Rv:CCAAAGCCGTCAAGTC	214

(continued)

Table 1
(continued)

Symbol	Sequence (5′-3′)	Amplicon size (bp)
AF052162	Fw:TTTCACTGTAGCCTAAACTCC Rv:ACATCCTCATCACCCTCC	282
C9orf30	Fw:GCCCACGAATACAACTC Rv:TTCTCATCATCGCACAG	305
FBXO31	Fw:GCCGTGAGGAGTATGGT Rv:TGGTCCGTCTGGTTGC	373
IGFBP5	Fw:AGGGATGCTGTCACTCG Rv:TTCGCTATTCCTCTTCGT	241
ESM1	Fw:TGGGAAACATGAAGAGCG Rv:CCTGAGACTGTGCGGTAG	220
RUNDC1	Fw:CACAGACAATGGGCTTTC Rv:TGCTGTAGTTCCTATCCTCC	315

3 Methods

3.1 Targets and Primers

For the evaluation, ten genes (AL080059, MMP9, EXT1, ORC6L, AF052162, C9orf30, FBXO31, IGFBP5, ESM1, and RUNDC1) selected from the prognostic markers of breast cancer used in MammaPrint™ kit were used as examples [1].

3.2 Reverse Transcription

1. Tumor tissues and normal tissues were snap frozen in liquid nitrogen within 1 h after surgery, and total RNA was isolated from the tissues with TRIzol reagent.

2. The purity and concentration of extracted RNA were determined by UV–Vis spectrophotometer (Naka Instruments, Japan).

3. Total RNA was dissolved in RNase-free water to a final concentration of 1 μg μL^{-1}.

4. Total RNA in RNase-free water was heated to 65 °C for 5 min and snap chilled on ice for at least 1 min.

5. A reaction mixture containing 0.5 mM of each dNTP, 1× RT buffer, 1 μM RT primer (see **Note 1**), 0.5 U/μL RNase inhibitor, and 10 U/μL SuperScript II Reverse Transcriptase was added to each tube containing RNA, mixed gently, collected by brief centrifugation, and incubated at 42 °C for 50 min, followed by incubation at 70 °C for 15 min to terminate the reaction.

6. Single-stranded cDNAs from different sources that had been labeled by the sequences tagged in RT primers were diluted 1:10. Aliquots of each source-specific cDNA were pooled and used as PCR templates.

3.3 PCR

1. Each 50 μL PCR mixture contained 1.5 mM MgCl$_2$, 0.2 mM of each dNTP, 0.3 μM of each gene-specific primer (GSP) and the common primer (bio-MP), 1 μL of template pool, and 1.25 units of DNA polymerase (see **Note 3**).

2. Amplification was performed on a PTC-225 thermocycler PCR system (MJ research) according to the following protocol: denatured at 94 °C for 15 min and followed by 35 cycles (94 °C for 40 s; 55 °C for 40 s; 72 °C for 1 min). After the reaction cycle, the product (*see* **Note 2**) was incubated at 72 °C for 10 min and held at 4 °C before us.

3.4 Pyrosequencing

1. Streptavidin-coated Dynabeads were used to prepare ssDNA template for pyrosequencing. Both immobilized biotinylated strands and nonbiotinylated strands were used as sequencing templates.

2. The reaction volume for pyrosequencing was 50 μL, containing 0.1 M Tris–acetate (pH 7.7), 2 mM EDTA, 10 mM magnesium acetate, 0.1 % BSA, 1 mM dithiothreitol (DTT), 2 μM adenosine 5′-phosphosulfate (APS), 0.4 mg mL^{-1} PVP, 0.4 mM D-luciferin, 200 mU/mL ATP sulfurylase, 3 μg mL^{-1} luciferase, 18 U/mL Klenow fragment, and 1.6 U/mL apyrase. Each of dNTPs was added in the reservoir of the micro-dispenser, and pyrosequencing reaction starts when the dispensed dNTP is complementary to the template sequence.

4 Method Validation

4.1 Construction of PD Array-Based Pyrosequencer for SRPP

The key instrument for SRPP is the pyrosequencer, which is used to quantitatively decode the tag sequences in amplicons. As pyrosequencing is based on the real-time monitoring of bioluminescence during a step-by-step primer extension reaction, a sensitive light sensor is necessary to the instrumentation. The possible light sensors which can be employed for sensitive detection are PMT, CCD, and PD for the moment. Unlike PMT, PD sensor is very small (6 W × 2 H × 8 D mm) and can be readily compacted and arrayed. We constructed a prototype of 8-channel pyrosequencer by using a PD array sensor. Figure 2a shows the schematic of the PD array-based pyrosequencer, which includes capillary-based micro-dispensers driven by air pressure, eight reaction chambers, and eight PD species specific to each chamber. To vibrate the chambers after the dispensing of dNTP into the pyrosequencing reaction, a motor used in a mobile phone was employed. As PD is very sensitive to noise (e.g., vibration), an electric shield film that could transmit visible light was used to coat the PD surface for suppressing the noise [6]. By carefully designing PD amplification circuit, the new pyrosequencer is as sensitive as 50 fmol of ssDNA template in a 50-μL pyrosequencing reaction. For an accurate DNA sequencing by the PD-based pyrosequencer, 5 μL of PCR products, which contains 0.1–1 pmol of target DNA, is routinely used in SRPP. Due to the small size of PD as well as the compacted capillary-based dNTP dispenser, the dimension of the pyrosequencer is as small as 140 W × 158 H × 250 D (mm), which is ideal for a portable usage.

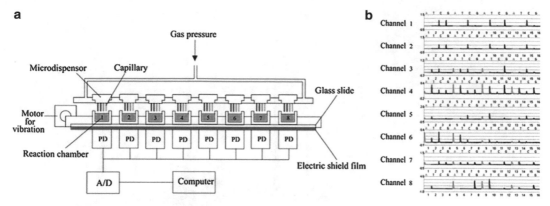

Fig. 2 Schematic of a photodiode array-based bioluminescence analyzer (8-channel) (**a**) and typical pyrograms from eight channels (**b**)

4.2 Comparison of SRPP Sensitivity among Various Light Sensors

Comparison of pyrograms from an artificial pooling sample (G:C = 1:2) by SRPP on a PD (S1133, Hamamatsu, Japan)-based pyrosequencer, a commercialized CCD (equipped in Biotage pyrosequencer, Sweden)-based pyrosequencer, and a PMT (R928, Hamamatsu, Japan)-based homemade pyrosequencer, shown in Fig. 3, indicates that all three pyrosequencers can give quantitative signals. The signal-to-noise ratios (S/N, S = signal intensity; N = SD of baseline fluctuation) calculated from the peak "G" in the pyrograms are about 20, 7, and 420 ($n=3$) for PD-, CCD-, and PMT-based pyrosequencers, respectively; thus, the PD pyrosequencer is about 20 times less sensitive than the PMT pyrosequencer but more sensitive than the CCD-based pyrosequencer.

4.3 Sensitivity Improvement of SRPP

Since PCR is used to amplify the sequence-labeled cDNAs, the sensitivity of SRPP should be very high even if the target genes are expressed at low levels. However, we found that some genes (such as MMP9, AF052162, and ESM1) cannot be detected with sensitivity in clinical samples when using the PD-based pyrosequencer. By trying several *Taq* DNA polymerases, including TaKaRa rTaq, Promega Taq, and Qiagen HotStarTaq, pyrosequencing results for clinical samples of the three genes, shown in Fig. 4, indicate that the HotStarTaq DNA polymerase (green curve) provides a three- to fivefold higher sensitivity than two other *Taq* polymerases (black and red curves). However, HotStarTaq DNA polymerase is very expensive; to obtain higher sensitivity with a less costly Taq polymerase, we have tried to use gene-specific RT primers instead of poly-T structured RT primers for reverse transcription (Fig. 1). Interestingly, this strategy significantly improved SRPP sensitivity. As shown in Fig. 4 (blue curve), the use of gene-specific RT primers increased the intensities of G-signals in the pyrograms by factors of 12.2, 24.2, and 11.6 for the respective MMP9, AF052162, and

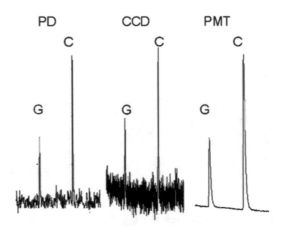

Fig. 3 SRPP results (G:C = 1:2) from pyrosequencers based on sensors of PD (S1133, Hamamatsu, Japan), CCD (equipped in Biotage pyrosequencer, Sweden), and PMT (R928, Hamamatsu, Japan), respectively

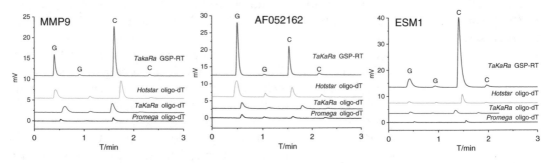

Fig. 4 Pyrograms of the MMP9, AF052162, and ESM1 gene expressed in a clinical sample by using different RT primers for reverse transcription and different polymerases for PCR. *Blue curve*: gene-specific RT primers and TaKaRa rTaq; *green curve*: universal RT primers (oligo-dT) and HotStarTaq; *red curve*: oligo-dT and TaKaRa rTaq; *black curve*: oligo-dT and Promega rTaq

ESM1 genes, almost compensating the sensitivity loss of an SRPP assay using the PD-based pyrosequencer.

4.4 Accuracy Evaluation

Based on the previously reported SRPP, poly-T structured RT primers did not yield any amplification bias on cDNA templates having different source-specific sequence tags. To investigate whether or not base labels in the proposed gene-specific RT primers cause an amplification bias on source-specific templates, the MMP9 gene from two aliquots of total RNA extracted from human mammary tissue was transcribed with two source-specific primers: RT-G and RT-C, respectively. Source sequence-tagged cDNAs were pooled individually at G:C ratios of 0:10, 1:9, 2:8, 3:7, 4:6, 5:5, 6:4, 7:3, 8:2, 9:1, and 10:0. After PCR on each pooled template, the amplicons were subjected to pyrosequencing. The relationship ($r = 0.9990$, $n = 3$) between the fold numbers indicated by pyrograms' signal intensities and the theoretical artificially pre-mixed fold number suggests that there is no significant bias of PCR on source-specific templates during amplification. Consequently, SRPP with gene-specific RT primers is very accurate in quantitatively detecting gene expression changes between samples by using PD-based pyrosequencer [10].

4.5 Gene Expression Analysis of Ten Breast Cancer Related Genes

The expression levels of ten prognostic marker genes (AL080059, MMP9, EXT1, ORC6L, AF052162, C9orf30, FBXO31, IGFBP5, ESM1, and RUNDC1) in the breast tumor tissues and normal tissues of ten patients were detected by the gene-specific RT primer-based SRPP method. At first, two kinds of RT primers (RT-G and RT-C) with source-specific tags in the middle were designed to individually reverse-transcribe normal tissue and breast cancer tissue, and the bases G and C, tagged in the cDNAs, were assigned to represent the normal tissue source and the tumor tissue source, respectively. Then SRPP on PD array-based pyrosequencer was carried out to quantify the relative levels of the ten genes expressed in two sources. The results clearly showed that the expression profiles of the ten markers differ among patients (Fig. 5). For instance, most of the ten prognostic genes were overexpressed (>threefold) in tumor tissues for patients 1–3, and expression of these genes was reduced inpatients 4–10, indicating a higher relative risk of metastasis for patients 1–3 [4, 9]. The accuracy of the proposed method was further confirmed by real-time PCR, the gold standard for quantitative gene expression analysis (Fig. 6).

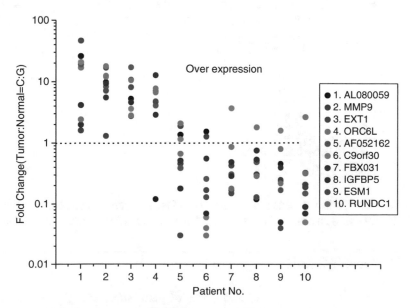

Fig. 5 Gene expression profiling of ten prognostic genes in ten breast cancer patients by SRPP ($n = 3$)

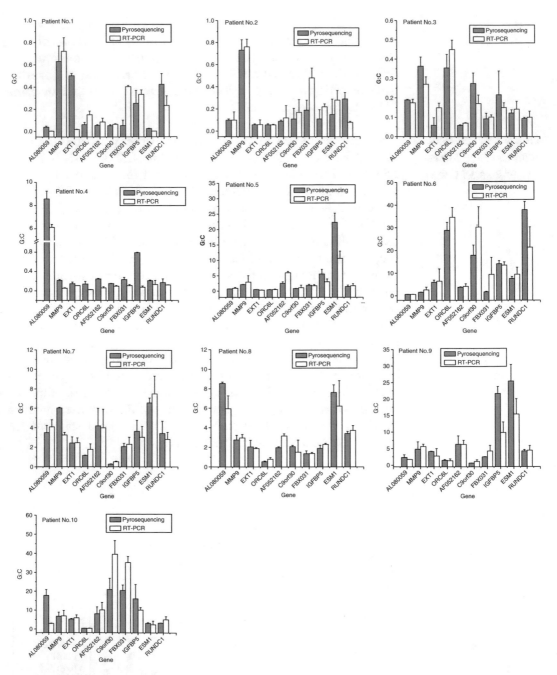

Fig. 6 Comparison of gene expression levels of ten breast prognostic genes in normal and tumor tissues from ten patients, as measured by portable bioluminescence analysis (*gray*) and real-time PCR (*white*)

5　Technical Notes

1. The use of gene-specific RT primers increased the intensities of G-signals in the pyrograms by factors of 12.2, 24.2, and 11.6 for the respective MMP9, AF052162, and ESM1 genes, almost compensating the sensitivity loss of an SRPP assay

using the PD-based pyrosequencer. SRPP with gene-specific RT primers is very accurate is quantitatively detecting gene expression changes between samples by using PD-based pyrosequencer [10].

2. HotStarTaq DNA polymerase provides a three- to fivefold higher sensitivity than two other Taq polymerases (TaKaRa rTaq, Promega Taq).

3. For an accurate DNA sequencing by the PD-based pyrosequencer, 5 μL of PCR products, which contains 0.1–1 pmol of target DNA, is routinely used in SRPP.

References

1. Van't Veer LJ, Dai H, Van de Vijver MJ, He YD, Hart AA, Mao M, Peterse HL, Van der Kooy K, Marton MJ, Witteveen AT, Schreiber GJ, Kerkhoven RM, Roberts C, Linsley PS, Bernards R, Friend SH (2002) Gene expression profiling predicts clinical outcome of breast cancer. Nature 415:530–536

2. Van de Vijver MJ, He YD, Van't Veer LJ, Dai H, Hart AA, Voskuil DW, Schreiber GJ, Peterse JL, Roberts C, Marton MJ, Parrish M, Atsma D, Witteveen A, Glas A, Delahaye L, Van der Velde T, Bartelink H, Rodenhuis S, Rutgers ET, Friend SH, Bernards R (2002) A gene-expression signature as a predictor of survival in breast cancer. N Engl J Med 347:1999–2009

3. Glas AM, Floore A, Delahaye LJ, Witteveen AT, Pover RC, Bakx N, Lahti-Domenici JS, Bruinsma TJ, Warmoes MO, Bernards R, Wessels LF, Van't Veer LJ (2006) Converting a breast cancer microarray signature into a high-throughput diagnostic test. BMC Genomics 7:278

4. Desmedt C, Ruiz-Garcia E, Andre F (2008) Gene expression predictors in breast cancer: current status, limitations and perspectives. Eur J Cancer 44:2714–2720

5. Zhang X, Wu H, Chen Z, Zhou G, Kajiyama T, Kambara H (2009) Dye-free gene expression detection by sequence-tagged reverse-transcription polymerase chain reaction coupled with pyrosequencing. Anal Chem 81:273–281

6. Zhou G, Kambara H (2009) DNA analysis with a photo-diode array sensor. Methods Mol Biol 503:337–360

7. Zhou G, Kamahori M, Okano K, Harada K, Kambara H (2001) Miniaturized pyrosequencer for DNA analysis with capillaries to deliver deoxynucleotides. Electrophoresis 22:3497–3504

8. Zhou G, Kajiyama T, Gotou M, Kishimoto A, Suzuki S, Kambara H (2006) Enzyme system for improving the detection limit in pyrosequencing. Anal Chem 78:4482–4489

9. Stadler Z, Come S (2009) Review of gene-expression profiling and its clinical use in breast cancer. Crit Rev Oncol Hematol 69:1–11

10. Kamahori M, Harada K, Kambara H (2002) A new single nucleotide polymorphisms typing method and device by bioluminometric assay coupled with a photodiode array. Meas Sci Technol 13:1779–1785

Chapter 28

MicroRNA Quantification by Pyrosequencing with a Sequence-Tagged Stem-Loop RT Primer

Hua Jing, Qinxin Song, Zhiyao Chen, Bingjie Zou, Guohua Zhou, and Hideki Kambara

Abstract

A novel dye-free method to quantify miRNA expression levels as low as fM is by using sequence-encoded miRNA-specific stem-loop RT primers coupled with pyrosequencing. We employed pyrosequencing technology to quantitate microRNAs by quantitatively decoding the sequence labels artificially tagged in RT products of miRNA. The miRNA was encoded by reverse transcription using sequence-tagged stem-loop RT primers. Pyrosequencing technology was employed to quantitate microRNAs by quantitatively decoding the sequence labels artificially tagged in RT products of miRNA. As no dye is used, the main merit of our method superior to the existing methods for miRNA quantification is the low cost of reagents and instrumentation. By using the sensitive pyrosequencer we developed by employing a cheap and compact photodiode array, a portable and inexpensive miRNA detector as a tool of point-of-care test (POCT) could be possible. Along with the discoveries of more disease-specific miRNA biomarkers, the detection of very limited number of miRNAs (<10) is enough for clinical diagnosis.

Key words miRNA, Pyrosequencing, Dye-free, Gene expression analysis, Sequence labels

1 Introduction

MicroRNAs (miRNAs) are a class of endogenous, ~ 22-nucleotide (nt) noncoding RNAs that play an important role in the control of the developmental processes of cells by negative regulation of protein-coding gene expression [1, 2]. To date, there are 17341 mature miRNAs, including 1048 human miRNAs, in the University of Manchester miRNA database (http://www.mirbase.org/) [3]. Although miRNAs represent a relatively abundant class of transcripts, their expression levels vary greatly in different tissue types and species [4]. Analyzing miRNA expression levels in tissues or cells can supply valuable information for investigating the biological functions of miRNAs; however conventional techniques to amplify miRNAs for detection and quantification present a

Guohua Zhou and Qinxin Song (eds.), *Advances and Clinical Practice in Pyrosequencing*, Springer Protocols Handbooks, DOI 10.1007/978-1-4939-3308-2_28, © Springer Science+Business Media New York 2016

significant challenge because of the short length of these molecules; thus, a number of straightforward methods without the use of amplification have been developed for miRNA detection [5–9]. Northern blotting [5, 10] is the widely used standard method for analyzing miRNAs; however, relatively large amounts of starting material (RNA) are required for an assay. To improve the sensitivityof miRNA quantification, a method based on splinted ligation was developed [11, 12]. This exhibits approximately 50 times greater sensitivity than Northern blotting, but radioactive 32P labels are needed. A single-molecule method, based on the hybridization of two spectrally distinguishable LNA–DNA oligonucleotide probes (for the miRNA of interest), offers a direct miRNA assay as sensitive as 500 fm, but an expensive single-molecule detection instrument is required [7]. For sensitive miRNA detection, amplification techniques are thus necessary. By skillfully designing detection probes, a modified "Invader" assay was developed for the quantification of miRNAs [13]. Although 20,000 miRNAs were detected, accurate quantification of miRNAs among samples is difficult because the initial target concentration is proportional to the steady-state reaction rate of "invasive" amplification.

In contrast, an miRNA assay based on real-time quantitative PCR with a stem–loop reverse transcription (RT) primer was much more quantitative, as the Ct (cycle threshold) value is inversely proportional to the amount of initial target [14–17]. However, PCRs of the sample and reference targets are performed separately, and a small difference in amplification efficiency between the sample and the reference yields a large difference in the amount of final product; this results in large inter-PCR variations [18]. Recently, a simple and sensitive miRNA quantification method that used branched rolling-circle amplification (BRCA) was reported [19], but quantification based on endpoint readout seems challengeable because of the time-dependent amplification efficiency of BRCA. To achieve accurate quantification of a target miRNA in a sample, real-time monitoring of signal intensities from both a sample and a reference (quantification standard) is necessary, because the reaction rate slows down as the reaction proceeds. As the real-time detection requires a sophisticated instrument, quantification using endpoint data is preferable. In this study, we have developed a pyrosequencing-based method for absolute quantification, and for comparing the relative miRNA expression levels in biological samples.

Pyrosequencing is a well-developed technology for DNA sequencing. It uses cascade enzymatic reactions to monitor the release of inorganic pyrophosphate that results from dNTP incorporation [20]. Because of its highly quantitative performance, pyrosequencing has been widely used for genotyping [21, 22], and the analysis of DNA methylation [23] and gene expression [24]. Here we employed pyrosequencing technology to quantify microRNAs by quantitatively detecting sequence labels that were artificially tagged into the RT products of miRNA. Unlike mRNA, miRNA is very short and can be easily synthesized; synthesized molecules with known concentration could thus be used as a reference for quantifying miRNA in a sample. As shown in Fig. 1, sequence labels for discriminating the sources of miRNA (sample or reference) are designed into the loop near to the 3′-end of the miRNA-specific RT primer, so that the 5′-end of the primer can offer a universal priming site for the following PCR. The structure of the miRNA-specific stem–loop RT primer is the same as that used by Chen's group [14]. After reverse transcription with the sequence-tagged RT primers, cDNA from the different sources (sample and reference) were similarly labeled with different sequences (thus, different colors in a fluorescence-based assay) (*see* **Note 1**). We labeled the sample-miRNA and the reference-miRNA with the sequences "**catg**" and "**gatc**," respectively; hence, in a

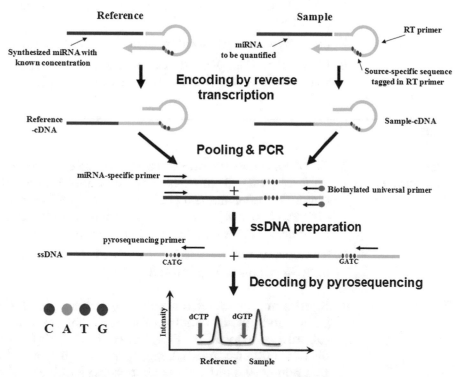

Fig. 1 miRNA quantification by pyrosequencing with sequence-tagged stem–loop RT primers. Three steps are involved: reverse transcription of target miRNA with sequence-tagged miRNA-specific stem–loop RT primer; amplification of the pooled sequence-labeled cDNA (1:1; sample, and synthesized miRNA reference); and decoding by pyrosequencing of the source-specific sequences tagged in the amplicons. The base order in the pyrogram represents the miRNA source, and the peak intensity reflects the relative miRNA expression level in the corresponding miRNA source. The abundance of the target miRNA can be deduced from the intensities of the "G" and "C" peaks

pyrogram (Fig. 1), signal intensities from the "C" and "G" peaks can exactly reflect the relative concentrations of a given miRNA between sample and reference (*see* **Note 2**).

2 Materials

1. An MMLV reverse-transcription kit was purchased from TransGen Biotech Co., Ltd. (Beijing, China).

2. DNA polymerase, SYBR Premix ExTaq Kit, and ribonuclease inhibitor were obtained from TaKaRa (Dalian, China).

3. Diethylpyrocarbonate (DEPC) was purchased from Shengxing Biotechnology Co. Ltd. (Nanjing, China).

4. Streptavidin-Sepharose HP Beads (about 34 mm) were purchased from GE Health-care Bio Sciences.

5. dGTP and dCTP were purchased from Amersham Pharmacia Biotech.

6. TRIzol and HPLC-purified oligonucleotides were obtained from Invitrogen.

7. miRNAs were synthesized by Gene-Pharma (Shanghai, China).

8. Other chemicals were of extra-pure commercial grade. All solutions were prepared in DEPC-treated deionized water.

3 Methods

3.1 Reverse Transcription Reaction

1. The reverse transcription reaction mixture consisted of 5× RT buffer (4 μL), TransScript reverse transcriptase (200 U), ribonuclease inhibitor (20 U μL^{-1}), stem–loop RT primer (1 μm), dNTPs (500 μM), and an appropriate amount of miRNA reference or RNA samples (reaction volume 20 μL).

2. The reaction mixture was incubated (16 °C, 30 min; 42 °C, 30 min; 85 °C, 5 min) and stored at 4 °C.

3.2 PCR

1. Equal amounts of reference-cDNA and sample-cDNA were pooled and used as templates for PCR. The reaction mixture (50 mL) contained 10× PCR buffer (5 μL), MgCl$_2$ (2 mM), dNTPs (600 μm), miRNA-specific primer (0.3 μm), biotinylated primer (0.3 μM), pooled templates (3 μL), and Taq DNA polymerase (1.25 U).

2. PCR (94 °C, 5 min; 35× (94 °C, 15 s; 55 °C, 15 s; 72 °C, 15 s); 72 °C, 10 min) was performed in an EDC-810 Thermal Cycler (Eastwin, China). The PCR tube was stored at 4 °C before use.

3.3 Pyrosequencing

After the preparation of ssDNA [14], pyrosequencing primer (1 μL, 10 μm) was added for the annealing reaction (95 °C, 30 s; 55 °C, 3 min). The pyrosequencing reaction mixture consisted of Tris–acetate (0.1 M, pH 7.7), EDTA (2 mM), magnesium acetate (10 mM), polyvinylpyrrolidone (PVP; 0.4 mg mL^{-1}), BSA (0.1 %), dithiothreitol (DTT, 1 mM), adenosine 5′-phosphosulfate (APS; 3 μM), D-luciferin (0.4 mM), ATP sulfurylase (0.3 % (v/v)), apyrase (1.6 U mL^{-1}), Klenow fragment (18 U mL^{-1}), and appropriate amount of luciferase. Real-time pyrosequencing was achieved on our homemade prototype pyrosequencer [26, 30].

4 Method Validation

4.1 Accuracy Evaluation

To investigate the accuracy of the miRNA assay, a series of artificial pools with known concentrations of the target miRNA were employed. The mir-16 miRNA was used as a target for the investigation. The synthesized mir-16 miRNA oligonucleotides were reverse-transcribed with two source-specific RT primers, mir-16-RT-G and mir-16-RT-C (Fig. 2a). After the RT reactions, pools were prepared by mixing the two RT products in different ratios. Within the mixing range, the ratios calculated from the signal intensities of peaks "G" and "C" were very close to the ratios of the theoretical concentrations of mir-16 miRNA in the artificial pools, with a correlation coefficient of 0.9984 ($n = 3$, Fig. 2b). In addition, no PCR bias due to different cycles was observed; this indicated that RT products tagged with different source-specific sequences exhibited identical PCR behavior— just like a single template.

4.2 Specificity Evaluation

There are some miRNA families whose members differ by only one or two nucleotide bases; it was necessary to determine the specificity of the proposed assay in discrimination among such family members. Three members of the let-7miRNA family (let-7a, let-7b, and let-7c) were artificially synthesized and used for the evaluation. As shown in Fig. 3a, the sequences of each member differ by only one or two bases (shown in bold). The RT-primer specific for let-7a miRNA was used to reverse-transcribe the three targets, let-7a, let-7b, and let-7c. Specificity was evaluated by comparing the RT products from let-7b and let-7c with that from let-7a. To simplify the detection, let-7a was assigned as the reference, and reverse-transcribed with the sequence-tagged RT primer, let-7a-RT-C; let-7b and let-7c were assigned as two different samples, and separately reverse-transcribed with let-7a-RT-G. After the RT reactions, RT products from the samples were separately pooled with the reference, and then PCR was performed on each of the two pools. Pyrograms of the single-stranded PCR products are

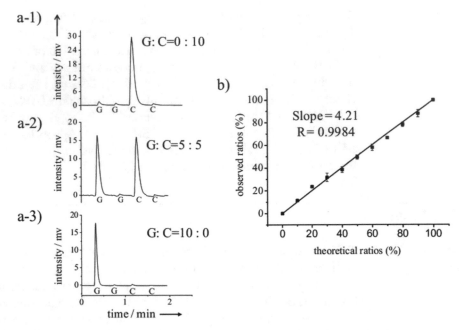

Fig. 2 Accuracy evaluation of the miRNA assay. (**a**) The typical pyrograms of artificial templates pooled with various amounts of source-specific RT products. The ratios (G:C) of source-specific RT products in the pools were 0:10 (*a-1*), 5:5 (*a-2*), and 10:0 (*a-3*), respectively. (**b**) Correlation between the expected ratios of the amounts of mir-16 in two sources and the observed ratios by the mir-16 assay (*n* = 3)

shown in Fig. 3b: the signal intensities from let-7a are 17-fold and 7-fold higher than that of let-7b and let-7c, respectively (Fig. 3c). The lower intensity from let-7b (compared to let-7c) is because let-7b has two bases that are noncomplementary to the let-7a-RT primer. These results suggest that the specificities of the RT primer and the miRNA-specific PCR primer are high enough to discriminate between the three let-7 family members. Because the discrimination power of the proposed assay mainly depends on the RT step, the contribution to the high specificity of the assay is believed to result from the structure of the stem–loop RT primers [8].

4.3 Sensitivity Evaluation

As PCR is used to amplify the sequence-tagged RT products, the sensitivity of the present miRNA quantification assay should be very high. To estimate the sensitivity, a series of mir-16 miRNA sample–reference pairs were synthesized, at concentration from 400 nm to 40 fm. To simplify the calculation, the ratio of the mir-16 miRNA concentration in each pair was fixed at 1:3. Each sample and the reference was reverse-transcribed with the sequence-tagged RT primers mir-16-RT-G and mir-16-RT-C, respectively. As showed in Fig. 4, the ratios of signal intensity (between peaks "G" and "C") are very close to 1:3 (average 1:2.9) for all tested pairs; this indicates that the present assay can detect miRNAs at sub-femtomolar concentrations—sufficient for the quantification of most miRNAs [27–29]. At the plateau of the amplification

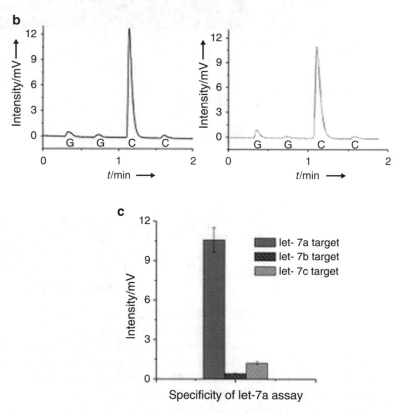

a

let-7a UGA GGU AGU AGG UUG UAU AGU U
let-7b UGA GGU AGU AGG UUG UGU GGU U
let-7c UGA GGU AGU AGG UUG UAU GGU U

Fig. 3 Specificity of the proposed assay in discrimination between let-7 family members (let-7a, let-7b, and let-7c). (**a**) The sequences of three closely related let-7 family members. (**b**) Pyrograms comparing the signals from RT products between let-7a and let-7b (*left*) or let-7c (*right*) when using the let-7a-specific RT primer. (**c**) Discrimination capability of the let-7a miRNA assay ($n=3$)

reaction, the signal intensities of amplicons are not in proportion to the starting template concentrations, but the ratio of "G" to "C" peaks from each pair remained at 1:3. This proves the unbiased feature of PCR on different sequence-tagged templates, even when the template concentration varies over a range of seven orders of magnitude.

4.4 Determination of the Expression Level of mir-16 in Breast Cancer Cells

For absolute quantification of an miRNA of interest in a sample, it is necessary to prepare a reference of synthesized miRNA at a given concentration. We employed the proposed assay to detect the expression level of mir-16 in breast cancer cells. First, total RNA was extracted from breast cancer cells, and 2 μg total RNA was used for reverse transcription with the RT primer (mir-16-RT-C). The reference was prepared by performing reverse transcription on

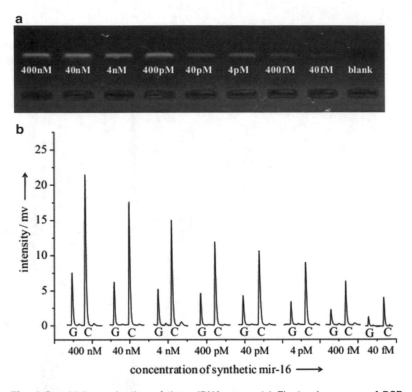

Fig. 4 Sensitivity evaluation of the miRNA assay. (**a**) Electropherogram of PCR products using pools with various concentrations (from 400 nM to 40 fm) of C-source mir-16 transcripts as staring targets. (**b**) Pyrograms of the PCR products. For the convenience, two sources were termed as source-G and source-C, respectively, and the ratio of the amount of mir-16 between two sources was simply expressed as G:C

a series of concentration of synthesized mir-16 with mir-16-RT-G. Typical pyrograms for the quantification (Fig. 5a) indicate that the expression level of this miRNA was 8.3 pmol in 2 μg total RNA (the RT products of the samples were diluted 100-fold before mixing).

4.5 Determination of Expression Level of gga-mir-206 and gga-mir-1b within Chicken Embryos at Different Development Stages

This method was also used to detect the expression level of gga-mir-206 and gga-mir-1b within chicken embryos at different development stages. These two miRNAs are expressed in skeletal muscles and have been shown to contribute to muscle development [25]. First, total RNA was extracted from 13 chicken embryos at different stages of development, and 50 ng total RNAs of each was used for reverse transcription with mir-206-RT-C or mir-1b-RT-C. Graphs of the results from different developmental stages (from days 8 to 20; $n = 3$, *see* Fig. 5b) clearly demonstrate the concentration variation of the two miRNAs during the development of chicken embryo. The accuracy of these results was confirmed by real-time quantitative PCR.

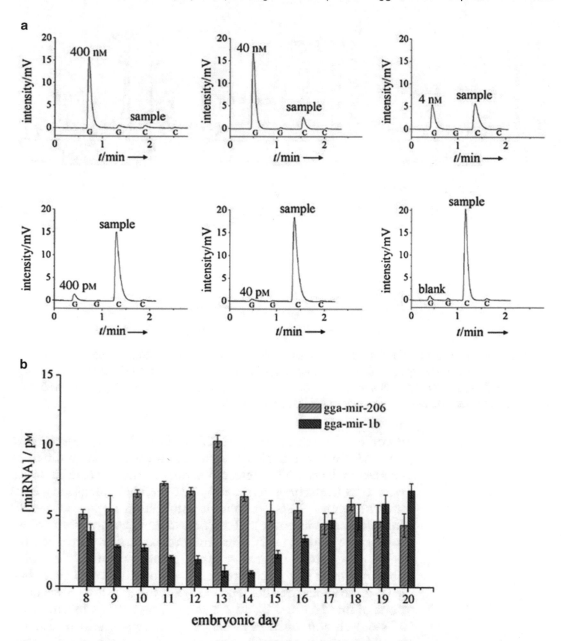

Fig. 5 Quantification of target miRNAs in total RNA sample by the proposed assay. (**a**) Pyrograms for absolute quantification of mir-16 in breast cancer cells with different concentrations of synthesized mir-16 (0, 0.04, 0.4, 4, 40, and 400 nM). The reference of the synthesized mir-16 and the sample of breast cancer cells were labeled "G" and "C," respectively. (**b**) Expression levels of gga-mir-206 and gga-mir-1b at different development stages in chicken embryo (day 8–20; $n = 3$)

4.6 Relative Quantification of mir-16 among Different Tissues of a Mouse

To demonstrate the applicability of the established method, relative expression levels of mir-16 miRNA—between right brain and left brain, cerebellum and spleen, heart and lungs, small intestine and stomach, and bladder and large intestine tissues of a mouse—were detected. Typical pyrograms for quantitatively

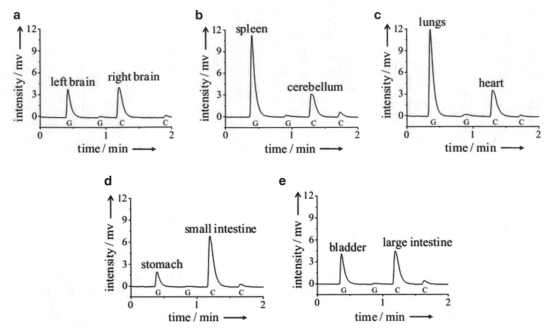

Fig. 6 The typical pyrograms for detecting the relative mir-16 expression levels between right brain and left brain (**a**), cerebellum and spleen (**b**), heart and lungs (**c**), small intestine and stomach (**d**), as well as large intestine and bladder (**e**) tissues of a mouse. "G" and "C" under the pyrogram mean the type of the dispensed dNTP and represent the tissue sources indicated in the top of each peak

decoding the sequence tags in RT products (Fig. 6) indicate that mir-16 is expressed in all ten organs of the mouse, but at different expression levels. The detected ratios of the expression levels were 1.03 (right brain:left brain), 0.23 (cerebellum:spleen), 0.29 (heart:lungs), 3.36 (small intestine:stomach), and 0.99 (bladder:large intestine). To confirm the accuracy of these results, we also analyzed the absolute expression levels of mir-16 in tissue from the ten organs. A comparison of the ratios obtained from the two detection methods indicates that they gave quite similar results. For example, the absolute concentrations of mir-16 are 0.7 and 2.8 fmol of total RNA in the tissue of stomach and small intestine, respectively: a ratio of 3:8 for small intestine to stomach—very close to the ratio of 3:4 for the relative quantification method.

5 Technical Notes

1. To avoid PCR bias resulting from Tm differences, the labels were designed from the same base species but with different base order.

2. As the concentration of the miRNA in a reference is known, the miRNA in a sample can be accurately quantified by using a

series of references. Usually three references are enough for a routine assay. If the aim is to compare the concentrations of a given miRNA in two different sources (e.g., in two tissues or cells) the assay can be simply performed by 1:1 pooling of the source-specific RT products; the relative expression levels of the given miRNA between the sources can be readily obtained by comparing the peak intensities of the source-specific bases "G" and "C" in a pyrogram.

References

1. Bartel DP (2004) MicroRNAs: genomics, biogenesis, mechanism, and function. Cell 116:281–297

2. Farh KK, Grimson A, Jan C, Lewis BP, Johnston WK, Lim LP, Burge CB, Bartel DP (2005) The widespread impact of mammalian MicroRNAs on mRNA repression and evolution. Science 310:1817–1821

3. Griffiths-Jones S, Saini HK, van Dongen S, Enright AJ (2008) miRBase: tools for microRNA genomics. Nucleic Acids Res 36:D154–D158

4. Kim J, Krichevsky A, Grad Y, Hayes GD, Kosik KS, Church GM, Ruvkun G (2004) Identification of many microRNAs that copurify with polyribosomes in mammalian neurons. Proc Natl Acad Sci U S A 101(1):360–365

5. Varallyay E, Burgyan J, Havelda Z (2007) Detection of microRNAs by northern blot analyses using LNA probes. Methods 43:140–145

6. Yang WJ, Li XB, Li YY, Zhao LF, He WL, Gao YQ, Wan YJ, Xia W, Chen T, Zheng H, Li M, Xu SQ (2008) Quantification of microRNA by gold nanoparticle probes. Anal Biochem 376:183–188

7. Neely LA, Patel S, Garver J, Gallo M, Hackett M, McLaughlin S, Nadel M, Harris J, Gullans S, Rooke J (2006) A single-molecule method for the quantitation of microRNA gene expression. Nat Methods 3:41–46

8. Qavi AJ, Bailey RC (2010) Multiplexed detection and label-free quantitation of microRNAs using arrays of silicon photonic microring resonators. Angew Chem Int Ed Engl 49:4608–4611

9. Yang H, Hui A, Pampalakis G, Soleymani L, Liu FF, Sargent EH, Kelley SO (2009) Direct, electronic microRNA detection for the rapid determination of differential expression profiles. Angew Chem Int Ed Engl 48:8461–8464

10. Varallyay E, Burgyan J, Havelda Z (2008) MicroRNA detection by northern blotting using locked nucleic acid probes. Nat Protoc 3:190–196

11. Maroney PA, Chamnongpol S, Souret F, Nilsen TW (2007) A rapid, quantitative assay for direct detection of microRNAs and other small RNAs using splinted ligation. RNA 13:930–936

12. Maroney PA, Chamnongpol S, Souret F, Nilsen TW (2008) Direct detection of small RNAs using splinted ligation. Nat Protoc 3:279–287

13. Allawi HT, Dahlberg JE, Olson S, Lund E, Olson M, Ma WP, Takova T, Neri BP, Lyamichev V (2004) Quantitation of microRNAs using a modified Invader assay. RNA 10:1153–1161

14. Chen C, Ridzon DA, Broomer AJ, Zhou Z, Lee DH, Nguyen JT, Barbisin M, Xu NL, Mahuvakar VR, Andersen MR, Lao KQ, Livak KJ, Guegler KJ (2005) Real-time quantification of microRNAs by stem-loop RT-PCR. Nucleic Acids Res 33, e179

15. Tang F, Hajkova P, Barton SC, Lao K, Surani MA (2006) MicroRNA expression profiling of single whole embryonic stem cells. Nucleic Acids Res 34, e9

16. Tang F, Hajkova P, Barton SC, O'Carroll D, Lee C, Lao K, Surani MA (2006) 220-plex microRNA expression profile of a single cell. Nat Protoc 1:1154–1159

17. Lao K, Xu NL, Sun YA, Livak KJ, Straus NA (2007) Real time PCR profiling of 330 human micro-RNAs. Biotechnol J 2:33–35

18. Pfaffl MW (2001) A new mathematical model for relative quantification in real-time RT-PCR. Nucleic Acids Res 29:e45

19. Cheng Y, Zhang X, Li Z, Jiao X, Wang Y, Zhang Y (2009) Highly sensitive determination of microRNA using target-primed and branched rolling-circle amplification. Angew Chem Int Ed Engl 48:3268–3272

20. Ronaghi M, Uhlen M, Nyren P (1998) A sequencing method based on real-time pyrophosphate. Science 281(363):365

338   Hua Jing et al.

21. Duffy KJ, Littrell J, Locke A, Sherman SL, Olivier M (2008) A novel procedure for genotyping of single nucleotide polymorphisms in trisomy with genomic DNA and the invader assay. Nucleic Acids Res 36:e145

22. Elahi E, Pourmand N, Chaung R, Rofoogaran A, Boisver J, Samimi-Rad K, Davis RW, Ronaghi M (2003) Determination of hepatitis C virus genotype by Pyrosequencing. J Virol Methods 109:171–176

23. Tost J, Gut IG (2007) DNA methylation analysis by pyrosequencing. Nat Protoc 2:2265–2275

24. Zhang X, Wu H, Chen Z, Zhou G, Kajiyama T, Kambara H (2009) Dye-free gene expression detection by sequence-tagged reverse-transcription polymerase chain reaction coupled with pyrosequencing. Anal Chem 81:273–281

25. Yuasa K, Hagiwara Y, Ando M, Nakamura A, Takeda S, Hijikata T (2008) MicroRNA-206 is highly expressed in newly formed muscle fibers: implications regarding potential for muscle regeneration and maturation in muscular dystrophy. Cell Struct Funct 33:163–169

26. Song Q, Jing H, Wu H, Zhou G, Kajiyama T, Kambara H (2010) Gene expression analysis on a photodiode array-based bioluminescence analyzer by using sensitivity-improved SRPP. Analyst 135:1315–1319

27. Asslaber D, Pinon JD, Seyfried I, Desch P, Stocher M, Tinhofer I, Egle A, Merkel O, Greil R (2010) microRNA-34a expression correlates with MDM2 SNP309 polymorphism and treatment-free survival in chronic lymphocytic leukemia. Blood 115:4191–4197

28. Ji J, Shi J, Budhu A, Yu Z, Forgues M, Roessler S, Ambs S, Chen Y, Meltzer PS, Croce CM, Qin LX, Man K, Lo CM, Lee J, Ng IO, Fan J, Tang ZY, Sun HC, Wang XW (2009) MicroRNA expression, survival, and response to interferon in liver cancer. N Engl J Med 361:1437–1447

29. Lee DY, Deng Z, Wang CH, Yang BB (2007) MicroRNA-378 promotes cell survival, tumor growth, and angiogenesis by targeting SuFu and Fus-1 expression. Proc Natl Acad Sci USA 104:20350–20355

30. Zhou G, Kamahori M, Okano K, Harada K, Kambara H (2001) Miniaturized pyrosequencer for DNA analysis with capillaries to deliver deoxynucleotides. Electrophoresis 22:3497–3504

Chapter 29

Analysis of Genetically Modified Organisms by Pyrosequencing on a Portable Photodiode-Based Bioluminescence Sequencer

Qinxin Song, Guijiang Wei, Bingjie Zou, and Guohua Zhou

Abstract

A portable bioluminescence analyzer for detecting the DNA sequence of genetically modified organisms (GMO) was developed by using a photodiode (PD) array. Pyrosequencing on eight genes (zSSIIb, Bt11, and Bt176 gene of genetically modified maize; Lectin, 35S-CTP4, CP4EPSPS, CaMV35S promoter, and NOS terminator of the genetically modified roundup ready soya) was successfully detected with this instrument. The corresponding limit of detection (LOD) was 0.01 % with 35 PCR cycles. The maize and soya available from three different provenances in China were detected. The results indicate that pyrosequencing using the small size of the detector is a simple, inexpensive, and reliable way in a farm/field test of GMO analysis.

Key words Genetically modified organisms (GMO), Bt-11 and Bt-176 maize, Roundup ready soya, Pyrosequencing, Portable bioluminescence analyzer

---

1 Introduction

With the development of genetically modified organisms (GMO) technology, many qualitative and quantitative detection methods have been established for safety assessment and risk management. Many countries have established their own thresholds for the content of genetically modified crops, such as 0.9 % in the EU; 3 % in Korea; 5 % in Taiwan; 1 % in Australia, New Zealand, and Brazil; and 5 % in Japan [1].

Many methods have also been developed for detecting GMO DNA using mainly PCR, which requires an instrument to heat and cool a reaction tube, and loop-mediated isothermal amplification (LAMP), which requires only a water bath to keep the reaction tube at a constant temperature [2]. Although LAMP is sensitive and easy to operate in the field, the detection of amplicons is nonspecific because the turbidity- (relying on sedimentation of magnesium with by-products of pyrophosphate) and

Guohua Zhou and Qinxin Song (eds.), *Advances and Clinical Practice in Pyrosequencing*, Springer Protocols Handbooks,
DOI 10.1007/978-1-4939-3308-2_29, © Springer Science+Business Media New York 2016

florescence-based (relying on intercalating of SYBR Green I with dsDNA) detection methods are also nonspecific. The most widely used method is PCR [3–7], which amplifies GMO components using a pair of GMO-specific primers, but the specificity of GMO detection is not satisfactory because the amplification products of GMO are usually identified by slab gel electrophoresis and ethidium bromide staining. These methods lack precision because they are based on the size of the amplicons for judgment rather than the real DNA sequence information [8–10]. As a result, nonspecific amplification of products of similar size may lead to erroneous interpretation. The replacement of gel electrophoresis with gold nanoparticle lateral-flow strips or DNA hybridization greatly facilitates the detection of PCR products, but the specificity of the detection is still low because sequencing information from amplicons is not provided. Although RFLP-PCR greatly improves the accuracy of qualitative detection, it is difficult to find a suitable endonuclease for all GMOs.

A straightforward way to achieve a highly specific detection of GMO is to sequence the GMO amplicons after PCR. Although DNA sequencing based on the Sanger principle and capillary electrophoresis is a state-of-the-art method for DNA sequencing, the size of the instrumentation limits its application for GMO detection in the field.

Pyrosequencing is a well-developed technology for DNA sequencing that employs coupled enzymatic reactions to detect the inorganic pyrophosphate (PPi) released during dNTP incorporation. This technology has the advantages of accuracy, flexibility, and parallel processing, and therefore has been widely used for DNA resequencing, genotyping, DNA methylation, and gene expression analysis. However, the optics subsystem usually consists of a CCD camera and a camera controller, which again are bulky. Recently, we developed an inexpensive bioluminescence analyzer using a photodiode (PD) array (see **Note 1**); pyrosequencing with this instrument was successful [11–13]. The corresponding limit of detection (LOD) was 0.01 % with 35 PCR cycles. The GMO test result and the small size of the detector have immense potential for use in farm/field testing.

2 Materials

2.1 GMO Materials

Certified Reference Materials (CRMs) produced by the European Union (EU) Joint Research Center, Institute for Reference Materials and Measurements (IRMM), were purchased from Fluka, Buchs, Switzerland. 1 % genetically modified Bt11 maize, 2 % genetically modified Bt176 maize, and 2 % genetically modified roundup ready soya were used. Non-transgenic maize was purchased from the local market in Nanjing, China.

2.2 Reagents	1. HotStarTaq DNA polymerase was purchased from Qiagen (Qiagen GmbH, Hilden, Germany).

2. TransStart Taq DNA Polymerase was purchased from TransGen Biotech (Beijing, China).

3. Exo⁻ Klenow Fragment, polyvinylpyrrolidone (PPV), and QuantiLum recombinant luciferase were purchased from Promega (Madison, WI).

4. Dynabeads M-280 Streptavidin (2.8 μm) was purchased from Dynal Biotech ASA (Oslo, Norway).

5. ATP sulfurylase, apyrase, D-luciferin, bovine serum albumin (BSA), and adenosine 5′-phosphosulfate (APS) were obtained from Sigma (St. Louis, MO).

6. 2′-Deoxyadenosine-5′-O-(1-thiotriphosphate) sodium salt (dATP-α-S) was purchased from Amersham Pharmacia Biotech (Amersham, UK).

7. dGTP, dTTP, and dCTP were purchased from Amersham Pharmacia Biotech (Piscataway, NJ).

8. Other solutions were prepared with deionized and sterilized H_2O.

3 Methods

3.1 DNA Extraction

1. Plant genomic DNA was extracted using a Biospin Plant Genomic DNA Extraction Kit according to the manufacturer's manual. 1–30 μg genomic DNA can be acquired from up to 100 mg plant tissue by using this Kit (*see* **Note 2**).

3.2 Targets and Primers

1. For the evaluation, eight genes (zSSIIb, Bt11, and Bt176 gene of the genetically modified maize; Lectin, 35S-CTP4, CP4EPSPS, CaMV35S promoter, and NOS terminator of the genetically modified roundup ready soya) were selected as "proof-of-concept" examples.

3.3 PCR

1. Each 50 μL PCR mixture contained 1.5 mmol/L $MgCl_2$, 0.2 mmol/L of each dNTP, 0.3 μmol/L of each primer, 1 μL of genome DNA template, and 1.25 U of DNA polymerase.

2. Amplification was performed on a PTC-225 thermocycler PCR system (MJ research) according to the following protocol: denatured at 94 °C for 15 min and followed by 35 cycles (94 °C for 40 s; 55 °C for 40 s; 72 °C for 1 min). After the cycle reaction, the product was incubated at 72 °C for 10 min (*see* **Note 3**).

3.4 Pyrosequencing	1. The reaction volume for pyrosequencing was 40 μL, containing 0.1 mol/L Tris–acetate (pH 7.7), 2 mmol/L EDTA, 10 mmol/L magnesium acetate, 0.1 % BSA, 1 mmol/L dithiothreitol (DTT), 2 μmol/L adenosine 5′-phosphosulfate (APS), 0.4 mg/mL PVP, 0.4 mmol/L D-luciferin, 200 mU/mL ATP sulfurylase, 3 μg/mL luciferase, 18 U/mL Klenow fragment, and 1.5 U/mL apyrase (*see* **Note 4**).

2. Each of the dNTPs was added in the reservoir of the microdispenser, and pyrosequencing reaction starts when the dispensed dNTP is complementary to the template sequence.

3. Ten microliters of PCR product was used for an assay (*see* **Note 5**).

---

4 Method Validation

4.1 Effect of Concentration of Apyrase on Pyrosequencing

The concentration of apyrase is critical in the reaction system especially when the concentration of polymerase, luciferase, and ATP sulfurylase are tailored to ensure high sensitivity and low background signal.

When the amount of apyrase is very low, insufficient dNTP degradation occurs where dNTPs stay in the reaction chamber for a long period. False signals and peak broadening are produced (as shown in Fig. 1a, b) when these dNTPs are incorporated with newly injected dNTP species. When the apyrase amount is high, dNTPs are degraded before extension of the DNA strand is complete. Correctly extended DNA strands, together with foreshortened DNA strands, are produced simultaneously in the reaction chamber. This heterogeneous reaction decreases peak intensity as shown in Figs. 1d, e. When the amount of apyrase and injected dNTP is correct, nucleotide incorporation is sufficient and residual dNTPs degraded by apyrase before further dNTPs are added to the reaction chamber producing a proper pyrogram as shown in Fig. 1c.

4.2 Pyrosequencing of Certified Reference Materials

Typical pyrograms for the zSSIIb, Bt-11, and Bt-176 genes from genetically modified maize are presented in Fig. 2a. Typical pyrograms for the lectin, 35S-CTP4, CP4EPSPS, CaMV35S promoter, and NOS terminator genes from genetically modified roundup ready soya are presented in Fig. 2b. Sequence lengths were between 25 and 40 bp and our results indicate that the different genes were accurately detected.

4.3 Pyrosequencing on Various Amounts of GMO in Non-GMO Products

Three GM mixes were tested containing 1, 0.1, and 0.01 % roundup ready soya, respectively. 35S-CTP4 was amplified and sequenced successfully in all cases. The pyrograms for the different GMO contents are shown in Fig. 3. The proposed method meets the 0.01 % sensitivity criterion for pooled samples.

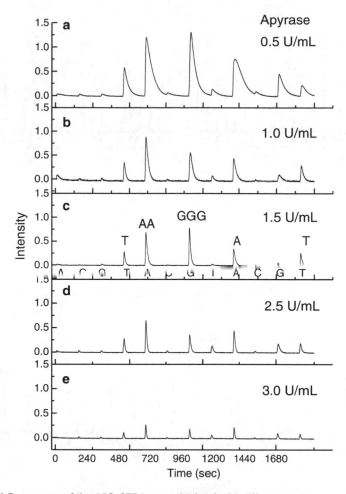

Fig. 1 Pyrograms of the 35S-CTP4 gene obtained with different apyrase concentration. Apyrase: (**a**) 0.5 U/mL, (**b**) 1.0 U/mL; (**c**) 1.5 U/mL; (**d**) 2.5 U/mL; (**e**) 3.0 U/mL. The detected sequence is on the top of each peak on (**c**). Each dNTP was dispensed with the order of A–C–G–T

4.4 Analysis of GMO Contents in Grains Available from Market

We have applied the proposed method using samples purchased on the market. GMO DNA sequences were detected in three batches of corn and soybean from Hebei, Shandong, and Heilongjiang Provinces of China. CRMs containing 1 % genetically modified Bt11 maize, 2 % genetically modified Bt176 maize, and 2 % genetically modified roundup ready soya were used as positive controls. The results showed that zSSIIb (Zea maize starch synthase isoform) and lectin (lectin is a major protein in soybean) genes were detected in all samples and CRMs. While Bt-11, Bt-176, 35S-CTP4, CP4EPSPS, CaMV35S, and NOS genes (transgenes) were only detected in the GMO CRMs by using portable pyrosequencer, the corresponding DNA fragment does not exist in the samples from market.

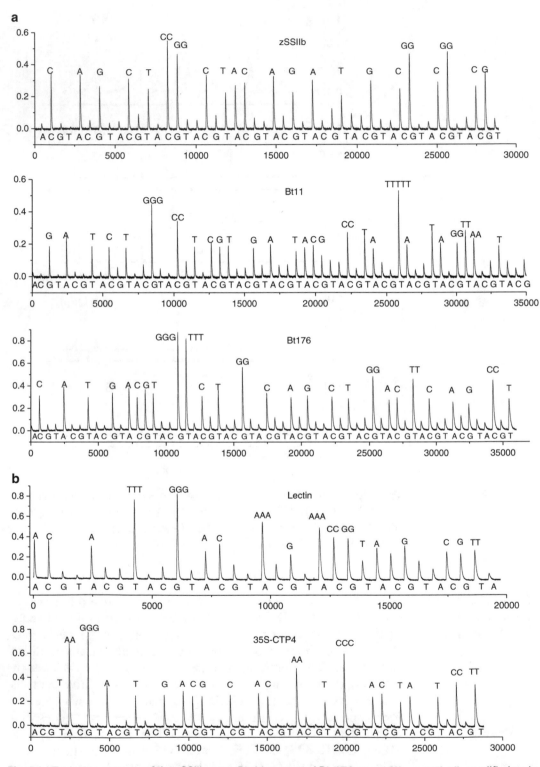

Fig. 2 (a) Typical pyrograms of the zSSIIb gene, Bt-11 gene, and Bt-176 gene of the genetically modified maize. (b) Typical pyrograms of the lectin gene, 35S-CTP4 gene, CP4EPSPS gene, CaMV35S promoter, and NOS terminator of the genetically modified roundup ready soya. The detected sequence is on the *top* of each peak. Each dNTP was dispensed with the order of A–C–G–T

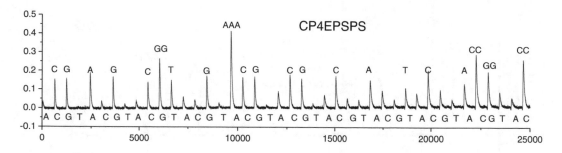

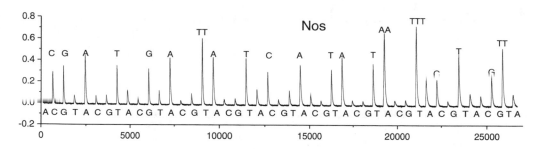

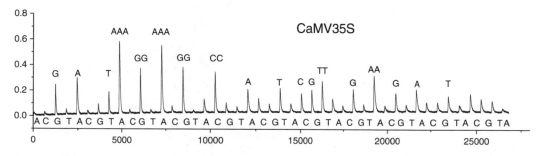

Fig. 2 (continued)

5 Technical Notes

1. A custom-built portable bioluminescence analyzer was constructed using a PD array sensor. Unlike PMT, the PD sensor is very small (6 W×2H×8D mm) and can be readily made smaller in an array format. Figure 4 shows the schematic of a single channel of the PD array-based pyrosequencer, which included capillary-based micro-dispensers driven by air pressure. A motor from a mobile phone was used to vibrate the chambers after the dispensing dNTPs into the reaction mixture. The working temperature was controlled at 28–30 °C, which is the most suitable temperature for the enzyme reaction. By carefully designing the PD amplification circuit, the new pyrosequencer is sensitive to

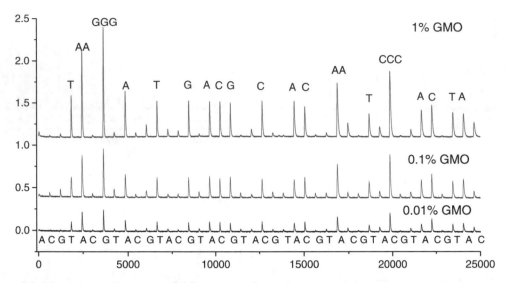

Fig. 3 Pyrograms of the different content GMO detection and the detection target is 35S-CTP4 gene

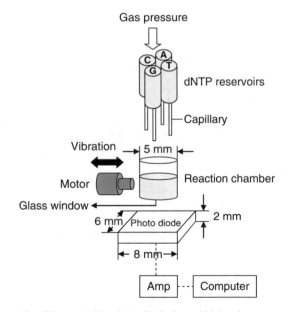

Fig. 4 Schematic of the portable photodiode-based bioluminescence analyzer

50 fmol of ssDNA template in a 50 μL pyrosequencing reaction. Due to the small size of PD as well as the compact capillary-based dNTP dispenser, the dimensions of a prototype of 8-channel pyrosequencer were 140 W × 158H × 250D (mm), which is ideal for portable device.

2. The quantity and quality of DNA in the samples should be measured and evaluated according to the absorbance measurements at 260 nm wavelength and 1 % agarose gel electrophoresis.

3. The product should be held at 4 °C before use.

4. The concentration of apyrase is critical in the reaction system especially when the concentration of polymerase, luciferase, and ATP sulfurylase are tailored to ensure high sensitivity and low background signal.

5. Streptavidin-coated Dynal beads were used to prepare ssDNA template for pyrosequencing. Both immobilized biotinylated strands and nonbiotinylated strands were used as sequencing templates.

References

1. Holst-Jensen A (2009) Testing for genetically modified organisms (GMOs): Past, present and future perspectives. Biotechnol Adv 27: 1071–1082

2. Kiddle G, Hardinge P, Buttigieg N, Gandelman O, Pereira C, McElgunn CJ, Rizzoli M, Jackson R, Appleton N, Moore C, Tisi LC, Murray JA (2012) GMO detection using a bioluminescent real time reporter (BART) of loop mediated isothermal amplification (LAMP) suitable for field use. BMC Biotechnol 12:15

3. Cankar K, Chauvensy-Ancel V, Fortabat MN, Gruden K, Kobilinsky A, Zel J, Bertheau Y (2008) Detection of nonauthorized genetically modified organisms using differential quantitative polymerase chain reaction: application to 35S in maize. Anal Biochem 376: 189–199

4. Chaouachi M, Chupeau G, Berard A, McKhann H, Romaniuk M, Giancola S, Laval V, Bertheau Y, Brunel D (2008) A high-throughput multiplex method adapted for GMO detection. J Agric Food Chem 56:11596–11606

5. Liu J, Xing D, Shen X, Zhu D (2004) Detection of genetically modified organisms by electrochemiluminescence PCR method. Biosens Bioelectron 20:436–441

6. Mavropoulou AK, Koraki T, Ioannou PC, Christopoulos TK (2005) High-throughput double quantitative competitive polymerase chain reaction for determination of genetically modified organisms. Anal Chem 77:4785–4791

7. Morisset D, Dobnik D, Hamels S, Zel J, Gruden K (2008) NAIMA: target amplification strategy allowing quantitative on-chip detection of GMOs. Nucleic Acids Res 36:e118

8. Liu J, Guo J, Zhang H, Li N, Yang I, Zhang D (2009) Development and in-house validation of the event-specific polymerase chain reaction detection methods for genetically modified soybean MON89788 based on the cloned integration flanking sequence. J Agric Food Chem 57:10524–10530

9. Peano C, Bordoni R, Gulli M, Mezzelani A, Samson MC, Bellis GD, Marmiroli N (2005) Multiplex polymerase chain reaction and ligation detection reaction/universal array technology for the traceability of genetically modified organisms in foods. Anal Biochem 346:90–100

10. Ujhelyi G, Dijk JP, Prins TW, Voorhuijzen MM, Hoef AM, Beenen HG, Morisset D, Gruden K, Kok EJ (2012) Comparison and transfer testing of multiplex ligation detection methods for GM plants. BMC Biotechnol 12:4

11. Song Q, Jing H, Wu H, Zhou G, Kajiyama T, Kambara H (2010) Gene expression analysis on a photodiode array-based bioluminescence analyzer by using sensitivity-improved SRPP. Analyst 135:1315–1319

12. Song Q, Wu H, Feng F, Zhou G, Kajiyama T, Kambara H (2010) Pyrosequencing on nicked dsDNA generated by nicking endonucleases. Anal Chem 82:2074–2081

13. Wu H, Wu W, Chen Z, Wang W, Zhou G, Kajiyama T, Kambara H (2011) Highly sensitive pyrosequencing based on the capture of free adenosine 5′ phosphosulfate with adenosine triphosphate sulfurylase. Anal Chem 83:3600–3605

Chapter 30

Genotyping of Pathogenic Serotypes of *S. suis* with Pyrosequencing

Huiyong Yang, Huan Huang, Haiping Wu, Bingjie Zou, Qinxin Song, Guohua Zhou, and Hideki Kambara

Abstract

Streptococcus suis (*S. suis* for short) can cause a variety of infections in pigs, and the infections have brought about great losses in the swine industry and some cases of deaths in human beings. In order to rapidly diagnose and control the infections of *S. suis*, we designed a pyrosequencing-based assay to identify the serotypes of *S. suis*. In the assay, pyrosequencing is used to genotype most of the pathogenic serotypes of *S. suis* by detecting five informative regions on the *Chaperonin 60* (*cpn60*) gene and one species-specific region on the 16S rRNA gene, and further a few undistinguished serotypes by pyrosequencing were finely discriminated by multiplex PCR of serotype-specific fragments on the *cps* gene as well as species-specific fragments on the 16S rRNA gene. Through carefully designing the dispensing order of dNTP for each pyrosequencing reaction, the serotypes of *S. suis* could be discriminated by four pyrosequencing reactions within 3 h. Five reference serotypes and three clinical strains were successfully detected and genotyped by our assay. The results indicated that our assay is a reliable, information-rich diagnostic method for the accurate detection of *S. suis* serotypes.

Key words *Streptococcus suis*, Pyrosequencing, Genotyping, Pathogenic serotypes

1 Introduction

S. suis, recognized as an important swine pathogen worldwide, can cause various diseases such as meningitis, pneumonia, arthritis, septicemia with sudden death, and so on. According to the standard capsular reaction test, *S. suis* has been classified into **35** serotypes which are named as 1 to 34 and **1/2** [1–4], and the serotype **2** is considered to be the most virulent serotype [5, 6], while some strains of the serotypes **1/2, 9, 7, 1**, and **14** have been isolated from diseased and dead animals in different areas [7, 8]. Recently, infections caused by *S. suis* have brought about a few cases of death in human beings, although no evidence shows that the infection transmits directly among human beings [9, 10]. For example, in the summer of 2005, a severe epidemic caused by *S. suis* serotype **2**

Guohua Zhou and Qinxin Song (eds.), *Advances and Clinical Practice in Pyrosequencing*, Springer Protocols Handbooks, DOI 10.1007/978-1-4939-3308-2_30, © Springer Science+Business Media New York 2016

broke out in Sichuan province of China. The epidemic killed 38 persons and more than 600 pigs within 2 months, and then the epidemic spread rapidly in four additional provinces of China [10, 11].

In order to prevent and control the epidemic of *S. suis*, bacteriological and immunology diagnostic techniques are routinely used, but some of the techniques are time-consuming and require labs with a high level of biosafety [12]. Now, various molecular diagnostic methods have been developed for detecting the *S. suis* pathogen, such as real-time PCR, DNA hybridization, and electrophoresis of amplified targets [13, 14]. Although gel electrophoresis of PCR amplicons is the most convenient and simple method, some important serotypes may be difficult to identify correctly or clearly due to the similar size of the amplicons, for example, serotype **1** from serotype **14** and serotype **1/2** from serotype **2** [14, 15].

DNA sequencing is regarded as a straightforward way for pathogen diagnosis, and the Sanger method is routinely applied to DNA sequencing for its low cost and high accuracy. However, it is not necessary to sequence a long segment for genotyping a known pathogen. Pyrosequencing is a newly developed sequencing-by-synthesis technology, which can accurately and reproducibly read 20 bases from the 3′ end of the sequencing primer [16]. Although the sequencing length is very short, pyrosequencing has been widely used to detect pathogens, sequence variations, DNA methylations, and so on [12, 17–20]. With a new inexpensive instrumentation of pyrosequencing developed by our group [21, 22], a straightforward and simple pyrosequencing-based approach for identifying microbial pathogens is proposed here. Based on the method, we have successfully identified the serotypes of five reference strains and three clinical strains isolated from swine of Jiangsu province of China; the results indicated that pyrosequencing-based diagnosis is a potential method for the detection of pathogenic serotypes of *S. suis*.

2   Materials

1. Deoxynucleotides (dNTPs, 10 mM), 10× buffer (Mg^{2+} free), Taq DNA polymerase, and $MgCl_2$ were purchased from TaKaRa Biotech (Dalian, China).

2. Klenow fragment (Exonuclease Minus), polyvinylpyrrolidone (PVP), and QuantiLum recombinant luciferase were purchased from Promega (Madison, WI).

3. Dynabeads M-280 Streptavidin was from Dynal Biotech ASA (Oslo, Norway).

4. Apyrase VI, ATP sulfurylase, D-luciferin, bovine serum albumin (BSA), and adenosine 5′-phosphosulfate (APS) were obtained from Sigma (St. Louis, MO).

5. Sodium 2′-deoxyadenosine-5′-O-(1-triphosphate) (dATP-α-S), 2′-deoxy-guanosine-5′-triphosphate(dGTP),2′-deoxythymidine-5′-triphosphate (dTTP), and 2′-deoxycytidine-5′-triphosphate (dCTP) were purchased from Amersham Pharmacia Biotech.

6. All genomic samples of *S. suis* were obtained from Dr Feng Zheng (Nanjing CDC).

7. Genomic DNAs of five *S. suis* serotypes were isolated from reference strains: strain 2651 (serotype **1/2**, reference **a**), strain 5428 (serotype **1**, reference **b**), strain 735 (serotype **2**, reference **c**), strain 22083 (serotype **9**, reference **d**), and strain 13730 (serotype **14**, reference **e**).

8. The three clinical strains were isolated from pigs: one (named 05H33, sample **a**) from diseased pigs and others (named 05S68 and 0682 for samples **b** and **c**, respectively) from healthy pigs.

3 Methods

3.1 PCR

1. 50 μL of PCR mixture contains 5 μL of 10× PCR buffer, 1.2 mM MgCl₂ (pH 8.8), 0.24 mM of each dNTP, 2.0 U of Taq DNA polymerase, 50 ng of DNA template, 0.2 μM forward primer, and 0.4 μM reverse primer.

2. In the case of multiplex PCR, 0.4 μM of two forward primers (16S–172F and cps2J-s) and two reverse primers (16S–469R and cps2J-as) were added, and 0.8 μM forward primers (cps2E-s) and reverse primers (cps2E-as) were also added.

3. The reaction procedure consisted of incubation at 94 °C for 5 min, 35cycles of denaturation at 94 °C for 30 s, primer annealing at 52 °C for 30 s, and extension at 72 °C for 40 s, and lastly extension at 72 °C for 10 min.

4. For the PCR products, the detection was performed by electrophoresis in a 2 % agarose gel consisting of 0.5 mg L⁻¹ ethidium bromide with 1× TAE buffer for 10 min at a constant voltage of 100 V.

3.2 Pyrosequencing

1. ssDNA was prepared from 50 μL of biotinylated PCR products by using the standard protocol of magnetic beads. Then 1 μL of 10 μM sequencing primer was added into the beaded ssDNA for the annealing (95 °C for 30 s and 55 °C for 3 min) [18].

2. 100 μL of the reaction mixture containing 0.1 M tris–acetate (pH 7.7), 2 mM EDTA, 10 mM magnesium acetate, 0.1 % BSA, 1 mM dithiothreitol (DTT), 2 μM adenosine 5′-phosphosulfate (APS), 0.4 g L⁻¹ PVP, 0.4 mM D-luciferin, 0.2 mU L⁻¹ ATP sulfurylase, 3 mg L⁻¹ luciferase, 18 U mL⁻¹ Klenow fragment, and 1.6 U mL⁻¹ apyrase, 65 μL of reaction mixture, and 3 μL of beaded ssDNA template were added for one pyrosequencing reaction.

3. The pyrosequencing reaction uses a four-enzyme cascade system to produce a visible light that was detected by a photosensitive device photomultiplier tube (PMT) and the prototype of a small pyrosequencer made by Hitachi Ltd., Japan.

4 Typical Examples

4.1 S. suis Species Identification

The 16S rRNA gene was used for the identification of *S. Suis* species. To select the suitable sequence part for the identification, a comparison of the sequences of the 16S rRNA gene between 35 *S. suis* serotypes and other 16 common species of *Streptococcus* was carried out [23]. The segment 172–183 bp (bold capitals) is a species-dependent region in the 16S rRNA gene, and most of the 35 *S. suis* serotypes have similar sequences in the region. So we used this segment as a pyrosequencing target region. If the sequence of segment 172–183 bp in the amplicon corresponds to the expected sequence of the 16S rRNA gene fragment, the detected sample can be identified as *S. suis* species.

After PCR, the forward primer (16S–151F) was also used as the pyrosequencing primer for sequencing the target segment 172–183 bp, which is enough for species identification. According to the sequences on the NCBI, the theoretical pattern of the pyrogram of this 12-bp segment was simulated in Fig. 1a. Five reference strains (references a, b, c, d, and e) and three clinical isolates (samples a, b, and c) from swine of Jiangsu province of China were detected (*see* Fig. 1b for the typical pyrograms of reference c and three clinical strains). This indicates that the tested strains have the *S. Suis* species-specific sequence of "CAGTATTTACCG" illustrated in Fig. 1a.

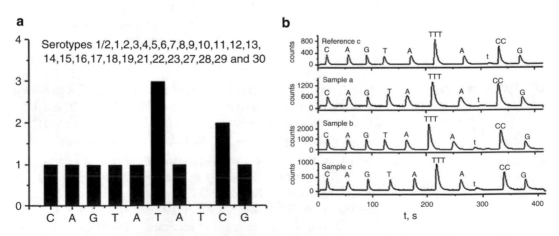

Fig. 1 Theoretical pattern (**a**) and pyrograms (**b**) obtained from pyrosequencing the 16S rRNA gene. The pyrogram of the samples showed that the samples all have the identical sequence "CAGTATTTACCG"

In comparison with the conventional PCR-based method, which directly used segments 172–193 bp and 469–490 bp as the target regions to design a pair of PCR primers for species identification, our sequencing-based assay is sensitive to all *S. suis* serotypes. This is because the segments 151–171 bp and 401–422 bp are highly conserved in *S. suis*, and all serotypes can be amplified by the primers. However, when using the conventional PCR for diagnosis, additional PCR primers are required for identifying serotypes 32, 33, and 34 as they have mutation sequences in the segment of 469–490 bp; in addition, it is very difficult to get positive results for serotypes 7 and 9 due to the mutated sequence in the segment of 469–490 bp.

4.2 S. suis Serotype Identification

It was reported that *S. suis* can be classified into 35 serotypes (types 1/2 and 1 through 34) according to capsular polysaccharide antigens [14]. The available sequence size of *cps* gene in GenBank with the accession numbers of AF237423 (serotype1) to AF237457 (serotype 34) is only 552 bp. In order to discriminate the serotypes by pyrosequencing, a 390-bp segment in this gene was selected as the target for serotype identification. After PCR amplification by the primer pair of cF-106 and cR-478, five regions (named CR177, CR248, CR418, CR443, and CR462) were sequenced by one multiplex pyrosequencing and two simplex pyrosequencing. Multiplex pyrosequencing was used to detect complementary sequences of CR462 and CR418 by annealing two sequencing primers simultaneously. The complexity of a pyrogram pattern in multiplex pyrosequencing is dependent on the dNTP dispensing order and the target sequences. As the reference sequences of CR462 and CR418 of all serotypes can be found from GenBank in advance, it is easy to design an optimal dNTP dispensing order for getting a simple pattern. By analyzing the GenBank sequences of all serotypes carefully, the optimum dispensing order of dNTP was designed as "A→G→C→A→T→A→T→C," and the dispensing order of the first four dNTPs ("A→G→C→A") is for pyrosequencing CR462, and the last four dNTPs ("T→A→T→C") is for pyrosequencing CR418. The possible serotype can be readily obtained by comparing the detected pyrograms with the sequencing patterns based on GenBank sequences. There are 13 different pyrogram patterns for all 35 serotypes. Serotypes 1, 7, 9, 16, 30, 32, 33, and 34 have unique patterns; thus, these serotypes can be specifically discriminated only by a multiplex pyrosequencing.

The protocol to detect the five reference strains and three clinical isolates by multiplex pyrosequencing was carried out. The comparison between the expected sequencing patterns (Fig. 2a) and the observed pyrograms (Fig. 2b) indicates that the reference strains b and d are serotypes 1 and 9, respectively, but no unique serotype can be identified for the other tested samples. In Fig. 2b, we found that not all peaks are proportional to the base numbers

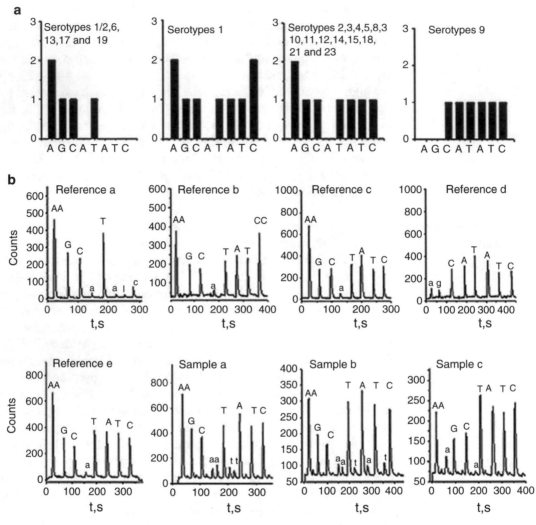

Fig. 2 Theoretical patterns (**a**) and pyrograms (**b**) obtained from multiplex pyrosequencing on CR466 and CR422 for the references a, b, c, d, and e and samples f, g, and h with the dispensing order of dNTP: "A→G→C→A→T→A→T→C"

in the homogeneous region; for example, in the pyrogram of sample b, the first three peaks give the sequence of "AAGC," while all the rest of the peaks are explained as the sequence of "TTAATTCC" based on the initial peak height ("AA"). This sequence is incorrect in comparison with the expected sequence of CR418. However, it is not a problem for getting a correct serotype if we read the pyrogram regions corresponding to two pyrosequencing primers individually. Although the final TATC peaks are actually higher than the initial one-base peaks, there is no difficulty to read a correct sequence of "TATC" only from TATC peak intensities. We believe that this issue is caused by the multiplexed pyrosequencing because an expected sequence was obtained when two simplex pyrosequencing was used [28–41].

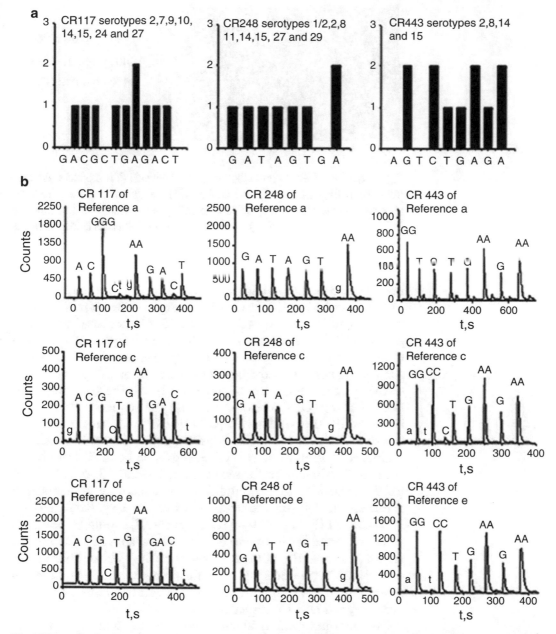

Fig. 3 Theoretical patterns (**a**) and pyrograms (**b**) of simplex pyrosequencing on CR117, CR248, and CR443 of the cpn60 gene for the references a, b, c, d, and e. The dNTP dispensing order on individual pyrosequencing is "G→A→C→G→C→T→G→A→G→A→C→T" for CR177, "A→T→A→G→T→G→A" for CR248, and "A→G→T→C→T→G→A→G→A" for CR443

For typing the reference stains that were not specifically identified in Fig. 2b, three simplex pyrosequencing was performed on the regions CR177, CR248, and CR443 of the cpn60 gene. By comparing the observed pyrograms of the three reference strains shown in Fig. 3b with the patterns from GenBank sequences (Fig. 3a), one of the reference strains (strain a) was concluded to

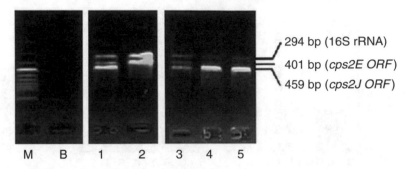

Fig. 4 Agarose gel electrophoretogram of the multiplex PCR products obtained from 16S rDNA, cps2E (ORF), and cps2J (ORF). *Lanes 1* and *2* were from the reference strains c and e, respectively; *lanes 3, 4,* and *5* were from three clinical isolates a, b, and c, respectively; *lane M* is a 100–1500-bp DNA ladder; *lane B* is blank control

be the serotype 1/2, while the two reference strains (strains c and e) could not be identified. They were only classified into a serotype group including serotypes 2, 14, and 15. Consequently, we need additional information for identifying the serotypes of the reference strains c and e. Based on the sequence data from GenBank, some serotypes have sequence deletions in serotype-specific ORFs of the cps gene. For example, serotype 14 has the sequence deletion of cps2J (ORF); serotype 15 has the sequence deletion of both cps2J (ORF) and cps2E (ORF); serotype 2 has no sequence deletion for cps2J (ORF) and cps2E (ORF). Therefore, a simple multiplex PCR on these two ORFs (cps2J and cps2E) can give an accurate discrimination for serotypes 2, 14, and 15. A 16S rRNA gene fragment was also amplified simultaneously as a control. Three amplicons with the sizes of 294 bp for 16S rRNA, 401 bp for cps2E (ORF), and 459 bp for cps2J (ORF) should be observed when the tested strain has no deletion of the above two ORFs. As shown in Fig. 4, the number of bands in the electrophoretogram of 3-plex PCR products was three for strains c (lane 1) and two for strains e (lane 2), suggesting that the reference strains c and e are of serotypes 2 and 14, respectively.

As the three clinical isolates were not classified into a unique serotype from the experiments shown in Fig. 2, simplex pyrosequencing was further performed on the regions of CR177 and CR248 in the cpn60 gene. As shown in Fig. 5, the three clinical isolates had the identical pyrogram patterns for both regions and were identified as one of the serotypes 2, 14, and 15 by GenBank sequences (Fig. 3a). For determining the serotypes of these three isolates precisely, the same 3-plex PCR as that used for finely genotyping reference strains c and e was carried out. As shown in Fig. 4 (lanes 3, 4, and 5), three bands were observed and indicated that all the three clinical isolates were of serotype 2. Consequently, the *S. suis* serotypes of five reference strains and three clinical isolates

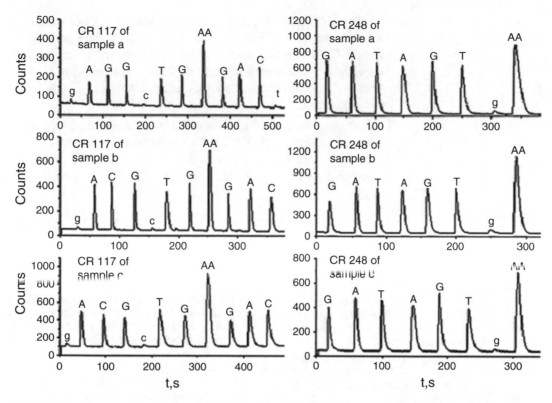

Fig. 5 The simplex pyrosequencing results in CR117 and CR248 of the cpn60 gene obtained from the clinical isolates a, b, and c. The dNTP dispensing order on individual pyrosequencing is "G→A→C→G→C→T→G →A→G→A→C→T" for CR 177 and "A→T→A→G→T→G→A" for CR24

were successfully identified by four pyrosequencing reactions coupled with a multiplex PCR assay.

As only 5 out of 35 serotypes of *S. suis* were detected by the proposed method, the work is preliminary, and more serotypes need to be tested in the future. Nevertheless, we believe that it is possible to identify most serotypes of *S. suis* with pyrosequencing according to the published sequences of all *S. suis* serotypes. Many serotypes have unique patterns according to the sequences of the target segments of 16SrRNA, CR177, CR248, CR418, CR443, and CR462. Although we do not think all bases of isolated strains meet the patterns from GenBank sequences, the results of the four pyrosequencing reactions can supply information on sequence variation in the samples and thus are very helpful for serotype identification.

5 Technical Notes

1. In order to design an efficient assay that can specifically discriminate the serotype of *S. suis*, the target regions selected for serotype detection should have serotype-specific sequences.

The 16SrRNA [24, 26] gene is considered as a gold standard for the broad identification of bacteria species; the Cpn60 gene [26, 27], which is found universally in bacteria and eukaryotes, has a characteristic that enables some regions to vary greatly between species; so this gene is suitable for serotype discrimination.

2. However, the Cpn60 gene is still not so sensitive to identification of all serotypes. We tried to use the *cps* gene for the fine discrimination of serotypes as the classification of *S. suis* serotypes is based on cps antigen reactions [25].

References

1. Perch B, Pedersen KB, Henrichsen J (1983) Serology of capsulated streptococci pathogenic for pigs: six new serotypes of Streptococcus suis. J Clin Microbiol 17:993–996

2. Higgins R, Gottschalk M, Boudreau M, Lebrun A, Henrichsen J (1995) Description of six new capsular types (29-34) of Streptococcus suis. J Vet Diagn Invest 7:405–406

3. Gottschalk M, Higgins R, Jacques M, Mittal KR, Henrichsen J (1989) Description of 14 new capsular types of Streptococcus suis. J Clin Microbiol 27:2633–2636

4. Gottschalk M, Higgins R, Jacques M, Beaudoin M, Henrichsen J (1991) Characterization of six new capsular types (23 through 28) of Streptococcus suis. J Clin Microbiol 29:2590–2594

5. Higgins R, Gottschalk M, Beaudoin M, Rawluk SA (1992) Distribution of Streptococcus suis capsular types in Quebec and western Canada. Can Vet J 33:27–30

6. Gottschalk M, Segura M (2000) The pathogenesis of the meningitis caused by Streptococcus suis: the unresolved questions. Vet Microbiol 76:259–272

7. Wisselink HJ, Smith HE, Stockhofe-Zurwieden N, Peperkamp K, Vecht U (2000) Distribution of capsular types and production of muramidase-released protein (MRP) and extracellular factor (EF) of Streptococcus suis strains isolated from diseased pigs in seven European countries. Vet Microbiol 74:237–248

8. Higgins R, Gottschalk M (1998) Distribution of Streptococcus suis capsular types in 1997. Can Vet J 39:299–300

9. Wangsomboonsiri W, Luksananun T, Saksornchai S, Ketwong K, Sungkanuparph S (2008) Streptococcus suis infection and risk factors for mortality. J Infect 57:392–396

10. Normile D (2005) Infectious diseases. WHO probes deadliness of China's pig-borne disease. Science 309:1308–1309

11. Ye C, Zhu X, Jing H, Du H, Segura M, Zheng H, Kan B, Wang L, Bai X, Zhou Y, Cui Z, Zhang S, Jin D, Sun N, Luo X, Zhang J, Gong Z, Wang X, Wang L, Sun H, Li Z, Sun Q, Liu H, Dong B, Ke C, Yuan H, Wang H, Tian K, Wang Y, Gottschalk MA, Xu J (2006) Streptococcus suis sequence type 7 outbreak, Sichuan, China. Emerg Infect Dis 12:1203–1208

12. Pourmand N, Diamond L, Garten R, Erickson JP, Kumm J, Donis RO, Davis RW (2006) Rapid and highly informative diagnostic assay for H5N1 influenza viruses. PLoS One 1, e95

13. Wisselink HJ, Joosten JJ, Smith HE (2002) Multiplex PCR assays for simultaneous detection of six major serotypes and two virulence-associated phenotypes of Streptococcus suis in tonsillar specimens from pigs. J Clin Microbiol 40:2922–2929

14. Marois C, Bougeard S, Gottschalk M, Kobisch M (2004) Multiplex PCR assay for detection of Streptococcus suis species and serotypes 2 and 1/2 in tonsils of live and dead pigs. J Clin Microbiol 42:3169–3175

15. Smith HE, Veenbergen V, van der Velde J, Damman M, Wisselink HJ, Smits MA (1999) The cps genes of Streptococcus suis serotypes 1, 2, and 9: development of rapid serotype-specific PCR assays. J Clin Microbiol 37:3146–3152

16. Ronaghi M (2001) Pyrosequencing sheds light on DNA sequencing. Genome Res 11:3–11

17. Wang C, Mitsuya Y, Gharizadeh B, Ronaghi M, Shafer RW (2007) Characterization of mutation spectra with ultra-deep pyrosequencing: application to HIV-1 drug resistance. Genome Res 17:1195–1201

18. Shaw RJ, Akufo-Tetteh EK, Risk JM, Field JK, Liloglou T (2006) Methylation enrichment pyrosequencing: combining the specificity of MSP with validation by pyrosequencing. Nucleic Acids Res 34:e78

19. Ronaghi M, Elahi E (2002) Pyrosequencing for microbial typing. J Chromatogr B Analyt Technol Biomed Life Sci 782:67–72

20. Innings A, Krabbe M, Ullberg M, Herrmann B (2005) Identification of 43 Streptococcus species by pyrosequencing analysis of the rnpB gene. J Clin Microbiol 43:5983–5991

21. Zhou GH, Gotou M, Kajiyama T, Kambara H (2005) Multiplex SNP typing by bioluminometric assay coupled with terminator incorporation (BATI). Nucleic Acids Res 33:e133

22. Zhou G, Kajiyama T, Gotou M, Kishimoto A, Suzuki S, Kambara H (2006) Enzyme system for improving the detection limit in pyrosequencing. Anal Chem 78:4482–4489

23. Rasmussen SR, Andresen LO (1998) 16S rDNA sequence variations of some Streptococcus suis serotypes. Int J Syst Bacteriol 48:1063–1065

24. Holden MT, Hauser H, Sanders M, Ngo TH, Cherevach I, Cronin A, Goodhead I, Mungall K, Quail MA, Price C, Rabbinowitsch E, Sharp S, Croucher NJ, Chieu TB, Mai NT, Diep TS, Chinh NT, Kehoe M, Leigh JA, Ward PN, Dowson CG, Whatmore AM, Chanter N, Iversen P, Gottschalk M, Slater JD, Smith HE, Spratt BG, Xu J, Ye C, Bentley S, Barrell BG, Schultsz C, Maskell DJ, Parkhill J (2009) Rapid evolution of virulence and drug resistance in the emerging zoonotic pathogen Streptococcus suis. PLoS One 4:e6072

25. Korczak B, Christensen H, EmLer S, Frey J, Kuhnert P (2004) Phylogeny of the family Pasteurellaceae based on rpoB sequences. Int J Syst Evol Microbiol 54:1393–1399

26. Hill JE, Gottschalk M, Brousseau R, Harel J, Hemmingsen SM, Goh SH (2005) Biochemical analysis, cpn60 and 16S rDNA sequence data indicate that Streptococcus suis serotypes 32 and 34, isolated from pigs, are Streptococcus orisratti. Vet Microbiol 107:63–69

27. Brousseau R, Hill JE, Prefontaine G, Goh SH, Harel J, Hemmingsen SM (2001) Streptococcus suis serotypes characterized by analysis of chaperonin 60 gene sequences. Appl Environ Microbiol 67:4828–4833

28. Marois C, Le Devendec L, Gottschalk M, Kobisch M (2007) Detection and molecular typing of Streptococcus suis in tonsils from live pigs in France. Can J Vet Res 71:14–22

29. Marois C, Le Devendec L, Gottschalk M, Kobisch M (2006) Molecular characterization of Streptococcus suis strains by 16S–23S intergenic spacer polymerase chain reaction and restriction fragment length polymorphism analysis. Can J Vet Res 70:94–104

30. Enright MC, Spratt BG, Kalia A, Cross JH, Bessen DE (2001) Multilocus sequence typing of Streptococcus pyogenes and the relationships between emm type and clone. Infect Immun 69:2416–2427

31. Enright MC, Spratt BG (1998) A multilocus sequence typing scheme for Streptococcus pneumoniae: identification of clones associated with serious invasive disease. Microbiology 144:3049–3060

32. Enright MC, Day NP, Davies CE, Peacock SJ, Spratt BG (2000) Multilocus sequence typing for characterization of methicillin-resistant and methicillin-susceptible clones of Staphylococcus aureus. J Clin Microbiol 38:1008–1015

33. Dingle KE, Colles FM, Wareing DR, Ure R, Fox AJ, Bolton FE, Bootsma HJ, Willems RJ, Urwin R, Maiden MC (2001) Multilocus sequence typing system for Campylobacter jejuni. J Clin Microbiol 39:14–23

34. Spratt BG (1999) Multilocus sequence typing: molecular typing of bacterial pathogens in an era of rapid DNA sequencing and the internet. Curr Opin Microbiol 2:312–316

35. Selander RK, Caugant DA, Ochman H, Musser JM, Gilmour MN, Whittam TS (1986) Methods of multilocus enzyme electrophoresis for bacterial population genetics and systematics. Appl Environ Microbiol 51:873–884

36. King SJ, Leigh JA, Heath PJ, Luque I, Tarradas C, Dowson CG, Whatmore AM (2002) Development of a multilocus sequence typing scheme for the pig pathogen Streptococcus suis: identification of virulent clones and potential capsular serotype exchange. J Clin Microbiol 40:3671–3680

37. Wu H, Wu W, Chen Z, Wang W, Zhou G, Kajiyama T, Kambara H (2011) Highly sensitive pyrosequencing based on the capture of free adenosine 5′ phosphosulfate with adenosine triphosphate sulfurylase. Anal Chem 83:3600–3605

38. Song Q, Wu H, Feng F, Zhou G, Kajiyama T, Kambara H (2010) Pyrosequencing on nicked dsDNA generated by nicking endonucleases. Anal Chem 82:2074–2081

39. Song Q, Jing H, Wu H, Zhou G, Kajiyama T, Kambara H (2010) Gene expression analysis on a photodiode array-based bioluminescence analyzer by using sensitivity-improved SRPP. Analyst 135:1315–1319

40. Kambara H, Zhou G (2009) DNA analysis with a photo-diode array sensor. Methods Mol Biol 503:337–360

41. Jing H, Song Q, Chen Z, Zou B, Chen C, Zhu M, Zhou G, Kajiyama T, Kambara H (2011) Dye-free microRNA quantification by using pyrosequencing with a sequence-tagged stem-loop RT primer. Chembiochem 12:845–849

Chapter 31

Differential Gene Expression Analysis of Breast Cancer by Combining Sequence-Tagged Reverse-Transcription PCR with Pyrosequencing

Xiaodan Zhang, Haiping Wu, Zhiyao Chen, Bingjie Zou, Qinxin Song, and Guohua Zhou

Abstract

It is an important way to understand the gene function by relatively comparing gene expression levels among different tissues or cells. For the moment, most of the methods for gene expression detection are based on dye labels. To establish a novel approach without using a dye label, a sequence-tagged reverse-transcription PCR coupled with pyrosequencing (SRPP) was proposed. In this technique, the gene from a source is labeled with a source-specific sequence by sequence-tagged reverse transcription (RT). Then PCR on the pools of each source-specific RT product was performed, and the source-specific amplicons were decoded by pyrosequencing. In the pyrogram, the sequence represents the gene source, and the peak intensity represents the relative expression level of the gene in the corresponding source. The accuracy of SRPP was confirmed by real-time quantitative PCR. Finally, the relative expression levels of the Egr1 gene among the diabetes model mice, obesity model mice, and normal mice were successfully detected. In comparison with real-time quantitative PCR, the advantages of SRPP include dye-free detection, inexpensive instruments, and simultaneous comparison of a given gene expressed in multiple sources.

Key words Sequence-tagged reverse transcription, Polymerase chain reaction, Pyrosequencing, Gene expression

1 Introduction

Differentially expressed genes are closely related to disease, and further study of gene expression levels among different tissues can reveal the pathogenesis of a disease. Up to now, main techniques developed for detecting gene expression levels include SAGE [1], real-time PCR [2, 3], microarray [4], and so on. However, these methods still have some drawbacks, such as the requirement of expensive equipments, the weak quantitative performance, and the limited number of sources which can be analyzed simultaneously. Pyrosequencing is a newly developed method for DNA sequencing, and it is based on a cascade of enzymatic reactions [5–8]. This

Guohua Zhou and Qinxin Song (eds.), *Advances and Clinical Practice in Pyrosequencing*, Springer Protocols Handbooks,
DOI 10.1007/978-1-4939-3308-2_31, © Springer Science+Business Media New York 2016

method does not require any fluorescent labels and has a good performance on quantification. For the moment, pyrosequencing has been used for single-nucleotide polymorphism (SNP) analysis, microbic genotyping, gene methylation analysis, and so on. Here, on the basis of pyrosequencing, a novel method, sequence-tagged reverse-transcription PCR coupled with pyrosequencing (SRPP), was developed to analyze the gene expression level. SRPP did not require the expensive equipments and could simultaneously detect the expression levels of a provided gene in multiple sources.

To quantitatively detect the gene expression level, sequence-tag labels were combined with pyrosequencing. There are two key points for the method: (1) to label and to distinguish the same gene from different sources with source-specific tags and (2) to quantitatively decode the sequence tags. In this study, a source-specific sequence labeled in an RT primer was used for discriminating a gene source and used pyrosequencing for quantitatively decoding the labeled sequences.

As shown in Fig. 1, the process includes the following steps: (1) Reverse transcription of mRNA extracted from different sources was carried out by the source-specific RT primers. There were four parts in the source-specific RT primers: a common tail in the 5′-end, a source-specific sequence with four bases (represented

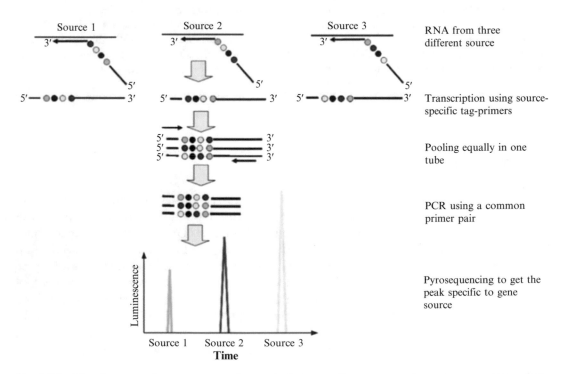

Fig. 1 Principle of comparative gene expression analysis by coupling sequence-tagged reverse-transcription PCR with pyrosequencing (SRPP)

by four circles with different colors in Fig. 1) in the middle, poly(T) n, plus two degenerate bases in the 3′-end. The function of these two degenerate bases is to fix the RT primer. Each source-specific sequence has the same base content but a different base order. (2) The sequence-labeled cDNAs from different sources were pooled in equal amount. (3) PCR amplification of the templates with a biotin gene-specific primer and a common primer was carried out. The other genes could be analyzed by simply changing the gene-specific primers. (4) The ssDNA templates were prepared by streptavidin-coated magnetic beads and by the pyrosequencing of labeled sequences. The base order in the pyrogram represents the gene source, and the peak intensity indicates the gene expression level in the corresponding gene source. The ratio of peak intensities is proportional to the relative abundance of the transcripts from different sources.

Because a same pair of primers was used to amplify the templates and the amplicons had the same base content except four bases with a different order, thus the TMs of cDNAs from different sources were completely identical. Unbiased PCR amplification on cDNA templates from different sources was achieved. Consequently, the relative ratios of SRPP peak intensities can accurately reflect the original expression levels of a given gene. In this study, the feasibility and accuracy of SRPP were investigated, and SRPP was applied to detect the differential expression level of the Egr1 gene in diabetes, obesity, and normal mouse.

2 Materials

1. Allegra 21R refrigerated centrifuge (Beckman Coulter, USA).

2. Gene Spec III spectrometer (Naka Instruments, Japan).

3. PTC-225 thermocycler PCR system (MJ Research, Inc., USA).

4. Opticon 2 System (MJ Research, Inc., USA)

5. A pyrosequencing device was developed in our laboratory [9, 10] (see Note 1).

6. Bioluminescence was detected by R6335 photomultiplier tube (Hamamatsu Photonics KK, Japan) and recorded by BPCL luminescence meter.

7. HotStarTaq DNA polymerase and Omniscript RT kit were purchased from Qiagen (Qiagen GmbH, Hilden, Germany).

8. TRIzol was purchased from Invitrogen (Shanghai, China).

9. D-luciferin, luciferase, ATP sulfurylase, apyrase, and adenosine 5′-phosphosulfate (APS) were purchased from Sigma (St. Louis, MO).

10. Dynabeads M-280 streptavidin (2.8 μm) was purchased from Dynal Biotech ASA (Oslo, Norway).

11. Exo⁻ Klenow fragment was purchased from Promega (Madison, WI).

12. All of the oligomers were synthesized and purified by Invitrogen (Shanghai, China).

13. The liver tissues of diabetes, obesity, and normal *Mus musculus* were provided by the College of Life Science, Nanjing Normal University.

3 Methods

3.1 RNA Extraction

1. Total RNA was extracted according to the standard procedures using TRIzol reagent. The purity and concentration of the extracted RNA were determined by a UV–vis spectrophotometer.

3.2 First-Strand cDNA Synthesis

1. 0.05–2.0 μg of total RNA was put into a nuclease-free tube, and DEPC–H_2O was added to the total volume of 12 μL (*see* **Note 2**).

2. The tube was incubated at 65 °C for 5 min and chilled on ice for 1 min.

3. Then a reaction mixture containing 0.5 mM of each dNTP, 1× RT buffer, 1 μM reverse- transcription primer, 0.5 U/μL RNase inhibitor, 10 U/μL omniscript reverse transcriptase, and DEPC–H_2O was added to the tube up to the total volume of 20 μL as mentioned earlier.

4. The reverse-transcription (RT) condition was at 37 °C for 60 min followed by 93 °C for 5 min to terminate the reaction.

3.3 Polymerase Chain Reaction for Specific Gene

1. First-strand cDNAs from different sources were mixed at equal proportion and used as templates of PCR. The common primer (CP, 5′-CCA TCT GTT CCC TCC CTG TC-3′) and a biotin-labeled gene-specific primer (GSP) were used for PCR.

2. Each 50 μL of PCR mixture contained 1 μL of template pool, 0.3 μM of each CP and GSP, 1.5 mM $MgCl_2$, 0.2 mM of each dNTP, 5 μL of 10× PCR buffer, 10 μL of 5 × Q solution, and 1.25 U of HotStarTaq DNA polymerase.

3. Amplification was performed according to the following protocol: denatured at 94 °C for 15 min, followed by 35 thermal reaction cycles (94 °C for 40 s; 60 °C for 40 s; 72 °C for 1 min). After the cycle reaction, the product was incubated at 72 °C for 10 min and held at 4 °C.

3.4 Preparation of Immobilized ssDNA Templates for Pyrosequencing

1. The immobilized ssDNA templates were prepared as follows: first, 5 μL of Dynabeads were washed by 100 μL of B&W buffer (10 mM tris–HCl, pH 7.5, 1 mM EDTA, 2.0 M NaCl) for twice and resuspended in 50 μL of B&W buffer, in which 50 μL of PCR products were added to a total volume of 100 μL.

2. Then the mixture was incubated at 37 °C for 30 min.

3. The Dynabeads immobilized with the PCR products were washed with 180 μL of H_2O for twice.

4. 20 μL of 0.1 M sodium hydroxide was added and left for 5 min, and ssDNA was obtained after denaturation.

5. The immobilized ssDNA templates were washed with 100 μL of B&W buffer and 100 μL of 1× annealing buffer, respectively, and resuspended in 8 μL of 1× annealing buffer.

6. Finally, 1 μM of sequencing primer was added into the aforementioned mixture and annealed at the following conditions: denatured at 94 °C for 30 s, followed by 55 °C for 3 min, and held at 4 °C for pyrosequencing.

3.5 Pyrosequencing

1. The pyrosequencing mixture contains 0.1 M tris–acetate (pH 7.7), 2 mM EDTA, 10 mM magnesium acetate, 0.1 % BSA, 1 mM dithiothreitol (DTT), 3 μM APS, 0.4 μg l^{-1} PVP, 0.4 mM D-luciferin, 0.2 μU/L ATP sulfurylase, 2×10^{-3} U/L apyrase, 18 μU/L Klenow fragment, and 14.6 mg/L luciferase.

---

4 Method Validation

4.1 Detection of the Levels of Egr1 Gene Expressed in the Livers of Diabetes Mice, Obese Mice, and Normal Mice

To evaluate the quantitative characteristics of pyrosequencing, an artificial single-strand template (5′-GGT TCC AAG TCA CCC CGC CCG C-3′) and a sequencing primer (5′-GCG GGC GGG G-3′) were designed. The 5′-end of the sequencing primer was completely complementary to the 3′-end of the single-strand template. After annealing, dNTPs were circularly added in an order of dTTP → dGTP → dATPα S → dCTP. The results indicated that the detected template sequence was "TGA CTT GGA ACC," and the signal intensity was proportional to the number of base pairs in the homogeneous area. It suggests that peak intensity is proportional to the amount of template. Therefore, the ratio of the peak heights can reflect the relative amount of templates. In this method, the relative gene expression was analyzed by measuring the ratios of the peak heights in the pyrograms based on the quantitative characteristics of pyrosequencing (*see* **Note 3**).

The key of SRPP assay in quantitative analysis is whether the PCR amplification of the templates produced by pooling sequence-labeled gene from different sources is unbiased. To investigate the quantitative characteristic of SRPP, we detected a series of three artificial sources from Actb gene, which was named as source-G, source-T, and source-C. The process was as follows: the total RNA was divided into three aliquots, which were transcribed with three source-specific primers RT-G (5′-CCG TCT GTT CCC TCC CTG TC *gatc* ttt ttt ttt ttt ttt VN-3′), RT-T (5′-CCA TCT GTT CCC TCC CTG TC *tacg* ttt ttt ttt ttt ttt VN-3′), and RT-C (5′-CCA TCT GTT CCC TCC CTG TC *catg* ttt ttt ttt ttt ttt VN-3′), respectively. As a result, the products were separately labeled with the source-specific sequence tags (the underlined italics) as source-G, source-T, and source-C. The PCR-template pools were prepared by mixing the three source-specific transcripts at the volume ratios of 1:1:1, 5:1:1, 1:5:1, and 1:1:5 (source-G/source-T/source-C). The pyrosequencing results are shown in Fig. 2; the bases "G," "T," and "C" represent source-G, source-T, and the source-C, respectively. The relative intensities of the three base signal peaks represent the relative expression of the Actb gene in three different sources. The difference in expression levels of the

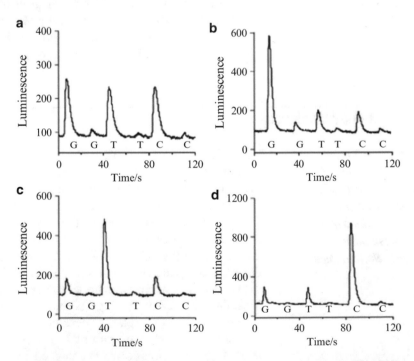

Fig. 2 Pyrograms of templates prepared by pooling three source-specific cDNAs at the ratios of 1:1:1 (**a**), 5:1:1 (**b**), 1:5:1 (**c**), and 1:1:5 (**d**), respectively. PCR was performed by using the common primer and the Actb gene-specific primer. Each dNTP was dispensed twice for detecting the background due to PPi impurity in dNTP solution

target gene in different sources could be obtained by calculating the ratio of the signal intensities (*see* **Note 4**).

The results of combination of the three source templates are shown in Fig. 2a; the signal peak intensity ratio is 1.1:1.0:1.0 (source-G/source-T/source-C), which is very close to the theoretical ratio of 1:1:1. As shown in Fig. 2b–d, the templates with the ratios of 5:1:1, 1:5:1, and 1:1:5 were determined as 5.1:1:10:1, 0.97:4.8:1, and 0.2:0.2:1, respectively. These results showed that the labeled templates mixed in different ratios were amplified equally, without any sequence bias. Therefore, the expression levels of the same gene from different sources can be detected by analyzing the ratio of amplified products.

To further evaluate the accuracy of the method, the results of SRPP were compared with those from real-time quantitative PCR. To evaluate the accuracy of the results, real-time quantitative PCR was used to detect the copies of the Actb gene in the kidney, the brain, and the heart tissues. The detected ratio was 37.8:22.0:40.2, which was very close to the results from SRPP, suggesting that SRPP is accurate enough for quantitatively comparing gene expression levels among different sources.

The SRPP was applied for investigating the Egr1 gene expression in model mice. The mice were divided into three groups as a, b, and c; each group has a diabetes mouse, an obese mouse, and a normal mouse. The RNA in the mouse liver was extracted and used as the RT template. By using the RT primers of RT-G, RT-C, and RT-T for the RT of each group, cDNAs from each group were labeled with the source-specific sequences, namely, diabetes-G, obese-T, and normal-C. After amplification with common primer CP and gene-specific primer bio-Egr1-GSP, pyrosequencing was performed for quantitative analysis. To eliminate difference in RNA yield, the quality and RT efficiency resulted from different sources, and the housekeeping gene Actb was used as an internal control gene to calibrate the difference. The three groups of mice were detected as mentioned earlier, and the results were showed in Fig. 3. The expression levels of the Egr1 gene and the Actb gene in the liver of diabetes mouse, obese mouse, and normal mouse were calculated by the content normalization. The relative expression ratios of the Egr1 gene among the three mice are 2.41:0.34:1.22 for group a, 0.78:0.49:2.18 for group b, and 0.54:0.90:1.56 for group c after the calibration of the Actb gene. The copy numbers of the Egr1 gene and the Actb gene in mice liver were detected by real-time PCR simultaneously, and the data were calibrated by the same way. The relative expression ratios were 2.50:0.39:1.08, 0.81:0.47:2.46, and 0.56:0.87:1.69 for the three groups, respectively. This experiment indicates that the SRPP can be effectively applied to differential gene expression profiling.

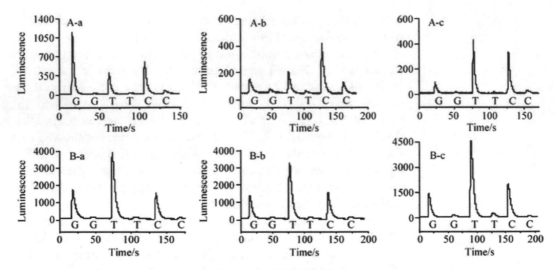

Fig. 3 Pyrograms for detecting the relative expression levels of the Egr1 gene (**a**) and the Actb gene (**b**) among the mouse livers of three different groups, a, b, and c. Bases G, T, and C represent sources from diabetic mouse, obese mouse, and normal mouse, respectively

5   Technical Notes

1. The instrument consisted of a reaction module, a photomultiplier tube (R6335, Hamamatsu Photonics KK, Japan), and a recorder (BPCL, the Institute of Biophysics, Chinese Academy of Sciences, China). The reaction chamber was located in the middle of the reaction module, which connected with four deoxynucleotide triphosphate (dNTP) reservoirs by capillary. A flow of dNTP was injected into the reaction chamber when adding a pressure through the syringe onto the dNTP reservoir.

2. The same amount of total RNA from different sources was used for cDNA synthesis by SuperScript II RNase H reverse transcriptase.

3. In the same pyrosequencing reaction system, the signal intensity is proportional to the amount of ATP, which is proportional to the number of incorporated dNTPs [11]; thus, the sequence of the DNA template can be determined from the signal intensity in the pyrograms.

4. dNTP is not so stable that a small amount of PPi due to dNTP degradation is produced. The noises by the unexpected PPi might interfere to the accuracy of SRPP. Accordingly, each dNTP was dispensed twice to obtain two peaks corresponding to the strand extension and background signals, respectively. The background should be deducted from the strand extension signals [12].

References

1. Velculescu VE, Zhang L, Vogelstein B, Kinzler KW (1995) Serial analysis of gene expression. Science 270:484–487

2. Karet FE, Charnock-Jones DS, Harrison-Woolrych ML, O'Reilly G, Davenport AP, Smith SK (1994) Quantification of mRNA in human tissue using fluorescent nested reverse-transcriptase polymerase chain reaction. Anal Biochem 220:384–390

3. Ginzinger DG (2002) Gene quantification using real-time quantitative PCR: an emerging technology hits the mainstream. Exp Hematol 30:503–512

4. Schena M, Shalon D, Davis RW, Brown PO (1995) Quantitative monitoring of gene expression patterns with a complementary DNA microarray. Science 270:107–470

5. Ronaghi M (2001) Pyrosequencing sheds light on DNA sequencing. Genome Res 11:3–11

6. Wang WP, Wu HP, Zhou GH (2008) Detection of avian influenza A virus using Pyrosequencing. Chinese J Anal Chem 36:775–780

7. Agah A, Aghajan M, Mashayekhi F, Amini S, Davis RW, Plummer JD, Ronaghi M, Griffin PB (2004) A multi-enzyme model for Pyrosequencing. Nucleic Acids Res 32(21):e166–e180

8. Yang HY, Xi T, Liang C, Chen ZY, Xu DB, Zhou GH (2009) Preparation of Single-Stranded DNA for Pyrosequencing by Linear-after-the-Exponential-Polymerase Chain Reaction. Chinese J Anal Chem 37:489–494

9. Zhou GH, Gu ZL, Zhang JB (2002) P53 gene mutation detection by bioluminometry assay. Acta Pharm Sin 37:41–45

10. Zhou GH, Kamahori M, Okano K, Harada K, Kambara H (2001) Miniaturized pyrosequencer for DNA analysis with capillaries to deliver deoxynucleotides. Electrophoresis 22:3497–3504

11. Aljada A, Ghanim H, Mohanty P, Kapur N, Dandona P (2002) Insulin inhibits the proinflammatory transcription factor early growth response gene-1 (Egr) expression in mononuclear cells (MNC) and reduces plasma tissue factor (TF) and plasminogen activator inhibitor-1 (PAI-1) concentrations. J Clin Endocrinol Metab 87:1419–1422

12. Hotamisligil GS, Shargill NS, Spiegelman BM (1993) Adipose expression of tumor necrosis factor-alpha: direct role in obesity-linked insulin resistance. Science 259:87–91

Chapter 32

Detection of Avian Influenza A Virus by Pyrosequencing

Weipeng Wang, Haiping Wu, Bingjie Zou,
Qinxin Song, and Guohua Zhou

Abstract

A pyrosequencing method was developed for rapidly detecting avian influenza A virus and predicting the pathogenicity. The avian influenza A virus and its subtype were preliminarily determined by PCR on a species-specific sequence of the *M* gene and a subtype-specific sequence of the *HA* gene containing a cleaving site, respectively. The results obtained by PCR were further validated via the pyrosequencing method. As apyrase and Klenow play an important role in pyrosequencing, their concentrations were optimized. The results indicate that the nonspecific signals were effectively suppressed using 1.6 U mL^{-1} apyrase and a readable sequence length of 33 bases was obtained with 90 U mL^{-1} Klenow. On the basis of the optimum pyrosequencing system, four specimens including an H5N1 subtype with high pathogenicity and three specimens of avian influenza A H9N2 subtype with low pathogenicity were confirmed. This method is accurate, fast, and can be used efficiently for identifying the pathogenicity of the avian influenza A virus.

Key words Avian influenza A virus, Subtype, Pathogenicity, Pyrosequencing

1 Introduction

Avian influenza is an avian acute infectious disease caused by *Orthomyxoviridae* influenza A virus and is ranked as class A potent infectious disease by the Office International Des Epizooties (OIE) and the Livestock and Poultry Epidemic Prevention of China. Tremendous economic losses in the poultry industry and serious threat to human health have been caused by the outbreak and spread of the highly pathogenic avian influenza A virus of subtypes H5 and H9 in China and many other countries. Thus, it is imperative to develop a fast and accurate method for detecting avian influenza A virus, which has become a much sought after research. At present, laboratory diagnosis of avian influenza virus is confirmed to be the only effective way, including the traditional detection methods and the molecular biologic detection method. Traditional detection methods mainly involve the isolation and culture of the virus [1], with serological diagnosis, such as enzyme-linked immunosorbent

Guohua Zhou and Qinxin Song (eds.), *Advances and Clinical Practice in Pyrosequencing*, Springer Protocols Handbooks,
DOI 10.1007/978-1-4939-3308-2_32, © Springer Science+Business Media New York 2016

assay (ELISA) [2], indirect hemagglutination inhibition test [3], and so on. However, these methods are tedious, time-consuming, and have poor reproducibility. In recent years, the methods based on molecular biology have been developed rapidly, including the PCR technique [4], real-time PCR [5], nucleic acid sequence-based amplification/electrochemiluminescent detection method (NASBA/ECL) [6], and DNA sequencing. By using the conventional PCR or real-time PCR technique, the golden standard of molecular diagnostics, the gene sequence information, cannot be obtained; DNA sequencing is not suitable to detect large-scale samples because of a long detection time and high cost. Pyrosequencing [7, 8] is a technique for DNA sequencing based on the bioluminescence analysis of pyrophosphate (PPi), that is, after each of the four different deoxyribonucleotide triphosphates (dNTP) is added in turn, extension occurs and equal molar PPi is released by the catalysis of DNA polymerase, if the dNTP is complementary to the base of the template. The released PPi can react with adenosine-5′-phosphosulfate (APS) to convert to adenosine triphosphate (ATP) under the enzyme catalysis of ATP sulfurylase. Then fluorescence is produced by luciferin and luciferase activated by ATP, and the fluorescence intensity is proportional to the number of combined dNTPs. If no dNTP is complementary to the template, no fluorescence will be produced. According to these procedures, the sequence of the target following the sequencing primer is determined. Apyrase is used in pyrosequencing for degradation of both the uncombined dNTPs and the produced ATP before the next extension. The pyrosequencing technique is very useful for real-time detection of a short sequence with advantages of quantitative accuracy and easy automation and to completely achieve high-throughput and rapid detection of large-scale samples. Here, pyrosequencing has been taken as a detecting platform to develop sequencing-based method for detecting avian influenza A virus and for discriminating the pathogenicity of the avian influenza A virus.

2 Materials

1. A cDNA sample of avian influenza A virus subtype H5N1 was provided by Yangzhou University, Yangzhou, China; three cDNA specimens of avian influenza A virus subtype H9N2 (A/HeNan/2/04, A/HeNan/3/04, and A/HeNan/5/04) were provided by the College of Veterinary Medicine, China Agricultural University, Beijing, China.

2. PTC-225 Thermal Cycler (MJ Research, Inc., Massachusetts, USA); POWER PAC1000 Electrophoresis System (Bio-Rad Laboratories, Inc., CA, USA); GeneGenius BioImaging Systems (Syngene, Co., Ltd., Cambridge, UK); Beads Combiner and Pyrosequencer (Homemade).

3. Taq DNA polymerase (TaKaRa Biotechnology (Dalian) Co. Ltd.).

4. Agarose (LP0028A, Oxoid Ltd., Hampshire, England).

5. Tris base and ethidium bromide (EtBr) (Sangon Biotech Co. Shanghai, China).

6. Washing buffer: 10 mM Tris–HCl, 1.0 mM EDTA, 1.0 M NaCl, pH 7.5.

7. Annealing buffer (1×): 10 mM Tris–HCl, 1.0 mM EDTA, pH 8.0.

8. Super paramagnetic beads (Dynabeads M-280 Streptavidin, Dynal AS, Oslo, Norway).

9. Polyvinylpyrrolidone (PVP), exonuclease-deficient (exo⁻) Klenow DNA polymerase, and deoxyribonucleotide triphosphate mixes (dNTPs) Promega (WI, USA).

10. D-luciferin, luciferase, ATP sulfurylase, apyrase, adenosine-5′-phosphosulfate (APS), and bovine serum albumin (BSA), Sigma (St. Louis, MO, USA).

11. 2′-Deoxyadenosine-5′-O-(1-thiotriphosphate) sodium salt (dATP-α-S) was purchased from Amersham Pharmacia Biotech (Amersham, UK).

3 Methods

3.1 Design of Gene-Specific Primers

1. Avian influenza A virus is classified as an *Orthomyxoviridae* influenza A virus, composed of an eight-segmented genome of single-stranded negative-sense RNA sequences, which are named PB2, PB1, PA, HA, NP, M, and NS according to the fragment sizes. As the *M* gene is a highly conserved sequence, a pair of primers specific to the *M* gene was designed for the preliminary determination of avian influenza A virus.

2. As there are many variations on the HA and NA genes, the avian influenza A virus is divided into 16 H subtypes (H1–H16) and nine N subtypes (N1–N9) [9]. The prerequisite for avian influenza A virus infecting cells is that the hemagglutinin (HA) protein can be cleaved into two peptides of HA1 and HA2, and the cleaving pathway is a key factor of the pathogenicity of avian influenza A virus. For the highly pathogenic avian influenza A virus, there are a number of alkaline amino acids near the cleaving site of the HA protein, which are more susceptible to be cleaved, but the lowly pathogenic avian influenza A virus does not have this characteristic.

3. Comparing the sequences of the HA gene of subtypes H5 and H9 with those published on the National Center for Biotechnology Information (NCBI) web (http://www.ncbi.nlm.nih.gov/sit es/entrez/) with a software of clustalwl.83.xp, it has been found that the HA1 segment (upstream of the

Table 1
The sequences of primers used for gene-specific PCR

Gene	Primer	Sequence (5′ → 3′)
M	Biotin-MF	Biotin-GTGCCCAGTGAGCGAGGAC
	MR	AGTTGCCATCTGTCTGTGAG
HA gene of subtype H5	Biotin-H5F	Biotin-TATGCATACAAAATTGTCAAG
	HR	ACCTGCTATAGCTCCAAATAG
HA gene of subtype H9	Biotin-H9F	Biotin-TTCAGGAGAGAGCCACGGAAG

cleaving site) of this gene is poorly homologous and the HA2 segment (downstream of the cleaving site) is highly homologous. Therefore, two primers hybridizing to the HA1 segment, each specific to subtype H5 or subtype H9, and a common primer hybridizing to the HA2 segment were designed to amplify a sequence fragment containing the cleaving site. The primer sequences are listed in Table 1.

3.2 Gene-Specific PCR Amplification

1. 100 μL of each PCR reaction mixture contained 20 μM each of primers, 0.5 mM of each dNTP, 3.0 mM $MgCl_2$ 1× buffer, 2.5 U of Taq DNA polymerase, and 100–500 ng of cDNA template (*see* **Note 1**).

2. PCR cycling was carried out as follows: 94 °C for 3 min, followed by 30 cycles of 94 °C for 10 s, 60 °C (for the *M* gene and the *HA* gene of subtype H5) or 55 °C (for the *HA* gene of subtype H9) for 20 s, and 72 °C for 40 s. Final extension was completed at 72 °C for 7 min.

3. PCR products of 2 μL were analyzed by electrophoresis on a 2.0 % agarose gel containing 0.5 mg L^{-1} ethidium bromide at 100 V for 15 min in 1× TAE buffer.

3.3 Preparation of Single-Stranded DNA Template

1. 10 μL of streptavidin-coated paramagnetic beads was washed in 100 μL of washing buffer twice, and the supernatants were removed.

2. 90 μL of the biotinylated products were immobilized on the streptavidin-coated paramagnetic beads and suspended in 90 μL washing buffer, which was incubated in a combiner of beads at 37 °C for 1 h. During this process, the PCR tubes were gently vibrated to keep the beads in a state of suspension.

3. The PCR products immobilized on the beads were washed with H_2O four to eight times and then were denatured with 0.1 M NaOH. The supernatant was discarded.

4. Washed with 100 μL of washing buffer twice and with 100 μL of 1× annealing buffer once.

5. Added pyrosequencing primer (20 pmol) to the captured strand that was annealed at 93 °C for 30 s and 55 °C for 3 min.

3.4 Pyrosequencing

1. Primed target DNA was added to the final volume of 100 μL, of the pyrosequencing reaction mixture containing 0.1 M Tris–acetate (pH 7.7), 2.0 mM EDTA, 10 mM Mg (Ac)$_2$, 0.1 % BSA, 1.0 mM dithiothreitol, 2.0 μM APS, 0.4 g L^{-1} PVP (360,000), 0.4 mM D-luciferin, 1.6 mU L^{-1} ATP sulfurylase, 1.6 U mL^{-1} apyrase (*see* **Note 2**), 27 U mL^{-1} of exonuclease-deficient (exo-) Klenow DNA polymerase (*see* **Note 3**), and 22.35 mg L^{-1} purified luciferase.

2. The pyrosequencing procedure was carried out by stepwise elongation of the primer strand upon sequential addition of dATP-α-S, dCTP, dTTP, and dGTP under the conditions of pH 7.7 and room temperature.

4   Method Validation

4.1 Evaluation of Specificity of Gene-Specific Primers

To evaluate the specificity of gene-specific primers, a human genomic DNA sample, a cDNA sample of avian influenza A virus subtype H5N1, and three cDNA specimens of avian influenza A virus subtype H9N2 were used as templates for amplification with each of the three primer-pairs of Biotin-MF/MR, Biotin-H5F/HR, and Biotin-H9F/HR, respectively. Blank control experiments were also performed in parallel. The electrophoretograms of the PCR products are shown in Fig. 1. The primer-pair of Biotin-MF/MR could specifically amplify the M gene of all the four avian influenza A virus specimens (*see* lanes 3–6 in Fig. 1a), indicating that the samples containing avian influenza A virus could be preliminarily discriminated

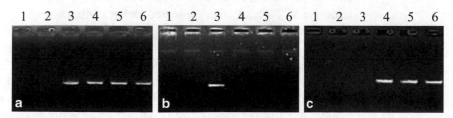

Fig. 1 The agarose gel electrophoretograms of the amplicons from gene-specific primers. (**a**) The amplicons from the primers specific to the *M* gene, (**b**) the amplicons from the primers specific to the *HA* gene of subtype H5, (**c**) the amplicons from the primers specific to the *HA* gene of subtype H9. *Lane 1*, blank control; *lane 2*, the amplicon of human genomic DNA; *lane 3*, the amplicon of H5N1 specimen; *lanes 4–6*, the amplicons of H9N2 specimens

by means of this pair of primers specific to the *M* gene. Moreover, the HA gene of avian influenza A virus subtypes H5N1 and H9N2 could be specifically amplified by the primer-pairs of Biotin-H5F/ HR (*see* lane 3 in Fig. 1b) and Biotin-H9F/HR (*see* lanes 4–6 in Fig. 1c), respectively. As shown in lanes 1 and 2 in Fig. 1, nonspecific amplicons were not found for the human genomic DNA sample and the blank controls. These results indicated that these three pairs of gene-specific primers were highly specific.

4.2 Effect of Concentration of Apyrase on Pyrosequencing

Apyrase plays a key role in pyrosequencing. First, the sequencing cycle is enabled by apyrase. In pyrosequencing, the residual dNTP in the previous reaction must be digested before the addition of dNTP; otherwise, the residual dNTP will participate in the next reaction, resulting in the failure of the sequencing cycle. As apyrase in the pyrosequencing reaction system can degrade the residual dNTP after the polymerization reaction, sequencing can be carried out continuously. Moreover, benefiting from apyrase, the sequencing signal is shaped into a peak. Without apyrase, much more ATP will be produced in the pyrosequencing reaction, resulting in the accumulation and overflow of the signal, which prevents the sequencing from being conducted. As apyrase can degrade both dNTPs and ATP, a peaked signal can be obtained.

Taking the pyrosequencing system for detecting the *M* gene of avian influenza A virus subtype H5N1 as an example, we have optimized the concentration of apyrase to 0.5, 1.0, 1.6, 2.0, 3.0, and 6.0 U mL^{-1}, respectively. The pyrosequencing results are shown in Fig. 2, indicating that the signal intensity decreases gradually with increasing the concentration of apyrase. Moreover, if a low concentration of apyrase is used, false signals will occur (Fig. 2a), because dNTPs are not completely digested by apyrase after each extension and the residual dNTPs participate in the next reaction. After increasing the concentration of apyrase, the residual dNTPs are almost totally degraded, and the signals of false extension are obviously decreased (Fig. 2b). However, in case the concentration of apyrase is too high, incomplete extension phenomenon will be found as reported before, because the added dNTPs have been digested before extension [10]. In this study, no incomplete extension phenomenon has been observed for 6.0 U mL^{-1} apyrase probably because a large amount of dNTPs have been used. The optimum concentration of apyrase not only relies on the concentration of dNTP but also on the concentration and extension efficiency of Klenow. It has been found that the concentration of apyrase in a large range is feasible, as long as the residual dNTP is completely degraded in the interval of each of the two consecutive dNTP injections. Considering the detection cost, 1.6 U mL^{-1} apyrase have been used for routine analysis.

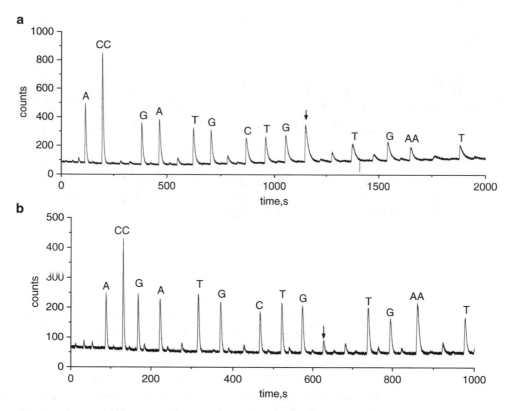

Fig. 2 Effect of concentration of apyrase on extension signal. Concentrations of apyrase are 0.5 and 2.0 U mL^{-1} in (**a**) and (**b**), respectively. dNTPs are added according to the order of "C-T-G-A." Additional dispensing of dNTP is performed after the occurrence of a peak to complete the extension reaction

4.3 Effect of Concentration of Klenow on Pyrosequencing

In pyrosequencing, the accuracy of a readout sequence relies on the extension reaction. The polymerase used in pyrosequencing is a key factor for the accurate extension reaction and must meet the following conditions: (1) It has a highly specific polymerizing ability for the complementary bases. No extension signal occurs if the added dNTP is not complementary to the target. If this is not the case, the consecutive extension reaction cannot be performed [11]. (2) It has no exonuclease activity, because the extended DNA strand can be digested by a polymerase with 3′–5′ exonuclease activity. (3) The extension by the polymerase can be carried out at room temperature as some heat-labile enzymes are used in pyrosequencing. There are two commercial polymerases, Klenow and Sequenase 2.0 [12], meeting these conditions. As Klenow is relatively cheap, the authors have used this for routine detection.

Taking the pyrosequencing system for detecting the M gene of avian influenza A virus subtypes H5N1 as an example, we optimized the concentration of Klenow to be 9.0, 27, 54 and 90 U mL^{-1}, respectively. As shown in Fig. 3, the concentration of Klenow had a great effect on the sequencing length, which was gradually increased

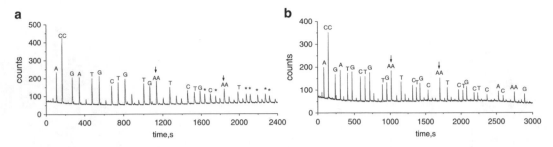

Fig. 3 The effect of the concentration of Klenow on extension signal. The concentrations of Klenow are 9 and 90 U/mL in **a** and **b**, respectively. The dNTPs were added according to the order of "C-T-G-A." More dNTP was added after the occurrence of peak to complete the extension reaction. The *arrows* represent the extension signals of double A; the *stars* represent the nonspecific signals

with increasing the concentration of Klenow. For example, the readable sequence length was 12 bases when the concentration of Klenow was 9.0 U/mL (Fig. 3a), and a readable sequence length of 33 bases was obtained when the concentration of Klenow was 90 U mL^{-1} (Fig. 3b). If the concentration of Klenow was too low, a number of nonspecific signals (Fig. 3a) would be produced, which would interfere with the accurate readout of the sequencing signals, resulting in the limitation of readable sequence length. In addition, the concentration of Klenow has the greatest effect on the extension efficiency of dATP-α-S. For example, the extension signal intensity of two repeated dATP-α-S can be clearly discriminated in Fig. 3b, but it is similar to that of the other single base as shown in Fig. 3a, indicating that the polymerization ability of Klenow is comparatively low for dATP-α-S. Therefore, an extension signal of dATP-α-S with an intensity proportional to the number of bases cannot be obtained when the concentration of Klenow is too low. This can be overcome using a high concentration of Klenow, which is beneficial for lengthening the readout sequence of pyrosequencing. Considering the detection cost, 27 U mL^{-1} Klenow have been used for routine analysis, with a readable sequence length of 24 bases.

4.4 Detection of M Gene and HA Gene of Avian Influence A Virus

By using the PCR amplification technique coupled with electrophoresis analysis, only the information of the length of PCR products can be obtained. For further accurate detection of avian influenza A virus, the DNA sequence of the gene-specific PCR products must be detected. Therefore, a pyrosequencing method has been established for the determination of the sequences of available samples. The sequence of a sample has been detected as 5′-ACC GAT GCT GTG AAT CTG CAA TCT-3′, and the sequences of the other three samples are all the same, 5′-ACC TAT GGT GTG AAT CAG CAA TCT-3′. To judge whether or not these samples are avian influenza A virus and to discriminate their subtypes, the detected sequences are compared with the sequences published in NCBI, by using BLAST program. It has been found that all four detected sequences have the character of the M gene of avian influenza A virus, indicating that all the four detected samples are avian influenza A virus. The sequence near the cleaving site of a sample has been determined as 5′-TCC TCT TTT TCT TCT TCT TTC TCT T-3′, and it is then compared with the sequences published in NCBI by right of the BLAST program. The result indicates that this sample is avian influenza A virus subtype H5. The detected sequence is translated into the amino acid sequence of RERRRKRG by virtue of a software, BioXM 2.2 (http://bioxm.go.nease.net/). According to the new pathogenicity identification standard of the avian influenza A virus, raised by the OIE, this sample has a potentially high pathogenicity. The sequences near the cleaving sites of the other three samples have been determined as being the same as 5′-TCC TCT ACT TGA TCT AGC AGG CAC ATT-3′. They are then compared with the sequences published in NCBI by right of the BLAST program. The results indicate that these samples are avian influenza A virus subtype H9. The detected sequences have been translated into the amino acid sequence of NVPARSSRG by means of BioXM 2.2, indicating that these samples have relatively low pathogenicity. For further confirmation, each sample has been detected by the Sanger's sequencing method. The typing results are completely consistent with those obtained by pyrosequencing.

5   Technical Notes

1. A 300 bp DNA fragment in the *M* gene, a 259 bp DNA fragment in the *HA* gene of subtype H5, and a 235 bp DNA fragment in the *HA* gene of subtype H9 were amplified by gene-specific PCR, respectively.

2. A low concentration of apyrase is used; false signals will occur, because dNTPs are not completely digested by apyrase after each extension; and the residual dNTPs participate in the next reaction. After increasing the concentration of apyrase, the residual dNTPs are almost totally degraded, and the signals of false extension are obviously decreased. However, in case the concentration of apyrase is too high, incomplete extension phenomenon will be found as reported before, because the added dNTPs have been digested before extension. Considering the detection cost, 1.6 U mL^{-1} apyrase have been used for routine analysis.

3. The concentration of Klenow had a great effect on the sequencing length, which was gradually increased with increasing the concentration of Klenow. In addition, the concentration of Klenow has the greatest effect on the extension efficiency of dATP-α-S. Considering the detection cost, 27 U mL^{-1} Klenow have been used for routine analysis, with a readable sequence length of 24 bases.

References

1. Cox NJ, Subbarao K (1999) Influenza. Lancet 354:1277–1282
2. Kaiser L, Briones MS, Hayden FG (1999) Performance of virus isolation and Directigen Flu A to detect influenza A virus in experimental human infection. J Clin Virol 14:191–197
3. Boivin G, Hardy I, Kress A (2001) Evaluation of a rapid optical immunoassay for influenza viruses (FLU OIA test) in comparison with cell culture and reverse transcription-PCR. J Clin Microbiol 39:730–732
4. Magnard C, Valette M, Aymard M, Lina B (1999) Comparison of two nested PCR, cell culture, and antigen detection for the diagnosis of upper respiratory tract infections due to influenza viruses. J Med Virol 59:215–220
5. Payungporn S, Chutinimitkul S, Chaisingh A, Damrongwantanapokin S, Buranathai C, Amonsin A, Theamboonlers A, Poovorawan Y (2006) Single step multiplex real-time RT-PCR for H5N1 influenza A virus detection. J Virol Methods 131:143–147
6. Lau LT, Banks J, Aherne R, Brown IH, Dillon N, Collins RA, Chan KY, Fung YW, Xing J, Yu AC (2004) Nucleic acid sequence-based amplification methods to detect avian influenza virus. Biochem Biophys Res Commun 313: 336–342
7. Zhou GH, Gu ZL, Zhang JB (2002) P53 gene mutation detection by bioluminometry assay. Acta Pharm Sin 37:41–45
8. Zhang XD, Wu HP, Zhou GH (2006) Pyrosequencing and its application in genetical analysis. Chinese J Anal Chem 34:582–586
9. Fouchier RA, Munster V, Wallensten A, Bestebroer TM, Herfst S, Smith D, Rimmelzwaan GF, Olsen B, Osterhaus AD (2005) Characterization of a novel influenza A virus hemagglutinin subtype (H16) obtained from black-headed gulls. J Virol 79:2814–2822
10. Zhou G, Kajiyama T, Gotou M, Kishimoto A, Suzuki S, Kambara H (2006) Enzyme system for improving the detection limit in pyrosequencing. Anal Chem 78:4482–4489
11. Frey MW, Sowers LC, Millar DP, Benkovic SJ (1995) The nucleotide analog 2-aminopurine as a spectroscopic probe of nucleotide incorporation by the Klenow fragment of Escherichia coli polymerase I and bacteriophage T4 DNA polymerase. Biochemistry 34:9185–9192
12. Derbyshire V, Freemont PS, Sanderson MR, Beese L, Friedman JM, Joyce CM, Steitz TA (1988) Genetic and crystallographic studies of the 3′,5′-exonucleolytic site of DNA polymerase I. Science 240:199–201

Chapter 33

Genotyping of Alcohol Dehydrogenase Gene by Pyrosequencing Coupled with Improved LATE-PCR Using Human Whole Blood as Starting Material

Zheng Xiang, Yunlong Liu, Xiaoqing Xing, Bingjie Zou, Qinxin Song, and Guohua Zhou

Abstract

Pyrosequencing is one of the important genetic polymorphism detection methods currently used, but the complicated preparatory work limits its application in clinical tests. In order to simplify the process of pyrosequencing, on the basis of the linear-after-the-exponential-polymerase chain reaction (LATE-PCR), we improved the primer design method of LATE-PCR, increased the length and the concentration of the excess primer, applied direct amplification technology with whole blood, and established a whole blood-improved LATE-PCR (imLATE-PCR) method based on common rTaq polymerase and "HpH Buffer." This study investigated the method of optimal amplification system, the influence of blood anticoagulant, and the amount of whole blood. Amplifying the PCR products using a single tube and one-step process, we successfully detected alcohol dehydrogenase gene polymorphisms of 24 clinical blood samples. The results can be used to guide clinical individualized medication. The genotypes of ADH1B locus of 24 samples are 6 cases of AA homozygote, 14 cases of AG heterozygote, and 4 cases of GG homozygote. The genotypes of ADH1C are 20 cases of GG homozygote, 4 cases of AG heterozygote, and 0 cases of AA homozygote.

Key words Whole blood polymerase chain reaction, Improved LATE-PCR, Pyrosequencing, Gene polymorphism, Ethanolic metabolism

1 Introduction

Pyrosequencing is a sequencing-by-synthesis method which is based on the bioluminometric detection of inorganic pyrophosphate (PPi) coupled with cascade enzymatic reactions [1–3]. Currently, pyrosequencing has been applied in the detection of gene polymorphisms [4], microbial typing [5], methylation analysis [6], and large-scale DNA sequencing [7], revolutionizing sequencing technology. Nowadays solid-phase microspheres are mainly used to prepare single-stranded templates for pyrosequencing [8], which has complicated procedures and lowered efficiency.

Guohua Zhou and Qinxin Song (eds.), *Advances and Clinical Practice in Pyrosequencing*, Springer Protocols Handbooks, DOI 10.1007/978-1-4939-3308-2_33, © Springer Science+Business Media New York 2016

In addition, biotin-labeled primers and streptavidin-coated microspheres increase the cost of detection, while this labor-intensive step has a possible risk of cross-contamination from amplicons. These deficiencies have caused a major bottleneck of pyrosequencing in clinical applications [9].

To solve the problem of template preparation, the asymmetry PCR can be taken to get single-stranded PCR products directly [10]. However, the conventional asymmetric PCR cannot be widely used because of the low efficiency in amplification. On the basis of asymmetric PCR, linear-after-the-exponential-polymerase chain reaction [11] (LATE-PCR) can give an amplification efficiency similar to symmetric PCR by optimizing primer concentration and T_m value. A high yield of single-stranded DNA (ssDNA) is obtained to meet the needs in single-stranded nucleic acid sequence hybridization and real-time PCR reactions [12]. However, LATE-PCR primer design requires strict criteria. Most importantly, the excess primer will compete with the amplicon strand. As the amplicon strand is increasing in concentration with the progress of PCR, while the excess primer is decreasing in concentration, the yield of ssDNA would not be high enough if the amplicon is longer. Improved LATE-PCR (imLATE-PCR) [13] employs a large amount of longer primer but a small amount of shorter primer; thus, T_m of the excess primer is much larger than that of the limiting primer. In contrast to LATE-PCR, the choice of primer sequences can be more, and the length of the amplicon can be longer, expanding the scope of its practical application.

In order to improve the detection speed and reduce the possibility of sample contamination, we used whole blood as PCR template directly. Compared with conventional PCR, whole blood PCR improves the detection speed by omitting DNA extraction and reduces the cost of detection by not using the variety of chemical reagents and equipment needed for DNA extraction. It also reduces the possibility of contamination by avoiding opening the lid repeatedly, adding the reagents, discarding the waste, and transferring the templates during the DNA extraction, so it is more suitable for clinical samples detection [14].

In this study, we coupled whole blood amplification directly with imLATE-PCR, establishing the whole blood-imLATE-PCR method with a common rTaq polymerase and "HpH Buffer." The advantages of this method are as follows: (1) Fast detection and easy operation. Whole blood PCR omits DNA extraction and single-stranded template preparation, which can greatly improve the detection speed, simplify the operation process, and save the detection time. (2) Low cost and environmentally friendly. Biotinylated primers and expensive magnetic microspheres can be avoided without single-stranded DNA preparation. Many organic reagents and test tubes can be saved without DNA extraction, thereby reducing detection costs. (3) Less contamination. This method avoids repeatedly opening the lid to add and transfer the reagents, so it reduces the possibility of cross-contamination when detecting multiple samples in parallel. and (4) High sensitivity. The results showed that 0.1 µL of whole blood can provide a successful sequencing result, as an accurate result can be obtained using fingertip blood, so this method can be easily and quickly applied to clinical detection.

We used this method to detect alcohol metabolism genes ADH1B and ADH1C polymorphisms. It can be used to rapidly assess alcohol metabolism and detect a variety of diseases associated with drinking behavior, which is of vital importance in the prevention of disease among heavy drinkers and also routine medical monitoring.

2   Materials

1. EDC-10 Gene amplification (Dongsheng Biological Technology Co. Ltd., China).

2. Portable bioluminescence analyzer for pyrosequencing (Hitachi Ltd., Central Research Laboratory, Japan).

3. ATP-sulfurylase and the Klenow fragment were obtained by gene engineering in our lab.

4. rTaq DNA polymerase and 500 bp DNA Ladder marker were purchased from TaKaRa (Dalian, China).

5. Polyvinylpyrrolidone (PVP) and QuantiLum Recombinant luciferase were purchased from Promega (Madison, USA).

6. Apyrase-VII, adenosine 5′-phosphosulfate (APS), and bovine serum albumin (BSA) were purchased from Sigma (St. Louis, USA).

7. Streptavidin Sepharose™ beads were purchased from GE Healthcare (New Jersey, USA).

8. dATPαS, dGTP, dTTP, and dCTP were purchased from Amersham Pharmacia (San Diego, USA).

9. Other chemicals were of commercially extra-pure grade. All solutions were prepared with deionized and sterilized water.

3   Methods

3.1   ImLATE-PCR Primer Design

1. Amplification primers were designed using the software Primer 5.0 (see **Note 1**).

2. Primer design principles: $T_m^E - T_m^L \geq 5$ °C; $T_m^A - T_m^E \leq 13$ °C (see **Note 2**). OligoAnalyzer 3.1 was used to calculate the T_m values of primers.

3.2 Whole Blood-imLATE-PCR Amplification

1. 1 μL anticoagulated peripheral whole blood was used to amplify the template directly of ADH1B and ADH1C locus (*see* **Note 3**).

2. Fifty microliters of PCR contained 5.35 μL of "HpH Buffer," 2 mM Mg^{2+}, 100 μM dNTPs, 1 μM excessive primer, 0.1 μM limited primer, 2.5 U of rTaq DNA polymerase, amount of PCR additive (10 % BSA and 5 % Tween-20), and 1 μL of whole blood.

3. The PCR program of ADH1B A227G was as follows: 3 cycles of 94 °C for 3 min, 55 °C for 3 min, followed by 65 cycles of 90 °C for 10 s, 53 °C for 20 s, and 72 °C for 20 s.

4. The PCR program of ADH1C G900A was as follows: 94 °C for 3 min, followed by 65 cycles of 90 °C for 10 s, 55 °C for 20 s, and 72 °C for 20 s.

3.3 Single-Stranded Amplicons Treatment

1. We used a self-prepared pyrosequencing mixture [15] to treat the products. The mixture contained 0.1 M Tris–acetate (pH 7.7), 2 mM EDTA, 10 mM Mg(Ac)$_2$, 0.1 % BSA, 1 mM DTT, 80 μM APS, 0.4 mM D-Luciferin, 60 U/mL ATP-sulfurylase, 1.6 U/mL Apyrase-VII, 18 U/mL Klenow polymerase, and some luciferase (*see* **Note 4**).

2. The specific operation was as follows: 3 μL imLATE-PCR amplicons were added into a tube containing the self-prepared pyrosequencing mixture, and then the tube was incubated at room temperature for 5 min (*see* **Note 5**).

3. Then 10 pmol of sequencing primers annealed at room temperature for 5 min were added (*see* **Note 6**).

3.4 Pyrosequencing

1. Pyrosequencing reaction mixture contained 0.1 M Tris–acetate (pH 7.7), 2 mM EDTA, 10 mM Mg(Ac)$_2$, 0.1 % BSA, 1 mM DTT, 80 μM APS, 0.4 mM D-Luciferin, 60 U/mL ATP-sulfurylase, 1.6 U/mL Apyrase-VII, 18 U/mL Klenow polymerase, and some luciferase.

2. Added the mixture and treated imLATE-PCR products to portable bioluminescence analyzer for pyrosequencing, then added dATPαS, dCTP, dTTP, and dGTP in turn to carry out the pyrosequencing reaction.

4 Method Validation

4.1 Detection of Alcohol Dehydrogenase ADH1B, ADH1C Gene SNP Locus

In order to use whole blood as a starting material for PCR amplification, the PCR system should be adjusted. A "HpH Buffer" system, previously developed in our lab, can largely reduce the effect of whole blood components on PCR amplification. Due to the high pH, the buffer system can make the protein surface negatively

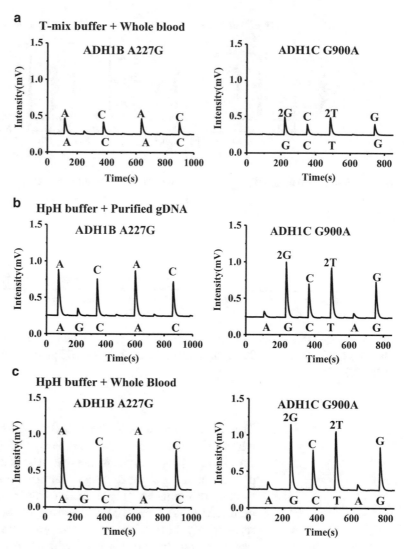

Fig. 1 Pyrosequencing results from the ADH1B A227G and ADH1C G900A with different kinds of PCR amplification buffer ((**a**) whole blood as a template, T-mix PCR amplification buffer; (**b**) genomic DNA as a template, HpH PCR amplification buffer; (**c**) whole blood as a template, HpH PCR amplification buffer)

charged, suppressing the electrostatic interaction between proteins and genomic DNA, thereby reducing the inhibitory effect on PCR reaction [16].

Figure 1 is the pyrosequencing result using whole blood and genomic DNA as template, respectively, with different kinds of PCR amplification buffer, a conventional PCR amplification system (T-mix Buffer), and "HpH Buffer" system for PCR amplification. T-mix Buffer contained 10× Buffer, 10 mM dNTP, and 25 mM MgCl₂; pH 8.5–8.8. "HpH Buffer" contained 100 mM

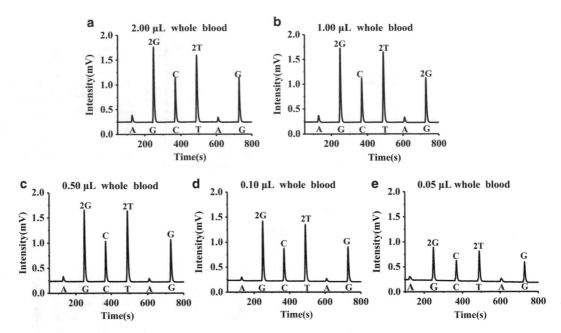

Fig. 2 Pyrosequencing results from the ADH1C G900A with different amounts of anticoagulated blood PCR amplicons ((**a**) 2.00 μL; (**b**) 1.00 μL; (**c**) 0.50 μL; (**d**) 0.10 μL; (**e**) 0.05 μL whole blood were used as template, separately)

Tris–HCl and 50 mM KCl; pH 9.3–9.5. As the results have shown, when using whole blood as template, conventional PCR amplification system (Fig. 1a) showed a low amplification efficiency and low pyrosequencing signals, which cannot make accurate SNP genotyping. When using "HpH Buffer" system for PCR amplification, genomic DNA (Fig. 1b) and whole blood (Fig. 1c) as template, respectively, both obtained better amplification results and stronger pyrosequencing signals, which can ensure accurate SNP genotyping.

We investigated the volume of whole blood required by this method for successful genotyping by pyrosequencing. In a 50 μL reaction, 0.05 μL, 0.10 μL, 0.50 μL, 1.00 μL, and 2.00 μL of a blood sample were individually added for imLATE-PCR. As shown in Fig. 2a–e, good pyrograms were obtained when the volume of a blood sample for an assay is larger than 0.10 μL. The average value of single nucleotide signals were 0.629, 0.794, 0.879, and 0.883, respectively, which can make accurate SNP genotyping. This proved that this method needed only 0.10 μL of whole blood to detect two SNP loci on alcohol dehydrogenase and greatly reduced the trauma for the patient.

According to the detection results of 24 cases of clinical blood samples (Fig. 3), this method can give good sequencing results and high sequencing signal intensity and make accurate

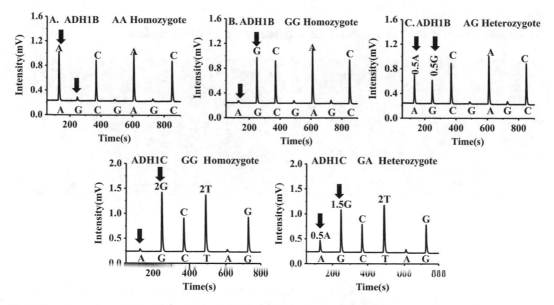

Fig. 3 Pyrograms from typical genotypes of ADH1B A227G polymorphisms ((**a**) AA homozygote; (**b**) GG homozygote; (**c**) AG heterozygote) and ADH1C G900A polymorphisms ((**d**) GG homozygote; (**e**) AG heterozygote)

SNP genotyping. 24 cases of genotype sequencing were shown in Table 1. In order to verify the accuracy of the pyrosequencing results, 10 cases from 24 cases were detected by Sanger sequencing. The same results proved the accuracy of this method.

5   Technical Notes

1. Two alcohol dehydrogenase (ADH) gene polymorphism loci common in Chinese people were selected to amplify, which were associated with alcohol metabolism.

2. T_m^E means the T_m value of excess primer, T_m^L means the T_m value of limiting primer, and T_m^A means the T_m value of amplicon [17].

3. Unless otherwise specified, anticoagulant used in this study is EDTA dipotassium.

4. In addition to a large amount of ssDNA used as a pyrosequencing template, the imLATE-PCR amplicons contained residual dNTPs, PPi, and incompletely extended products. These ingredients affected the subsequent pyrosequencing reactions. Therefore, the amplicons had to be treated before pyrosequencing [18–19].

5. APS in the mixture can react with PPi to produce ATP and excessive dNTPs, and the amount of ATP can be degraded by

Table 1
Genotyping results of two SNPs in 24 clinical samples by the proposed method

Genes	SNPs	Genotypes	Sample numbers (n)
ADH2*2 (ADH1B*2)	A227G	Homozygote (AA)	$n = 6$
		Homozygote (GG)	$n = 14$
		Heterozygote (AG)	$n = 4$
ADH3*2 (ADH1C*2)	G900A	Homozygote (GG)	$n = 20$
		Homozygote (AA)	$n = 0$
		Heterozygote (GA)	$n = 4$

Aprase-VII, thereby the effects of these ingredients on pyrosequencing reaction can be reduced [20].

6. The sequencing primers were ADH1B A227G (5′-ATGGT GGCTGTAGGAATCTGTC-3′) and ADH1C G900A (5′-TT TCGTTTGAAG TCATCGGTC-3′).

References

1. Ronaghi M, Uhlen M, Nyren P (1998) A sequencing method based on real-time pyrophosphate. Science 281:363–365
2. Chen ZY, Zhou GH (2008) Advances in pyrosequencing. Prog Mod Biomed 8:1573–1576
3. Zhang XD, Wu HP, Chen ZY, Zhou GH (2009) Differential gene expression analysis by combining sequence-tagged reverse-transcription polymerase chain reaction with pyrosequencing. Chinese J Anal Chem 37:1107–1112
4. Chen ZY, Fu XY, Zhang XD, Liu XQ, Zou BJ, Wu HP, Song QX, Li JH, Kajiyama T, Kambara H, Zhou GH (2012) Pyrosequencing-based barcodes for a dye-free multiplex bioassay. Chem Commun 48:2445–2447
5. Yang HY, Huang H, Wu HP, Zou BJ, Zhou GH, Kajiyama T, Kambara H (2011) A pyrosequencing-based method for genotyping pathogenic serotypes of S. suis. Anal Methods 3:2517–2523
6. Brakensiek K, Wingen LU, Langer F, Kreipe H, Lehmann U (2007) Quantitative high-resolution CpG island mapping with pyrosequencing reveals disease-specific methylation patterns of the CDKN2B gene in myelodysplastic syndrome and myeloid leukemia. Clin Chem 53:17–23
7. Schuster SC (2008) Next-generation sequencing transforms today's biology. Nat Methods 5:16–18
8. Diggle MA, Clarke SC (2003) A novel method for preparing single-stranded DNA for pyrosequencing. Mol Biotechnol 24:221–224
9. Royo JL, Hidalgo M, Ruiz A (2007) Pyrosequencing protocol using a universal biotinylated primer for mutation detection and SNP genotyping. Nat Protoc 2:1734–1739
10. Yang HY, Xi T, Liang C, Chen ZY, Xu DB, Zhou GH (2009) Preparation of single-stranded DNA for pyrosequencing by linear-after-the-exponential-polymerase chain reaction. Chinese J Anal Chem 2009(37):489–494
11. Salk JJ, Sanchez JA, Pierce KE, Rice JE, Soares KC, Wangh LJ (2006) Direct amplification of single-stranded DNA for pyrosequencing using linear-after-the-exponential (LATE)-PCR. Anal Biochem 353:124–132
12. Liu YL, Wu HP, Ye H, Chen ZY, Song QX, Zou BJ, Rui GJ, Zhou GH (2014) A simplified pyrosequencing protocol based on linear-after-the-exponential (LATE)-PCR using whole blood as the starting material directly. Anal Methods 6:1384–1390
13. Song QX, Yang HY, Zou BJ, Kajiyama T, Kambara H, Zhou GH (2013) Improvement of LATE-PCR to allow single-cell analysis by pyrosequencing. Analyst 38:4991–4997
14. Liu YL, Chen ZY, Wu HP, Zhou GH (2014) Establishment of cloning and sequencing method for high-resolution HLA-B genotype assay. Chinese J Anal Chem 40:1037–1042

15. Wu HP, Wu WJ, Chen ZY, Wang WP, Zhou GH, Kajiyama T, Kambara H (2011) Highly sensitive pyrosequencing based on the capture of free adenosine 5′ phosphosulfate with adenosine triphosphate sulfurylase. Anal Chem 83:3600–3605

16. Bu Y, Huang H, Zhou GH (2008) Direct polymerase chain reaction (PCR) from human whole blood and filter-paper-dried blood by using a PCR buffer with a higher pH. Anal Biochem 375:370–372

17. Zeng FF, Liu SY, Wang BY (2008) Progress in the study of alcohol dehydrogenase polymorphism and drinking behavior as well as alcohol related diseases. Chin J Dis Control Prev 12:164–167

18. Yamauchi M, Maezawa Y, Mizuhara Y, Ohata M, Hirakawa J, Nakajima H, Toda G (1995) Polymorphisms in alcohol metabolizing enzyme genes and alcoholic cirrhosis in Japanese patients: a multivariate analysis. Hepatology 22:1136–1142

19. Zhang ZM, Bian JC (2001) Progress in researches on the relationship between genetic polymorphisms of alcohol-metabolizing enzymes and cancers. Chin J Med Gentet 18:62–65

20. Royo JL, Galan JJ (2009) Pyrosequencing for SNP genotyping. Methods Mol Biol 578:123–133

Chapter 34

Pyrosequencing on a Single Cell

Qinxin Song, Huiyong Yang, Bingjie Zou,
Hideki Kambara, and Guohua Zhou

Abstract

Nucleic acid analysis in a single cell is very important, but the extremely small amount of template in a single cell requires a detection method more sensitive than the conventional method. In this paper, we describe a novel assay allowing a single-cell genotyping by coupling improved linear-after-the-exponential-PCR (imLATE-PCR) on a modified glass slide with highly sensitive pyrosequencing. Due to the significantly increased yield of ssDNA in imLATE-PCR amplicons, it is possible to employ pyrosequencing to sequence the products from 1 μL chip PCR which directly used a single cell as starting material. As a proof of concept, the 1555A>G mutation (related to inherited deafness) on mitochondrial DNA and the SNP 2731 C>T of the BRCA1 gene on genome DNA from a single cell were successfully detected, indicating that our single-cell-pyrosequencing method has high sensitivity, simple operation, and low cost. It is a promising approach in the fields of diagnosis of genetic disease from a single cell, for example, preimplantation genetic diagnosis (PGD).

Key words Single-cell analysis (SCA), Pyrosequencing, imLATE (improved linear-after-the-exponential-PCR), Low volume PCR, Nucleic acid analysis

1 Introduction

Single-cell analysis (SCA) is the new frontier in omics. One important aspect of SCA is nucleic acid analysis in a single cell, for example, preimplantation genetic diagnosis (PGD) [1–3]. However, it is very difficult to sequence a single cell due to a small amount of DNA template in a cell. Usually a step of preamplification by whole-genome amplification (WGA) is employed to supply enough amounts of templates for further sequencing. It is recently found that a loss of alleles during WGA frequently occurs [4]. Therefore, an approach enabling direct DNA sequencing without any use of WGA is preferred.

To achieve a sensitive PCR detection with a small amount of DNA template, a low volume (around 1 mL) PCR on a chemically structured chip was developed for the analysis of mitochondrial

Guohua Zhou and Qinxin Song (eds.), *Advances and Clinical Practice in Pyrosequencing*, Springer Protocols Handbooks, DOI 10.1007/978-1-4939-3308-2_34, © Springer Science+Business Media New York 2016

DNA at single-cell levels. However, it is difficult to prepare a single-stranded DNA (ssDNA) from this low volume PCR product for pyrosequencing, which is a very suitable tool for genetic analysis [5]. To allow pyrosequencing on this small amount of amplicons directly, it is necessary to escape the step of ssDNA preparation. If amplicons from PCR contains enough amount of ssDNA, no ssDNA preparation is needed. Conventionally, ssDNA can be directly generated by asymmetric PCR with regular PCR primers at unequal concentrations [6]. However, asymmetric PCR is inefficient, and it is difficult to get an optimized amplification condition for templates with different sequences.

In this paper, we describe a novel assay allowing a single-cell genotyping by coupling improved linear-after-the-exponential-PCR (imLATE-PCR) on a modified glass slide with highly sensitive pyrosequencing. Due to the significantly increased yield of ssDNA in imLATE-PCR amplicons, it is possible to employ pyrosequencing to sequence the products from 1 μL chip PCR which directly used a single cell as starting material (Fig. 1) (*see* **Notes 1** and **2**). As a proof of concept, the 1555A>G mutation related to inherited deafness on

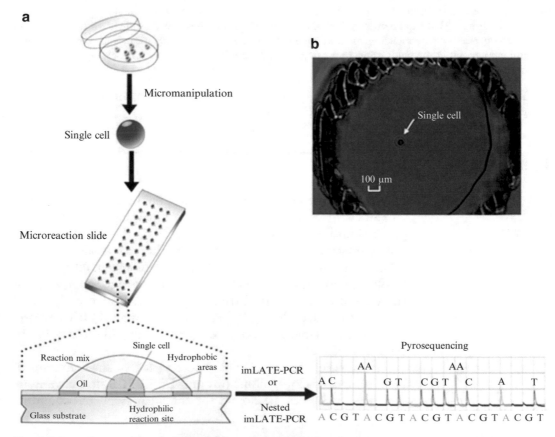

Fig. 1 Schematic overview of single-cell pyrosequencing (**a**) and micrographs (40 × magnifications) of the surface of a single reaction site supplied with one mouse oocyte (**b**)

mitochondrial DNA and the SNP 2731 C>T of the BRCA1 gene on genome DNA from a single cell were successfully detected, indicating that our single-cell-pyrosequencing method has high sensitivity, simple operation, and low cost. The approach has promise for efficient usage in the fields of diagnosis of genetic disease from a single cell, for example, preimplantation genetic diagnosis (PGD).

2   Materials

1. AmpliTaq Gold DNA Polymerase (Applied Biosystems, CA).

2. TransStart Taq DNA Polymerase (TransGen Biotech, China).

3. Exo-Klenow Fragment, QuantiLum recombinant luciferase (Promega, WI).

4. ATP sulfurylase apyrase, D-luciferin, and adenosine 5′-phosphosulfate (APS) (Sigma, MO).

5. 2′-Deoxyadenosine-5′-O-(1-thiotriphosphate)   sodium   salt (dATP-a-S) (Amersham Pharmacia Biotech, UK).

6. dGTP, dTTP, and dCTP (Amersham Pharmacia Biotech, NJ).

7. All the other reagents were analytical reagents or guaranteed reagents. All the solutions were prepared with deionized and sterilized H_2O.

8. AmpliGrid AG480 (Fa. Advalytix, Brunnthal, Germany).

9. SMZ1000 dissection microscope (Nikon, Japan).

10. ECLIPSE TE2000-S inverted microscope (Nikon, Japan).

11. PTC-225 Peltier Thermal Cycler (MJ Research, Watertown, MA, USA).

12. Homemade PD array 8-channel pyrosequencer [7].

3   Methods

3.1   Cell Lines

1. Hep G2 human liver cancer cell line, leukocyte in peripheral blood of nonsyndromic hearing impairment (NSHI) patients, ICR mice oocyte were used.

3.2   Primers

1. The sequences near the SNP (2731C>T) of human BRCA1 (breast cancer susceptibility gene 1) gene (NT_010755.15) was selected as examples to compare imLATE-PCR and LATE-PCR. The primers for 1555A>G mutation of inherited deafness on mitochondrial DNA are excess primer 5′-TCGCCTGA GTGTAAGTTGGGTGCTTTGTGTT-3′ and limiting primer (annealprimer)5′-AACCCCTACGCATTTATATAGAGGAG-3′, the amplicon length is 117 bp. All of the oligomers were synthesized and purified by Invitrogen (Shanghai, China).

3.3 Collect Single Cell by Using Glass Capillaries

1. The sterilized watch glass (or glass slides) was placed on microscope stage, and 30 µL of cell suspension was then added on the surface of the watch glass (*see* **Note 3**).

2. The watch glass was sit for 2 min to let cells precipitate completely to the surface of the watch glass.

3. With the SMZ1000 microscope under its 4×10 magnifications (Nikon, Japan), the capillary tip was adjusted into the cells suspension and was located at the central of the microscopic vision and then manually and slightly adjusted the pressure button of the manipulator to make a well-dispersed, full-membrane, and contour-cleared single cell [8].

4. Then, the capillary was lifted off the surface of cell suspension, and the captured single cell was transferred to the reaction locus of the AmpliGrid slides (AG480F). The image was obtained using ECLIPSE TE2000-S inverted microscope under its 10×10 magnifications (*see* **Note 4**).

3.4 Single-Cell Lysis and On-Chip imLATE-PCR

1. A volume of 0.5 µL of proteinase K (0.4 mg/mL) was pipetted to the reaction site of an AmpliGrid slide containing a single cell and covered immediately with 5 µL of sealing oil (*see* **Note 5**).

2. After complete loading, the AmpliGrid slide was incubated for 40 min at 56 °C and 10 min at 99 °C.

3. 0.5 µL of PCR master mix was added pierce through the sealing oil. So a total volume of 1 µL PCR reaction mix, containing 0.1 µL AmpliTaq Gold (5 U/µL), 0.1 µL GeneAmp $10 \times$ PCR Gold Buffer (both: Applied Biosystems), 0.04 µL dNTPs (2.5 mM each), 0.06 µL $MgCl_2$ (25 mM), 0.1 µL PX (10 µM), and 0.1 µL PL (1 µM).

4. On-chip imLATE-PCR program: initial heating step at 95 °C for 10 min, followed by 30 cycles (denaturation at 95 °C for 10 s, annealing at 54 °C for 10 s, elongation at 72 °C for 40 s), then followed by another 30 cycles (denaturation at 95 °C for 10 s, annealing at 65 °C for 10 s, elongation at 72 °C for 40 s), and followed by a final 10 min elongation step at 72 °C. Negative controls were performed on different positions on the chip using the same reagent solutions without cell or DNA.

5. After the amplification, joining of 1 µL aqueous phase and 4 µL loading dye (1.25×), total 5 µL of each mixture, was transferred to a 6 % PAGE gel and separated for 40 min at 100 V.

6. Silver staining was performed with 0.1 % $AgNO_3$ solution for 30 min, followed by a 10 s washing step in DI water and development in 2 % Na_2CO_3/0.1 % formaldehyde for 2 min.

3.5 Removal of PPi in dNTPs by Biotinylated PPase

1. The biotinylated PPase was immobilized onto streptavidin-coated M280 Dynabeads (37 °C, 30 min) and washed with $1 \times$ annealing buffer (4 mM Tris–HCl, pH 7.5, 2 mM $MgCl_2$, 5 mM NaCl) and then dissolved in $1 \times$ annealing buffer.

2. 10 mmol/L dNTPs (dATPαS, dCTP, dTTP, dGTP) were diluted by dNTPs diluent (5 mmol/L Tris–Ac, 25 mmol/L Mg(AC)$_2$, pH 7.7) to 200 µmol/L.

3. Then 0.5 µL Beads–PPase were added to each kind of 200 µL dNTPs and incubated at room temperature for 5 min.

4. The beads were focused with a magnet, and supernatant was aspirated carefully and added to the micro-dispenser of pyrosequencer separately. The signal of biotinylated PPase-treated dNTPs was detected by the pyrosequencer, and compared with the signal of untreated dNTPs.

3.6 Pyrosequencing

1. We constructed a prototype of 8-channel pyrosequencer by using a PD array sensor [7]. The reaction volume in every well for pyrosequencing was 40 µL, containing 0.1 M Tris–acetate (pH 7.7), 2 mM EDTA, 10 mM magnesium acetate, 0.1 % BSA, 1 mM dithiothreitol (DTT), 2 µM adenosine 50 phosphosulfate (APS), 0.4 mg/mL PVP, 0.4 mM D-LUCIFERIN, 200 mU/mL ATP sulfurylase, 3 µg/mL luciferase, 18 U/mL Klenow fragment, and 1.6 U/mL apyrase.

2. Each of biotinylated PPase-treated dNTPs was added in the reservoir of the micro-dispenser, and pyrosequencing reaction starts when the dispensed dNTP is complementary to the template sequence.

4   Method Validation

4.1   Single-Cell Analysis of the SNP 2731 C>T in the BRCA1 Gene on Genome DNA

To investigate the possibility of the proposed method in the sequencing of gDNA from a single cell, genotyping of 2731 C>T in the BRCA1 gene was used as a proof of concept with the protocol similar to mitochondrial DNA amplification. Although around ten bases were accurately pyrosequenced, the sensitivity is very low [9–10] (Fig. 2a). The sensitivity was significantly increased by nest PCR which was based on preamplification on a slide with a regular PCR primer pair, followed by imLATE-PCR in a tube (Fig. 2b).

4.2   Single-Cell Analysis of 1555A>G Mutation on Mitochondrial DNA

To further investigate the feasibility of the method for single-cell genotyping, a series of a single leukocyte were picked up from the peripheral blood of two healthy persons and two nonsyndromic hearing impairment (NSHI) patients who were diagnosed by Deafness Gene Mutation Detection Array Kit (CapitalBio, Beijing, China) in advance, respectively. A single leukocyte was picked up in triplicate from each blood sample and positioned at different sites on the slide. The typical pyrograms of a single cell from two healthy persons and two NSHI patients indicate that the genotype of a single leukocyte is GG for a NSHI patient but AA for a health person (Fig. 3). No signal was observed from the blank (no cell) and a

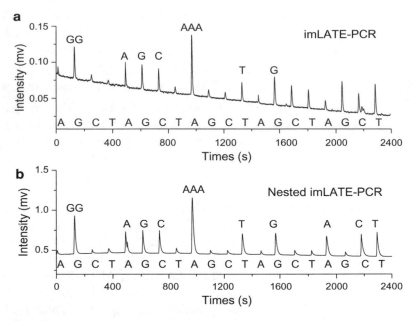

Fig. 2 Typical pyrograms for typing the SNP 2731 C>T on the BRCA1 gene in a single cell by pyrosequencing amplicons from imLATE-PCR (**a**) and nested imLATE-PCR (**b**). The nested imLATE-PCR was achieved with a regular PCR on a slide, followed by imLATE-PCR in a tube

negative control (ICR mice oocyte). Therefore, the pyrogram pattern from a single cell can clearly distinguish the mutant 1555A>G from the wild type. These promising results suggest that it is possible to use the proposed method to type a single cell for PGD

5   Technical Notes

1. AmpliGrid AG480 chips (Fa. Advalytix, Brunnthal, Germany) were used as the platform of 1 μL PCR. Each chip contains 48 independent hydrophilic reaction sites surrounded by a hydrophobic circle which holds aqueous reaction solutions, such as enzyme buffers, in place. Cells were deposited on the slide surface by a mouth tube to control an attached micropipette (glass capillaries) during cell sorting. Before each experiment, the correct deposition of single cells on the reaction sites can be easily verified with a microscope [11].

2. To investigate whether or not a single cell can be genotyped by pyrosequencing amplicons from low volume imLATE-PCR, one, three, and eight cells from Hep G2 human liver cancer cell lines were tested. The result showed that the quality of the pyrogram from one cell is as good as those from three cells and eight cells, indicating that it is successful to perform pyrosequencing on a single cell.

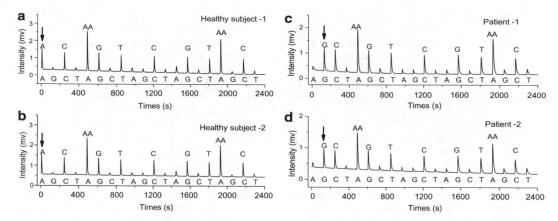

Fig. 3 Pyrograms for typing the 1555A>G mutation in a single cell from two healthy subjects (**a**, **b**) and two NSHI patients (**c**, **d**). The wild-type A and the mutant G were indicated by *arrows*

3. For picking up and transferring individual cells, we usually use a mouth tube to control an attached micropipette (glass capillaries) under a dissection microscope, which permits swift and efficiently control of individual cell collection and release. The glass pipette is connected by a flexible plastic pipe to the mouth of the researcher. If the pipette size is right, it is readily feasible to control the pressure inside the pipette and collect individual cells with minimum volume of extracellular solution (≪0.1 μL).

4. As a control for contamination and inhibition of downstream reactions, 1 μL of the buffer or medium surrounding the cells should be collected and analyzed together with the single-cell samples.

5. Low volume PCR was performed with chips (AG480F AmpliGrid slide) on PTC-225 Peltier Thermal Cycler Flat Block. These are chemically structured glass slides, originally developed for single-cell analysis and quantification of single genome equivalents. Biochemical reactions proceed on 48 lithographically defined hydrophilic anchor spots, each framed by a hydrophobic ring. Each of the reaction compartments can hold up to 2 μL of aqueous solution.

References

1. Kalisky T, Quake SR (2011) Single-cell genomics. Nat Methods 8:311–314
2. Schroeder T (2011) Long-term single-cell imaging of mammalian stem cells. Nat Methods 8:S30–S35
3. Zeevi DA, Renbaum P, Ron-El R, Eldar-Geva T, Raziel A, Brooks B, Strassburger DE, Margalioth J, Levy-Lahad E, Altarescu G (2013) Preimplantation genetic diagnosis in genomic regions with duplications and pseudogenes: long-range PCR in the single-cell assay. Hum Mutat 34:792–799
4. Kroneis T, Geigl JB, El-Heliebi A, Auer M, Ulz P, Schwarzbraun T, Dohr G, Sedlmayr P (2011) Combined molecular genetic and cytogenetic analysis from single cells after isothermal whole-genome amplification. Clin Chem 57:1032–1041

5. Sanchez JA, Pierce KE, Rice JE, Wangh LJ (2004) Linear-after-the-exponential (LATE)-PCR: an advanced method of asymmetric PCR and its uses in quantitative real-time analysis. Proc Natl Acad Sci U S A 101:1933–1938

6. Pierce KE, Sanchez JA, Rice JE, Wangh LJ (2005) Linear-After-The-Exponential (LATE)-PCR: primer design criteria for high yields of specific single-stranded DNA and improved real-time detection. Proc Natl Acad Sci U S A 102:8609–8614

7. Song Q, Jing H, Wu H, Zhou G, Kajiyama T, Kambara H (2010) Gene expression analysis on a photodiode array-based bioluminescence analyzer by using sensitivity-improved SRPP. Analyst (Cambridge, U K) 135:1315–1319

8. Ahmadian A, Ehn M, Hober S (2006) Pyrosequencing: history, biochemistry and future. Clin Chim Acta 363:83–94

9. Schmidt U, Lutz-Bonengel S, Weisser HJ, Sanger T, Pollak S, Schon U, Zacher T, Mann W (2006) Low-volume amplification on chemically structured chips using the PowerPlex16 DNA amplification kit. Int J Legal Med 120:42–48

10. Wu H, Wu W, Chen Z, Wang W, Zhou G, Kajiyama T, Kambara H (2011) Highly sensitive pyrosequencing based on the capture of free adenosine 5' phosphosulfate with adenosine triphosphate sulfurylase. Anal Chem 83:3600–3605

11. Song Q, Wu H, Feng F, Zhou G, Kajiyama T, Kambara H (2010) Pyrosequencing on nicked dsDNA generated by nicking endonucleases. Anal Chem 82:2074–2081

INDEX

Guohua Zhou and Qinxin Song (eds.), *Advances and Clinical Practice in Pyrosequencing*, Springer Protocols Handbooks,
DOI 10.1007/978-1-4939-3308-2, © Springer Science+Business Media New York 2016

Printed in the United States
By Bookmasters